PLANT BASED DIET COOKBOOK 2021

The New Complete Guide With 800 Easy and Delicious Plant-Based Recipes to Meet All The Nutritional Needs for a Modern, Healthy and Active Life.

The Kookerz

Table of Contents

Chapter 7: Drinks 237

Chapter 8: Dressings, Dips, and Sauces

Chapter 9: Bonus Recipes

Introduction

A plant-based diet is a diet based primarily on whole plant foods. It is identical to the regular diet we're used to already, except that it leaves out foods that are not exclusively from plants. Hence, a plant-based diet does away with all types of animal-sourced foods, hydrogenated oils, refined sugars, and processed foods. A whole food plant-based diet comprises not just fruits and vegetables; it also consists of unprocessed or barely processed oils with healthy monounsaturated fats (like extra-virgin olive oil), whole grains, legumes (essentially lentils and beans), seeds and nuts, as well as herbs and spices.

What makes a plant-based meal (or any meal) fun is the manner with which you make them; the seasoning process; and the combination process that contributes to a fantastic flavor and makes every meal unique and enjoyable. There are lots of delicious recipes (all plant-centered), which will prove helpful when you intend to make mouthwatering, healthy plant-based dishes for personal or household consumption. Provided you're eating these plant-based foods regularly, you'll have very problems with fat or diseases that result from bad dietary habits, and there would be no need for excessive calorie tracking.

Plant-based diet recipes are versatile; they range from colorful Salads to Lentil Stews, and Bean Burritos. The recipes also draw influences from around the globe, with Mexican, Chinese, European, Indian cuisines all part of the vast array of plant-based recipes available to choose from.

Why You Ought to Reduce Your Intake of Processed and Animal-Based Foods

You have likely heard over and over that processed food has adverse effects on your health. You might have also been told repeatedly to stay away from foods with lots of preservatives; nevertheless, nobody ever offered any genuine or concrete facts about why you ought to avoid these foods and why they are unsafe. Consequently, let us properly dissect it to help you properly comprehend why you ought to stay away from these healthy eating offenders.

They have massive habit-forming characteristics

Humans have a predisposition towards being addicted to some specific foods; however, the reality is that the fault is not wholly ours.

Every one of the unhealthy treats we relish now and then triggers the dopamine release in our brains. This creates a pleasurable effect in our brain, but the excitement is usually short-lived. The discharged dopamine additionally causes an attachment connection gradually, and this is the reason some people consistently go back to eat certain unhealthy foods even when they know it's unhealthy and unnecessary. You can get rid of this by taking out that inducement completely.

They are sugar-laden and plenteous in glucose-fructose syrup

Animal-based and processed foods are laden with refined sugars and glucose-fructose syrup which has almost no beneficial food nutrient. An ever-increasing number of studies are affirming what several people presumed from the start; that genetically modified foods bring about inflammatory bowel disease, which consequently makes it increasingly difficult for the body to assimilate essential nutrients. The disadvantages that result from your body being unable to assimilate essential nutrients from consumed foods rightly cannot be overemphasized.

Processed and animal-based food products contain plenteous amounts of refined carbohydrates. Indeed, your body requires carbohydrates to give it the needed energy to run body capacities.

In any case, refining carbs dispenses with the fundamental supplements; in the way that refining entire grains disposes of the whole grain part. What remains, in the wake of refining, is what's considered as empty carbs or empty calories. These can negatively affect the metabolic system in your body by sharply increasing your blood sugar and insulin quantities.

They contain lots of synthetic ingredients

At the point when your body is taking in non-natural ingredients, it regards them as foreign substances. Your body treats them as a health threat. Your body isn't accustomed to identifying synthetic compounds like sucralose or these synthesized sugars. Hence, in defense of your health against this foreign "aggressor," your body does what it's capable of to safeguard your health. It sets off an immune reaction to tackle this "enemy" compound, which indirectly weakens your body's general disease alertness, making you susceptible to illnesses. The concentration and energy expended by your body in ensuring your immune system remains safe could instead be devoted somewhere else.

They contain constituent elements that set off an excitable reward sensation in your body

A part of processed and animal-based foods contain compounds like glucose-fructose syrup, monosodium glutamate, and specific food dyes that can trigger some addiction. They rouse your body to receive a benefit in return whenever you consume them. Monosodium glutamate, for example, is added to many store-bought baked foods. This additive slowly conditions your palates to relish the taste. It gets mental just by how your brain interrelates with your taste sensors.

This reward-centric arrangement makes you crave it increasingly, which ends up exposing you to the danger of overconsuming calories

For animal protein, usually, the expression "subpar" is used to allude to plant proteins since they generally have lower levels of essential amino acids as against animal-sourced protein. Nevertheless, what the vast majority don't know is that large amounts of essential amino acids can prove detrimental to your health. Let me break it down further for you.

Animal-Sourced Protein has no Fiber

In their pursuit to consume animal protein increasingly, the vast majority wind up dislodging the plant protein that was previously available in their body. Replacing the plant proteins with its animal variant is wrong because, in contrast to plant protein, animal proteins typically have fiber deficiency, phytonutrients, and antioxidant properties. Fiber insufficiency is a regular feature across various regions and societies on the planet. In America, for example, according to the National Academy of Medicine, the typical adult takes in roughly 15 grams of dietary fiber daily rather than the recommended daily quantity of 25 to 30 grams. A deficiency in dietary fiber often leads to a heightened risk of breast and colorectal cancers, in addition to constipation, inflammatory bowel disease, and cardiovascular disease.

Animal Protein Leads to a Jump in IGF-1 Levels

Insulin-like growth factor 1 (IGF-1) is a vital growth hormone identical in molecular geometry to insulin which contributes significantly to the growth of children and impacts adults in an anabolic manner. It fuels cell division and development, which may seemingly seem positive; however, it correspondingly triggers the development of cancer cells. Hence, an increased level of IGF-1 in the blood is connected to a heightened risk of cancer, malignant tumor, and spread.

Animal protein brings about an upsurge in Phosphorus levels in the body

Animal protein has significant levels of Phosphorus. Our bodies stabilize these plenteous amounts of Phosphorus by producing and discharging a hormone known as fibroblast growth factor 23 (FGF23). Studies have shown that this hormone is dangerous to our veins. FGF23 also causes asymmetrical expansion of heart muscles – a determinant for congestive heart failure and even mortality in some advanced cases.

Having discussed the many problems associated with animal protein, it becomes more apt to replace its "high quality" perception with the tag, "highly hazardous." In contrast to caffeine, which has a withdrawal effect if it's discontinued abruptly, you can stop taking processed and animal-based foods right away without any withdrawals. Possibly the only thing that you'll give up is the ease of some meals taking little-to-no time to prepare.

Chapter 1: Breakfast

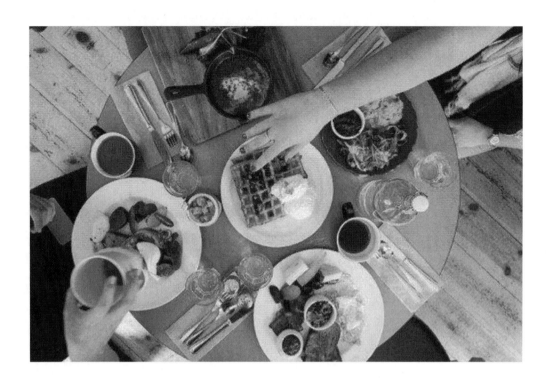

1. Dark Chocolate Quinoa Breakfast Bowl

Preparation Time: 15-30 minutes | **Cooking Time:** 30 minutes | **Servings:** 4

Ingredients:

Uncooked white quinoa: 1 cup	Unsweetened almond milk: 1 cup
Coconut milk: 1 cup	Sea salt: 1 pinch
Unsweetened cocoa powder: 2 tbsp	Maple syrup: 2-3 tbsp
Pure vanilla extract: 1/2 tsp	Vegan dark chocolate: 3-4 squares

Directions:

Rinse quinoa in a strainer
Heat the pan and add rinsed quinoa and dry them up
Add coconut milk, almond milk, and salt
Lower the heat to medium and stir gently for 20 minutes
Remove from heat after quinoa is tender
Add vanilla and maple syrup and serve

Nutrition:
Carbs: 40. 9 Protein: 7. 5g Fats: 6. 7g Calories: 236 Kcal

2. Quinoa Black Beans Breakfast Bowl

Preparation Time: 5-15 minutes | **Cooking Time:** 25 minutes | **Servings:** 4

Ingredients:

1 cup brown quinoa, rinsed well	Salt to taste
3 tbsp plant-based yogurt	½ lime, juiced
2 tbsp chopped fresh cilantro	1 (5 oz) can black beans, drained and rinsed
3 tbsp tomato salsa	¼ small avocado, pitted, peeled, and sliced
2 radishes, shredded	1 tbsp pepitas (pumpkin seeds)

Directions:

Cook the quinoa with 2 cups of slightly salted water in a medium pot over medium heat or until the liquid absorbs, 15 minutes.

Spoon the quinoa into serving bowls and fluff with a fork.

In a small bowl, mix the yogurt, lime juice, cilantro, and salt. Divide this mixture on the quinoa and top with the beans, salsa, avocado, radishes, and pepitas.

Serve immediately.

Nutrition:

Calories 131 Fats 3. 5g Carbs 20 Protein 6. 5g

3. Corn Griddle Cakes With Tofu Mayonnaise

Preparation Time: 5-15 minutes | **Cooking Time:** 35 minutes | **Servings:** 4

Ingredients:

1 tbsp flax seed powder + 3 tbsp water	1 cup water or as needed
2 cups yellow cornmeal	1 tsp salt
2 tsp baking powder	4 tbsp olive oil for frying
1 cup tofu mayonnaise for serving	

Directions:

In a medium bowl, mix the flax seed powder with water and allow thickening for 5 minutes to form the flax egg.

Mix in the water and then whisk in the cornmeal, salt, and baking powder until soup texture forms but not watery.

Heat a quarter of the olive oil in a griddle pan and pour in a quarter of the batter. Cook until set and golden brown beneath, 3 minutes. Flip the cake and cook the other side until set and golden brown too.

Plate the cake and make three more with the remaining oil and batter.

Top the cakes with some tofu mayonnaise before serving.

Nutrition:

Calories 896 Fats 50. 7g Carbs 91. 6g Protein 17. 3g

4. Savory Breakfast Salad

Preparation Time: 15-30 minutes | **Cooking Time:** 20 minutes | **Servings:** 2

Ingredients:

For the sweet potatoes:	Sweet potato: 2 small
Salt and pepper: 1 pinch	Coconut oil: 1 tbsp
For the Dressing:	Lemon juice: 3 tbsp
Salt and pepper: 1 pinch each	Extra virgin olive oil: 1 tbsp
For the Salad: Mixed greens: 4 cups	For Servings:
	Hummus: 4 tbsp
Blueberries: 1 cup	Ripe avocado: 1 medium
Fresh chopped parsley	Hemp seeds: 2 tbsp

Directions:

Take a large skillet and apply gentle heat

Add sweet potatoes, coat them with salt and pepper and pour some oil

Cook till sweet potatoes turns browns

Take a bowl and mix lemon juice, salt, and pepper

Add salad, sweet potatoes, and the serving together

Mix well and dress and serve

Nutrition:

Carbs: 57. 6g Protein: 7. 5g Fats: 37. 6g Calories: 523 Kcal

5. Almond Plum Oats Overnight

Preparation Time: 15-30 minutes | **Cooking Time:** 10 minutes plus overnight | **Servings:** 2

Ingredients:

Rolled oats: 60g	Plums: 3 ripe and chopped
Almond milk: 300ml	Chia seeds: 1 tbsp
Nutmeg: a pinch	Vanilla extract: a few drops
Whole almonds: 1 tbsp roughly chopped	

Directions:

Add oats, nutmeg, vanilla extract, almond milk, and chia seeds to a bowl and mix well

Add in cubed plums and cover and place in the fridge for a night

Mix the oats well next morning and add into the serving bowl
Serve with your favorite toppings

Nutrition:
Carbs: 24. 7g Protein: 9. 5g Fats: 10. 8g Calories: 248Kcal

6. High Protein Toast

Preparation Time: 15-30 minutes | **Cooking Time:** 15 minutes | **Servings:** 2

Ingredients:

White bean: 1 drained and rinsed	Cashew cream: ½ cup
Miso paste: 1 ½ tbsp	Toasted sesame oil: 1 tsp
Sesame seeds: 1 tbsp	Spring onion: 1 finely sliced
Lemon: 1 half for the juice and half wedged to serve	Rye bread: 4 slices toasted

Directions:
In a bowl add sesame oil, white beans, miso, cashew cream, and lemon juice and mash using a potato masher
Make a spread
Spread it on a toast and top with spring onions and sesame seeds
Serve with lemon wedges

Nutrition:
Carbs: 44. 05 g Protein: 14. 05 g Fats: 9. 25 g Calories: 332 Kcal

7. Hummus Carrot Sandwich

Preparation Time: 15-30 minutes | **Cooking Time:** 25 minutes | **Servings:** 2

Ingredients:

Chickpeas: 1 cup can drain and rinsed	Tomato: 1 small sliced
Cucumber: 1 sliced	Avocado: 1 sliced
Cumin: 1 tsp	Carrot: 1 cup diced
Maple syrup: 1 tsp	Tahini: 3 tbsp
Garlic: 1 clove	Lemon: 2 tbsp
Extra-virgin olive oil: 2 tbsp	Salt: as per your need
Bread slices: 4	

Directions:
Add carrot to the boiling hot water and boil for 15 minutes
Blend boiled carrots, maple syrup, cumin, chickpeas, tahini, olive oil, salt, and garlic together in a blender
Add in lemon juice and mix
Add to the serving bowl and you can refrigerate for up to 5 days
In between two bread slices, spread hummus and place 2-3 slices of cucumber, avocado, and tomato and serve

Nutrition:
Carbs: 53. 15 g Protein: 14. 1 g Fats: 27. 5 g Calories: 490 Kcal

8. Overnight Oats

Preparation Time: 15-30 minutes | **Cooking Time:** 15 minutes plus overnight | **Servings:** 6

Ingredients:

Cinnamon: a pinch	Almond milk: 600ml
Porridge oats: 320g	Pumpkin seeds 1 tbsp
Maple syrup: 1 tbsp	
Chia seeds: 1 tbsp	

Directions:
Add all the ingredients to the bowl and combine well
Cover the bowl and place it in the fridge overnight
Pour more milk in the morning Serve with your favorite toppings

Nutrition:
Carbs: 32. 3 g Protein: 10. 2 g Fats: 12. 7 g Calories: 298 Kcal

9. Avocado Miso Chickpeas Toast

Preparation Time: 15-30 minutes | **Cooking Time:** 15 minutes | **Servings:** 2

Ingredients:

Chickpeas: 400g drained and rinsed	Avocado: 1 medium
Toasted sesame oil: 1 tsp	White miso paste: 1 ½ tbsp
Sesame seeds: 1 tbsp	Spring onion: 1 finely sliced

Lemon: 1 half for the juice and half wedged to serve

Rye bread: 4 slices toasted

Directions:
In a bowl add sesame oil, chickpeas, miso, and lemon juice and mash using a potato masher
Roughly crushed avocado in another bowl using a fork
Add the avocado to the chickpeas and make a spread
Spread it on a toast and top with spring onion and sesame seeds
Serve with lemon wedges

Nutrition:
Carbs: 33. 3 g Protein: 14. 6 g Fats: 26. 6 g Calories: 456 Kcal

10.   Banana Malt Bread

Preparation Time: 15-30 minutes | **Cooking Time:** 1 hour 20 minutes and Maturing Time | **Servings:** 12 slices

Ingredients:

Hot strong black tea: 120ml	Malt extract: 150g plus extra for brushing Bananas: 2 ripe mashed
Sultanas: 100g Pitted dates: 120g chopped	Plain flour: 250g Soft dark brown sugar: 50g Baking powder: 2 tsp

Directions:
Preheat the oven to 140C
Line the loaf tin with the baking paper
Brew tea and include sultanas and dates to it
Take a small pan and heat the malt extract and gradually add sugar to it
Stir continuously and let it cook
In a bowl, add flour, salt, and baking powder and now top with sugar extract, fruits, bananas, and tea
Mix the batter well and add to the loaf tin
Bake the mixture for an hour
Brush the bread with extra malt extract and let it cool down before removing from the tin
When done, wrap in a foil; it can be consumed for a week

Nutrition:
Carbs: 43. 3 g Protein: 3. 4 g Fats: 0. 3 g Calories: 194 Kcal

11.   Banana Vegan Bread

Preparation Time: 15-30 minutes | **Cooking Time:** 1 hour 15 minutes | **Servings:** 1 loaf

Ingredients:

Overripe banana:	3 large mashed
All-purpose flour: 200 g Unsweetened non-dairy milk: 50 ml	White vinegar: ½ tsp
Ground flaxseed: 10 g	Granulated sugar: 140
Ground cinnamon: ¼ tsp	g Vanilla: ¼ tsp
Baking powder: ¼ tsp	Baking soda: ¼ tsp
Salt: ¼ tsp	Canola oil: 3 tbsp
Chopped walnuts: ½ cup	

Directions:
Preheat the oven to 350F and line the loaf pan with parchment paper
Mash bananas using a fork
Take a large bowl, and add in mash bananas, canola oil, oat milk, sugar, vinegar, vanilla, and ground flax seed
Also whisk in baking powder, cinnamon, flour, and salt
Add batter to the loaf pan and bake for 50 minutes
Remove from pan and let it sit for 10 minutes
Slice when completely cooled down

Nutrition:
Carbs: 40. 3g Protein: 2. 8g Fats: 8. 2g Calories: 240Kcal

12.   Berry Compote Pancakes

Preparation Time: 15-30 minutes | **Cooking Time:** 30 minutes | **Servings:** 2

Ingredients:

Mixed frozen berries: 200g	Plain flour: 140 g
Unsweetened almond milk: 140ml	Icing sugar: 1 tbsp
Lemon juice: 1 tbsp	Baking powder: 2 tsp
Vanilla extract: a dash	Salt: a pinch
Caster sugar: 2 tbsp	Vegetable oil: ½ tbsp

Directions:

Take a small pan and add berries, lemon juice, and icing sugar

Cook the mixture for 10 minutes to give it a saucy texture and set aside

Take a bowl and add caster sugar, flour, baking powder, and salt and mix well

Add in almond milk and vanilla and combine well to make a batter

Take a non-stick pan, and heat 2 teaspoons oil in it and spread it over the whole surface

Add ¼ cup of the batter to the pan and cook each side for 3-4 minutes

Serve with compote

Nutrition:

Carbs: 92 g Protein: 9. 4 g Fats: 5. 2 g Calories: 463 Kcal

13.   Southwest Breakfast Bowl

Preparation Time: 15-30 minutes | **Cooking Time:** 15 minutes | **Servings:** 1

Ingredients:

Mushrooms: 1 cup sliced	Chopped cilantro: ½ cup
Chili powder: 1 tsp	Red pepper: 1/2 diced
Zucchini: 1 cup diced	Green onion: 1/2 cup chopped
Onion: 1/2 cup	Vegan sausage: 1 sliced
Garlic powder: 1 tsp	Paprika: 1 tsp
Cumin: 1/2 tsp	Salt and pepper: as per your taste
Avocado: for topping	

Directions:

Put everything in a bowl and apply gentle heat until vegetables turn brown

Pour some pepper and salt as you like and serve with your favorite toppings

Nutrition:

Carbs: 31. 6g Protein: 33. 8g Fats: 12. 2g Calories: 361

14.   Buckwheat Crepes

Preparation Time: 15-30 minutes | **Cooking Time:** 25 minutes | **Servings:** 12

Ingredients:

Raw buckwheat flour: 1 cup	Light coconut milk: 1 and 3/4 cups
Ground cinnamon: 1/8 tsp	Flaxseeds: 3/4 tbsp
Melted coconut oil: 1 tbsp	Sea salt: a pinch
Any sweetener: as per your taste	

Directions:

Take a bowl and add flaxseed, coconut milk, salt, avocado, and cinnamon

Mix them all well and fold in the flour

Now take a nonstick pan and pour oil and provide gentle heat

Add a big spoon of a mixture

Cook till it appears bubbly, then change side

Perform the task until all crepes are prepared

For enhancing the taste, add the sweetener of your liking

Nutrition:

Carbs: 8g Protein: 1g Fats: 3g Calories: 71Kcal

15.   Chickpeas Spread Sourdough Toast

Preparation Time: 15-30 minutes | **Cooking Time:** 15 minutes | **Servings:** 4

Ingredients:

Chickpeas: 1 cup rinsed and drained	Pumpkin puree: 1 cup
Vegan yogurt: ½ cup	Salt: as per your need
Sourdough: 4 slices toasted	

Directions:

In a bowl add chickpeas and pumpkin puree and mash using a potato masher

Add in salt and yogurt and mix

Spread it on a toast and serve

Nutrition:

Carbs: 33. 7g Protein: 8. 45g Fats: 2. 5g Calories: 187Kcal

16. Chickpeas with Harissa

Preparation Time: 15-30 minutes | **Cooking Time:** 20 minutes | **Servings:** 2

Ingredients:

Chickpeas: 1 cup can rinse and drained well	Onion: 1 small diced
Cucumber: 1 cup diced	Tomato: 1 cup diced
Salt: as per your taste	Lemon juice: 2 tbsp
Harissa: 2 tsp	Olive oil: 1 tbsp
Flat-leaf parsley: 2 tbsp chopped	

Directions:

Add lemon juice, harissa, and olive oil in a bowl and whisk

Take a serving bowl and add onion, cucumber, chickpeas, salt and the sauce you made

Add parsley from the top and serve

Nutrition:

Carbs: 55. 6 g Protein: 17. 8g Fats: 11. 8g Calories: 398Kcal

17. Chocolate Chip Pancake

Preparation Time: 15-30 minutes | **Cooking Time:** 30 minutes | **Servings:** 6 pancakes

Ingredients:

All-purpose flour: 140g Melted coconut oil: 1 tbsp	Vegan sugar: 2 tbsp
Warm almond milk: 250ml	Baking powder: 1 tbsp
Sea salt: ¼ tsp	Chocolate chips: 2 tbsp

Directions:

Combine together flour, salt, and baking powder and add in chocolate chips

Warm almond milk in the microwave and add sugar and coconut oil and mix well

There should be no lump in the batter

Combine together now dry ingredients and the wet ingredients

Add oil to the non-stick pan on medium heat

Add ¼ cup of the batter to the pan and cook each side for 3-4 minutes

Serve with vegan butter or any topping you like

Nutrition:

Amount Per 1 Pancake

Carbs: 29. 4 g Protein: 3. 1 g Fats: 5 g Calories: 167 Kcal

18. Coconut, Raspberry, and Chocolate Porridge

Preparation Time: 15-30 minutes | **Cooking Time:** 20 minutes | **Servings:** 2

Ingredients:

Almond milk: 300 ml	Quinoa: 80 g Coconut water: 100ml
Raspberries: 100g Cocoa powder: 1 tbsp	Coconut sugar: 2 tbsp
Cocoa nibs: 2 tbsp	Vegan coconut chips: 2 tbsp toasted

Directions:

Take a small pan and add coconut water, quinoa, coconut sugar, almond milk, and cocoa powder

Heat the pan for 20 minutes over medium heat

Stir continuously in between

Top with cocoa nibs, coconut chips, and raspberries and serve

Nutrition:

Carbs: 45. 3 g Protein: 10. 3 g Fats: 19. 3 g Calories: 415 Kcal

19. Toasted Rye with Pumpkin Seed Butter

Preparation Time: 15-30 minutes | **Cooking Time:** 25 minutes and the cooling time | **Servings:** 4

Ingredients:

Pumpkin seeds: 220g	Avocado oil: 2 tbsp
Date nectar: 1 tsp	
Rye bread: 4 slices toasted	

Directions:

Toast the pumpkin seed on a frying pan on low heat for 5-7 minutes and stir in between

Let them turn golden and remove from pan

Add to the blender, when they cool down and make fine powder

Add in avocado oil and salt and then again blend to form a paste

Add date nectars too and blend

On the toasted rye, spread one tablespoon of this butter and serve with your favorite toppings

Nutrition:

Carbs: 3 g Protein: 5 g Fats: 10. 3 g Calories: 127 Kcal

20.   Vegan Breakfast Hash

Preparation Time: 15-30 minutes | **Cooking Time:** 25 minutes | **Servings:** 4

Ingredients:

Bell Pepper: 1	Smoked Paprika: ½ tsp
Potatoes: 3 medium	Mushrooms: 8 oz
Yellow Onion: 1	Zucchini: 1
Cumin Powder: ½ tsp	Garlic Powder: ½ tsp
Salt and Pepper: as per your taste	Cooking oil: 2 tbsp (optional)

Directions:

Heat a large pan on medium flame, add oil and put the sliced potatoes
Cook the potatoes till they change color
Cut the rest of the vegetables and add all the spices
Cooked till veggies are soften

Nutrition:

Carbs: 29. 7g Protein: 5. 5g Fats: 10g Calories: 217 Kcal

21.   Vegan Muffins Breakfast Sandwich

Preparation Time: 15-30 minutes | **Cooking Time:** 20 minutes | **Servings:** 2

Ingredients:

Romesco Sauce: 3-4 tablespoons	Fresh baby spinach: ½ cup
Tofu Scramble: 2	Vegan English muffins: 2
Avocado: ½ peeled and sliced	Sliced fresh tomato: 1

Directions:

In the oven, toast English muffin
Half the muffin and spread romesco sauce
Paste spinach to one side, tailed by avocado slices
Have warm tofu followed by a tomato slice
Place the other muffin half onto to the preceding one

Nutrition:

Carbs: 18g Protein: 12g Fats: 14g Calories: 276 Kcal

22.   Almond Waffles With Cranberries

Preparation Time: 5-15 minutes | **Cooking Time:** 20 minutes | **Servings:** 4

Ingredients:

2 tbsp flax seed powder + 6 tbsp water	2/3 cup almond flour
2 ½ tsp baking powder	A pinch salt
1 ½ cups almond milk	2 tbsp plant butter
1 cup fresh almond butter	2 tbsp pure maple syrup
1 tsp fresh lemon juice	

Directions:

In a medium bowl, mix the flax seed powder with water and allow soaking for 5 minutes.
Add the almond flour, baking powder, salt, and almond milk. Mix until well combined.
Preheat a waffle iron and brush with some plant butter. Pour in a quarter cup of the batter, close the iron and cook until the waffles are golden and crisp, 2 to 3 minutes.
Transfer the waffles to a plate and make more waffles using the same process and ingredient proportions.
Meanwhile, in a medium bowl, mix the almond butter with the maple syrup and lemon juice. Serve the waffles, spread the top with the almond-lemon mixture, and serve.

Nutrition:

Calories 533 Fats 53g Carbs 16. 7g Protein 1. 2g

23.   Chickpea Omelet With Spinach And Mushrooms

Preparation Time: 5-15 minutes | **Cooking Time:** 25 minutes | **Servings:** 4

Ingredients:

1 cup chickpea flour	½ tsp onion powder
½ tsp garlic powder	¼ tsp white pepper
¼ tsp black pepper	1/3 cup nutritional yeast

½ tsp baking soda

3 scallions, chopped

½ cup chopped fresh spinach

1 tbsp fresh parsley leaves

1 small green bell pepper, deseeded and chopped

1 cup sautéed sliced white button mushrooms

1 cup halved cherry tomatoes for serving

Directions:
In a medium bowl, mix the chickpea flour, onion powder, garlic powder, white pepper, black pepper, nutritional yeast, and baking soda until well combined.

Heat a medium skillet over medium heat and add a quarter of the batter. Swirl the pan to spread the batter across the pan. Scatter a quarter each of the bell pepper, scallions, mushrooms, and spinach on top, and cook until the bottom part of the omelet sets and is golden brown, 1 to 2 minutes. Carefully, flip the omelet and cook the other side until set and golden brown.

Transfer the omelet to a plate and make the remaining omelets using the remaining batter in the same proportions.

Serve the omelet with the tomatoes and garnish with the parsley leaves. Serve.

Nutrition:
Calories 147 Fats 1. 8g Carbs 21. 3g Protein 11. 6g

24. Sweet Coconut Raspberry Pancakes

Preparation Time: 5-15 minutes | **Cooking Time:** 25 minutes | **Servings:** 4

Ingredients:

2 tbsp flax seed powder + 6 tbsp water

¼ cup fresh raspberries, mashed

1 tsp baking soda

1 tbsp coconut sugar

½ tsp cinnamon powder

2 tsp plant butter

½ cup of coconut milk

½ cup oat flour

A pinch salt

2 tbsp pure date syrup

2 tbsp unsweetened coconut flakes

Fresh raspberries for garnishing

Directions:
In a medium bowl, mix the flax seed powder with the water and allow thickening for 5 minutes.

Mix in the coconut milk and raspberries.

Add the oat flour, baking soda, salt, coconut sugar, date syrup, and cinnamon powder. Fold in the coconut flakes until well combined.

Working in batches, melt a quarter of the butter in a non-stick skillet and add ¼ cup of the batter. Cook until set beneath and golden brown, 2 minutes. Flip the pancake and cook on the other side until set and golden brown, 2 minutes. Transfer to a plate and make the remaining pancakes using the rest of the ingredients in the same proportions.

Garnish the pancakes with some raspberries and serve warm!

Nutrition:
Calories 412 Fats 28. 3g Carbs 33. 7g Protein 7. 6g

25. Pumpkin-Pistachio Tea Cake

Preparation Time: 5-15 minutes | **Cooking Time:** 70 minutes | **Servings:** 4

Ingredients:

2 tbsp flaxseed powder + 6 tbsp water

¾ cup canned unsweetened pumpkin puree

3 tbsp pure date sugar

½ tsp cinnamon powder

¼ tsp cloves powder

½ tsp nutmeg powder

2 tbsp chopped pistachios

3 tbsp vegetable oil

½ cup pure corn syrup

1 ½ cups whole-wheat flour

½ tsp baking powder

½ tsp allspice powder

A pinch salt

Directions:
Preheat the oven to 350 F and lightly coat an 8 x 4-inch loaf pan with cooking spray. In a medium bowl, mix the flax seed powder with water and allow thickening for 5 minutes to make the flax egg.

In a bowl, whisk the vegetable oil, pumpkin puree, corn syrup, date sugar, and flax egg. In another bowl, mix the flour, cinnamon powder, baking powder, cloves powder, allspice powder, nutmeg powder, and salt. Add this mixture to the wet batter and mix until well combined.

Pour the batter into the loaf pan, sprinkle the pistachios on top, and gently press the nuts onto the batter to stick.

Bake in the oven for 50 to 55 minutes or until a toothpick inserted into the cake comes out clean. Remove the cake onto a wire rack, allow cooling, slice, and serve.

Nutrition:
Calories 330 Fats 13. 2g Carbs 50. 1g Protein 7g

26.   Carrot And Chocolate Bread

Preparation Time: 5-15 minutes | **Cooking Time:** 75 minutes | **Servings:** 4

Ingredients:
For the dry mix:

1 ½ cup whole-wheat flour	¼ cup almond flour
¼ tsp salt	¼ tsp cloves powder
¼ tsp cayenne pepper	1 tbsp cinnamon powder
½ tsp nutmeg powder	½ tsp baking soda
1 ½ tsp baking powder	

For the wet batter:

2 tbsp flax seed powder + 6 tbsp water	½ cup pure date sugar
¼ cup pure maple syrup	¾ tsp almond extract
1 tbsp grated lemon zest	½ cup unsweetened applesauce
¼ cup olive oil	

For folding into the batter:

4 carrots, shredded	3 tbsp unsweetened chocolate chips
2/3 cup black raisins	

Directions:
Preheat the oven to 375 F and line an 8x4 loaf tin with baking paper.

In a large bowl, mix all the flours, salt, cloves powder, cayenne pepper, cinnamon powder, nutmeg powder, baking soda, and baking powder.

In another bowl, mix the flaxseed powder, water, and allow thickening for 5 minutes. Mix in the

date sugar, maple syrup, almond extract, lemon zest, applesauce, and olive oil.

Combine both mixtures until smooth and fold in the carrots, chocolate chips, and raisins.

Pour the mixture into a loaf pan and bake in the oven until golden brown on top or a toothpick inserted into the bread comes out clean, 45 to 60 minutes.

Remove from the oven, transfer the bread onto a wire rack to cool, slice, and serve.

Nutrition:
Calories 524 Fats 15. 8g Carbs 94. 3g Protein 7. 9g

27.   Pineapple French Toasts

Preparation Time: 5-15 minutes | **Cooking Time:** 55 minutes | **Servings:** 4

Ingredients:

2 tbsp flax seed powder + 6 tbsp water	1 ½ cups unsweetened almond milk
½ cup almond flour	2 tbsp pure maple syrup + extra for drizzling
2 pinches salt	½ tbsp cinnamon powder
½ tsp fresh lemon zest	1 tbsp fresh pineapple juice
8 whole-grain bread slices	

Directions:
Preheat the oven to 400 F and lightly grease a roasting rack with olive oil. Set aside.

In a medium bowl, mix the flax seed powder with water and allow thickening for 5 to 10 minutes.

Whisk in the almond milk, almond flour, maple syrup, salt, cinnamon powder, lemon zest, and pineapple juice.

Soak the bread on both sides in the almond milk mixture and allow sitting on a plate for 2 to 3 minutes.

Heat a large skillet over medium heat and place the bread in the pan. Cook until golden brown on the bottom side. Flip the bread and cook further until golden brown on the other side, 4 minutes in total.

Transfer to a plate, drizzle some maple syrup on top and serve immediately.

Nutrition:
Calories 294 Fats 4. 7g Carbs 52. 0g Protein 11. 6g

28. Pimiento Cheese Breakfast Biscuits

Preparation Time: 5-15 minutes | **Cooking Time:** 30 minutes | **Servings:** 4

Ingredients:

2 cups whole-wheat flour	2 tsp baking powder
1 tsp salt	½ tsp baking soda
½ tsp garlic powder	¼ tsp black pepper
¼ cup unsalted plant butter, cold and cut into 1/2-inch cubes	¾ cup of coconut milk
1 cup shredded cashew cheese	1 (4 oz) jar chopped pimientos, well-drained
1 tbsp melted unsalted plant butter	

Directions:
Preheat the oven to 450 F and line a baking sheet with parchment paper. Set aside. In a medium bowl, mix the flour, baking powder, salt, baking soda, garlic powder, and black pepper. Add the cold butter using a hand mixer until the mixture is the size of small peas.

Pour in ¾ of the coconut milk and continue whisking. Continue adding the remaining coconut milk, a tablespoonful at a time, until dough forms.

Mix in the cashew cheese and pimientos. (If the dough is too wet to handle, mix in a little bit more flour until it is manageable). Place the dough on a lightly floured surface and flatten the dough into ½-inch thickness.

Use a 2 ½-inch round cutter to cut out biscuits' pieces from the dough. Gather, re-roll the dough once and continue cutting out biscuits. Arrange the biscuits on the prepared pan and brush the tops with the melted butter. Bake for 12-14 minutes, or until the biscuits are golden brown. Cool and serve.

Nutrition:
Calories 1009 Fats 71. 8g Carbs 74. 8g Protein 24. 5g

29. Breakfast Naan Bread With Mango Saffron Jam

Preparation Time: 5-15 minutes | **Cooking Time:** 40 minutes | **Servings:** 4

Ingredients:

For the naan bread:	¾ cup almond flour
1 tsp salt + extra for sprinkling	1 tsp baking powder
1/3 cup olive oil	2 cups boiling water
2 tbsp plant butter for frying	For the mango saffron jam:
4 cups heaped chopped mangoes	1 cup pure maple syrup
1 lemon, juiced	A pinch of saffron powder
1 tsp cardamom powder	

Directions:
For the naan bread:
In a large bowl, mix the almond flour, salt, and baking powder. Mix in the olive oil and boiling water until smooth, thick batter forms. Allow the dough to rise for 5 minutes.

Form 6 to 8 balls out of the dough, place each on a baking paper and use your hands to flatten the dough.

Working in batches, melt the plant butter in a large skillet and fry the dough on both sides until set and golden brown on each side, 4 minutes per bread. Transfer to a plate and set aside for serving.

For the mango saffron jam
Add the mangoes, maple syrup, lemon juice, and 3 tbsp of water in a medium pot and cook over medium heat until boiling, 5 minutes.

Mix in the saffron and cardamom powders and cook further over low heat until the mangoes are softened.

Mash the mangoes with the back of the spoon until fairly smooth with little chunks of mangoes in the jam.

Turn the heat off and cool completely. Spoon the jam into sterilized jars and serve with the naan bread.

Nutrition:
Calories 766 Fats 42. 7g Carbs 93. 8g Protein 7. 3g

30. Cauliflower And Potato Hash Browns

Preparation Time: 5-15 minutes | **Cooking Time:** 35 minutes | **Servings:** 4

Ingredients:

3 tbsp flax seed powder + 9 tbsp water	2 large potatoes, peeled and shredded
1 big head cauliflower, rinsed and riced	½ white onion, grated
1 tsp salt	1 tbsp black pepper
4 tbsp plant butter, for frying	

Directions:
In a medium bowl, mix the flaxseed powder and water. Allow thickening for 5 minutes for the flax egg.
Add the potatoes, cauliflower, onion, salt, and black pepper to the flax egg and mix until well combined. Allow sitting for 5 minutes to thicken. Working in batches, melt 1 tbsp of plant butter in a non-stick skillet and add 4 scoops of the hash brown mixture to the skillet. Make sure to have 1 to 2-inch intervals between each scoop.
Use the spoon to flatten the batter and cook until compacted and golden brown on the bottom part, 2 minutes. Flip the hashbrowns and cook further for 2 minutes or until the vegetables are cooked and golden brown. Transfer to a paper towel-lined plate to drain grease.
Make the remaining hashbrowns using the remaining ingredients.
Serve warm.

Nutrition:
Calories 265 Fats 11. 9g Carbs 36. 7g Protein 5. 3g

31. Raspberry Raisin Muffins With Orange Glaze

Preparation Time: 5-15 minutes | **Cooking Time:** 40 minutes | **Servings:** 4

Ingredients:

For the muffins:	
	2 tbsp flax seed powder + 6 tbsp water
2 cups whole-wheat flour	1½ tsp baking powder
A pinch salt	½ cup plant butter, room temperature
1 cup pure date sugar	½ cup oat milk
2 tsp vanilla extract	1 lemon, zested
1 cup dried raspberries	For the orange glaze:
2 tbsp orange juice	1 cup pure date sugar

Directions:
Preheat the oven to 400 F and grease 6 muffin cups with cooking spray. In a small bowl, mix the flax seed powder with water and allow thickening for 5 minutes to make the flax egg. In a medium bowl, mix the flour, baking powder, and salt. In another bowl, cream the plant butter, date sugar, and flax egg. Mix in the oat milk, vanilla, and lemon zest.
Combine both mixtures, fold in raspberries, and fill muffin cups two-thirds way up with the batter. Bake until a toothpick inserted comes out clean, 20-25 minutes.
In a medium bowl, whisk orange juice and date sugar until smooth. Remove the muffins when ready and transfer them to a wire rack to cool. Drizzle the glaze on top to serve.

Nutrition:
Calories 700 Fats 25. 5g Carbs 115. 1g Protein 10. 5g

32. Berry Cream Compote Over Crepes

Preparation Time: 5-15 minutes | **Cooking Time:** 35 minutes | **Servings:** 4

Ingredients:

For the berry cream:	
1 knob plant butter	2 tbsp pure date sugar
1 tsp vanilla extract	½ cup fresh blueberries
½ cup fresh raspberries	½ cup whipped coconut cream
For the crepes:	
2 tbsp flax seed powder + 6 tbsp water	1 tsp vanilla extract
1 tsp pure date sugar	¼ tsp salt
2 cups almond flour	1 ½ cups almond milk
1 ½ cups water	3 tbsp plant butter for frying

Directions:

Melt butter in a pot over low heat and mix in the date sugar, and vanilla. Cook until the sugar melts and then toss in berries. Allow softening for 2 3 minutes. Set aside to cool.

In a medium bowl, mix the flax seed powder with water and allow thickening for 5 minutes to make the flax egg. Whisk in the vanilla, date sugar, and salt.

Pour in a quarter cup of almond flour and whisk, then a quarter cup of almond milk, and mix until no lumps remain. Repeat the mixing process with the remaining almond flour and almond milk in the same quantities until exhausted.

Mix in 1 cup of water until the mixture is runny like that of pancakes and add the remaining water until the mixture is lighter. Brush a large non-stick skillet with some butter and place over medium heat to melt.

Pour 1 tablespoon of the batter into the pan and swirl the skillet quickly and all around to coat the pan with the batter. Cook until the batter is dry and golden brown beneath, about 30 seconds.

Use a spatula to carefully flip the crepe and cook the other side until golden brown too. Fold the crepe onto a plate and set aside. Repeat making more crepes with the remaining batter until exhausted. Plate the crepes, top with the whipped coconut cream, and the berry compote. Serve immediately.

Nutrition:

Calories 339 Fats 24. 5g Carbs 30g Protein 2. 3g

33.   Irish Brown Bread

Preparation Time: 5-15 minutes | **Cooking Time:** 50 minutes | **Servings:** 4

Ingredients:

4 cups whole-wheat flour	¼ tsp salt
½ cup rolled oats	1 tsp baking soda
1 ¾ cups coconut milk, thick	2 tbsp pure maple syrup

Directions:

Preheat the oven to 400 F.

In a bowl, mix flour, salt, oats, and baking soda. Add in coconut milk, maple syrup, and whisk until dough forms. Dust your hands with some flour and knead the dough into a ball. Shape the dough into a circle and place on a baking sheet. Cut a deep cross on the dough and bake in the oven for 15 minutes at 450 F. Then, reduce the temperature to 400 F and bake further for 20 to 25 minutes or until a hollow sound is made when the bottom of the bread is tapped. Slice and serve.

Nutrition:

Calories 963 Fats 44. 4g Carbs 125. 1g Protein 22. 1g

34.   Apple Cinnamon Muffins

Preparation Time: 5-15 minutes | **Cooking Time:** 40 minutes | **Servings:** 4

Ingredients:

For the muffins:

1 flax seed powder + 3 tbsp water	1 ½ cups whole-wheat flour
¾ cup pure date sugar	2 tsp baking powder
¼ tsp salt	1 tsp cinnamon powder
1/3 cup melted plant butter	1/3 cup flax milk
2 apples, peeled, cored, and chopped	

For topping:

1/3 cup whole-wheat flour	½ cup pure date sugar
½ cup cold plant butter, cubed	1 ½ tsp cinnamon powder

Directions:

Preheat the oven to 400 F and grease 6 muffin cups with cooking spray. In a bowl, mix the flax seed powder with water and allow thickening for 5 minutes to make the flax egg.

In a medium bowl, mix the flour, date sugar, baking powder, salt, and cinnamon powder. Whisk in the butter, flax egg, flax milk, and then fold in the apples. Fill the muffin cups two-thirds way up with the batter.

In a small bowl, mix the remaining flour, date sugar, cold butter, and cinnamon powder. Sprinkle the mixture on the muffin batter. Bake for 20-minutes. Remove the muffins onto a wire rack, allow cooling, and serve warm.

Nutrition:
Calories 1133 Fats 74. 9g Carbs 104. 3g Protein 18g

35.   Mixed Berry Walnut Yogurt

Preparation Time: 5-15 minutes | **Cooking Time:** 10 minutes | **Servings:** 4

Ingredients:

4 cups almond milk Dairy-Free yogurt, cold	2 tbsp pure malt syrup
2 cups mixed berries, halved or chopped	¼ cup chopped toasted walnuts

Directions:
In a medium bowl, mix the yogurt and malt syrup until well-combined. Divide the mixture into 4 breakfast bowls.
Top with the berries and walnuts.
Enjoy immediately.

Nutrition:
Calories 326 Fats 14. 3g Carbs 38. 3g Protein 12. 5g

36.   Orange Butter Crepes

Preparation Time: 5-15 minutes | **Cooking Time:** 30 minutes | **Servings:** 4

Ingredients:

2 tbsp flax seed powder + 6 tbsp water	1 tsp vanilla extract
1 tsp pure date sugar	¼ tsp salt
2 cups almond flour	1½ cups oat milk
½ cup melted plant butter	3 tbsp fresh orange juice
3 tbsp plant butter for frying	

Directions:
In a medium bowl, mix the flax seed powder with 1 cup water and allow thickening for 5 minutes to make the flax egg. Whisk in the vanilla, date sugar, and salt.
Pour in a quarter cup of almond flour and whisk, then a quarter cup of oat milk, and mix until no lumps remain. Repeat the mixing process with the remaining almond flour and almond milk in the same quantities until exhausted.

Mix in the plant butter, orange juice, and half of the water until the mixture is runny like that of pancakes. Add the remaining water until the mixture is lighter. Brush a large non-stick skillet with some butter and place over medium heat to melt.
Pour 1 tablespoon of the batter into the pan and swirl the skillet quickly and all around to coat the pan with the batter. Cook until the batter is dry and golden brown beneath, about 30 seconds.
Use a spatula to carefully flip the crepe and cook the other side until golden brown too. Fold the crepe onto a plate and set aside. Repeat making more crepes with the remaining batter until exhausted. Drizzle some maple syrup on the crepes and serve.

Nutrition:
Calories 379 Fats 35. 6g Carbs 14. 8g Protein 5. 6g

37.   Creole Tofu Scramble

Preparation Time: 5-15 minutes | **Cooking Time:** 20 minutes | **Servings:** 4

Ingredients:

2 tbsp plant butter, for frying	1 (14 oz) pack firm tofu, pressed and crumbled
1 medium red bell pepper, deseeded and chopped	1 medium green bell pepper, deseeded and chopped
1 tomato, finely chopped	2 tbsp chopped fresh green onions
Salt and black pepper to taste	1 tsp turmeric powder
1 tsp Creole seasoning	½ cup chopped baby kale
¼ cup grated plant-based Parmesan cheese	

Directions:
Melt the plant butter in a large skillet over medium heat and add the tofu. Cook with occasional stirring until the tofu is light golden brown while making sure not to break the tofu into tiny bits but to have scrambled egg resemblance, 5 minutes.

Stir in the bell peppers, tomato, green onions, salt, black pepper, turmeric powder, and Creole seasoning. Sauté until the vegetables soften, 5 minutes.

Mix in the kale to wilt, 3 minutes and then, half of the plant-based Parmesan cheese. Allow melting for 1 to 2 minutes and then turn the heat off.

Dish the food, top with the remaining cheese, and serve warm.

Nutrition:
Calories 258 Fats 15. 9g Carbs 12. 8g Protein 20. 7g

38.   Mushroom Avocado Panini

Preparation Time: 5-15 minutes | **Cooking Time:** 30 minutes | **Servings:** 4

Ingredients:

1 tbsp olive oil	1 cup sliced white button mushrooms
Salt and black pepper to taste	1 ripe avocado, pitted, peeled, and sliced
2 tbsp freshly squeezed lemon juice	1 tbsp chopped parsley
½ tsp pure maple syrup	8 slices whole-wheat ciabatta
4 oz sliced plant-based Parmesan cheese	1 tbsp olive oil

Directions:
Heat the olive oil in a medium skillet over medium heat and sauté the mushrooms until softened, 5 minutes. Season with salt and black pepper. Turn the heat off.

Preheat a panini press to medium heat, 3 to 5 minutes.

Mash the avocado in a medium bowl and mix in the lemon juice, parsley, and maple syrup.

Spread the mixture on 4 bread slices, divide the mushrooms and plant-based Parmesan cheese on top.

Cover with the other bread slices and brush the top with olive oil.

Grill the sandwiches one after another in the heated press until golden brown and the cheese melted.

Serve warm.

Nutrition:
Calories 338 Fats 22. 4g Carbs 25. 5g Protein 12. 4g

39.   Avocado Toast with Herbs and Peas

Preparation Time: 10 minutes | **Cooking Time:** 0 minute | **Servings:** 4

Ingredients:

½ of a medium avocado, peeled, pitted, mashed	6 slices of radish
2 tablespoons baby peas	¼ teaspoon ground black pepper
1 teaspoon chopped basil	¼ teaspoon salt
1/2 lemon, juiced	1 slice of bread, whole-grain, toasted

Directions:
Spread mashed avocado on one side of the toast and then top with peas, pressing them into the avocado.

Layer the toast with radish slices, season with salt and black pepper, sprinkle with basil and drizzle with lemon juice.

Serve straight away.

Nutrition:
Calories: 250 Cal Fat: 12 g Carbs: 22 g Protein: 7 g Fiber: 9 g

40.   Small Sweet Potato Pancakes

Preparation Time: 20 minutes | **Cooking Time:** 0 minutes | **Servings:** 2

Ingredients:

1 clove of garlic	3 tablespoon wholemeal rice flour
1 pinch of nutmeg	3 tablespoons of water
150 g sweet potato	1 pinch of chili flakes
1 teaspoon oil	Salt

Directions:
Peel the garlic clove and mash it with a fork. Peel the sweet potato and grate it into small sticks with a grater.

Knead the sweet potato and garlic in a bowl with the rice flour and water, then season with chili flakes, salt, and nutmeg.

Heat the oil in a pan and form small buffers.
Fry these in the pan on both sides until golden brown.
Goes perfectly with tzatziki and other fresh dips.

Nutrition:
Calories: 209 Fat: 15.4g Carbs: 10.5g Protein: 8.1g Fiber: 3.2g

41.   Tomato and Pesto Toast

Preparation Time: 5 minutes | **Cooking Time:** 0 minute | **Servings:** 4

Ingredients:

1 small tomato, sliced	¼ teaspoon ground black pepper
1 tablespoon vegan pesto	2 tablespoons hummus
1 slice of whole-grain bread, toasted	Hemp seeds as needed for garnishing

Directions:
Spread hummus on one side of the toast, top with tomato slices and then drizzle with pesto. Sprinkle black pepper on the toast along with hemp seeds and then serve straight away.

Nutrition:
Calories: 214 Cal Fat: 7.2 g Carbs: 32 g Protein: 6.5 g Fiber: 3 g

42.   Avocado and Sprout Toast

Preparation Time: 5 minutes | **Cooking Time:** 0 minute | **Servings:** 4

Ingredients:

1/2 of a medium avocado, sliced	1 slice of whole-grain bread, toasted
2 tablespoons sprouts	2 tablespoons hummus
¼ teaspoon lemon zest	½ teaspoon hemp seeds
¼ teaspoon red pepper flakes	

Directions:
Spread hummus on one side of the toast and then top with avocado slices and sprouts. Sprinkle with lemon zest, hemp seeds, and red pepper flakes, and then serve straight away.

Nutrition:
Calories: 200 Cal Fat: 10.5 g Carbs: 22 g Protein: 7 g Fiber: 7 g

43.   Apple and Honey Toast

Preparation Time: 5 minutes | **Cooking Time:** 0 minute | **Servings:** 4

Ingredients:

½ of a small apple, cored, sliced	1 slice of whole-grain bread, toasted
1 tablespoon honey	2 tablespoons hummus
1/8 teaspoon cinnamon	

Directions:
Spread hummus on one side of the toast, top with apple slices and then drizzle with honey. Sprinkle cinnamon on it and then serve straight away.

Nutrition:
Calories: 212 Cal Fat: 7 g Carbs: 35 g Protein: 4 g Fiber: 5.5 g

44.   Zucchini Pancakes

Preparation Time: 10 minutes | **Cooking Time:** 15 minutes | **Servings:** 4

Ingredients:

2 cups zucchini	1/4 cup onion
1 tablespoon all-purpose white flour	1 teaspoon herb seasoning
1 egg 1 tablespoon olive oil	1/8 teaspoon salt

Directions:
Grate onion and zucchini into a bowl and stir to combine. Place the zucchini mixture on a clean kitchen towel. Twist and squeeze out as much liquid as possible. Return to the bowl.
Mix flour, salt, and herb seasoning in a small bowl. Add egg and mix; stir into zucchini and onion mixture. Form 4 patties.
Heat oil over high heat in a large non-stick frying pan. Lower heat to medium and place zucchini patties into the pan. Sauté until brown, turning once.

Nutrition:
Calories 65, Total Fat 4.7g, Saturated Fat 0.9g, Cholesterol 41mg, Sodium 97mg, Total Carbohydrate 4.1g, Dietary Fiber 0.8g, Total Sugars 1.4g, Protein 2.3g, Calcium 16mg, Iron 1mg, Potassium 175mg, Phosphorus 24mg

45. Savory Spinach and Mushroom Crepes

Preparation Time: 60 minutes | **Cooking Time:** 30-120 minutes | **Servings:** 4

Ingredients:

For the crepes:	1 ¾ cup rolled oats
1 tsp pink Himalayan salt	1 ½ cup of soy milk
2 tbsp olive oil	1 tbsp almond butter
½ tsp nutmeg	2 tbsp egg replacement
For the filling:	1 lb button mushrooms
10 oz fresh spinach, finely chopped	4 oz crumbled tofu
1 tbsp chia seeds	1 tbsp fresh rosemary, finely chopped
1 garlic clove, crushed	2 tbsp olive oil

Directions:

First, prepare the crepes. Combine all dry ingredients in a large bowl. Add milk, butter, nutmeg, olive oil, and egg replacement. Mix well with a hand mixer on high speed. Transfer to a food processor and process until completely smooth.

Grease a large non-stick pancake pan with some oil. Pour 1 cup of the mixture into the pan and cook for one minute on each side.

Plug your instant pot and press the 'Sauté' button. Grease the stainless steel insert with some oil and add mushrooms. Cook for 5 minutes, stirring constantly.

Now add spinach, tofu, rosemary, and garlic. Continue to cook for another 5 minutes.

Remove the mixture from the pot and stir in chia seeds. Let it sit for 10 minutes.

Meanwhile, grease a small baking pan with some oil and line with parchment paper.

Divide the mushroom mixture between crepes and roll-up. Gently transfer to a prepared baking pan.

Wrap the pan with aluminum foil and set aside.

Pour 1 cup of water into your instant pot and set the steam rack. Put the pan on top and seal the lid. Press the 'Manual' button and set the timer for 10 minutes.

When done, release the pressure naturally, and open the lid.

Optionally, sprinkle with some dried oregano before serving.

Nutrition:
Calories:680, Total Fat:71.8g, Saturated Fat:20.9g, Total Carbs:10g, Dietary Fiber:7g, Sugar:2g, Protein:3g, Sodium:525mg

Chapter 2: Main Dishes

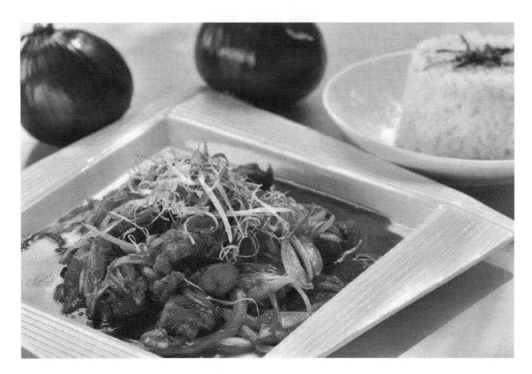

46.   Spinach Pesto Pasta

Preparation Time:05 minutes | **Cooking Time:** 10 minutes | **Servings:** 2

Ingredients:

1cup pasta	2 cups spinach, chopped
¼ cup of coconut oil	½ large lemon
¼ teaspoon garlic powder	1/8 cup chopped pecans
¼ cup goat cheese, grated	¼ teaspoon salt
Freshly cracked pepper to taste	2 oz. mozzarella (optional

Directions:

Add the chopped and washed spinach to a food processor along with the coconut oil, 1/4 cup juice from the lemon, garlic powder, pecans, goat cheese, salt, and pepper. Purée the mixture until smooth and bright green. Add more oil if needed to allow the mixture to become a thick, smooth sauce. Taste the pesto and adjust the salt, pepper, or lemon juice to your liking. Set the pesto aside.

Add pasta, water, and pesto, coconut oil into Instant Pot. Place lid on Instant Pot and lock into place to seal. Pressure Cook on High Pressure for 4 minutes. Use Quick Pressure Release.
Add mozzarella cheese and serve.

Nutrition:
Calories 534, Total Fat 35. 8g, Saturated Fat 27. 7g, Cholesterol 65mg, Sodium 514mg, Total Carbohydrate 39g, Dietary Fiber 1. 2g, Total Sugars 0. 7g, Protein 17. 5g

47.   Paprika Pumpkin Pasta

Preparation Time:05 minutes | **Cooking Time:** 10 minutes | **Servings:** 2

Ingredients:

¼ cup of coconut oil	½ onion
½ tablespoon butter	½ teaspoon garlic
¼ teaspoon paprika	1 cup pumpkin purée
1. 5 cups vegetable broth	¼ teaspoon salt
Freshly cracked pepper	1 cup pasta
1/8 cup coconut cream	1/4 cup grated mozzarella cheese

Directions:

Add the coconut oil to the Instant Pot, hit "Sauté", Add butter and onion until it is soft and transparent. Add the garlic and paprika to the onion and sauté for about one minute more. Finally, add the pumpkin purée, vegetable broth, salt, and pepper to the Instant Pot and stir until the ingredients are combined and smooth.

Add pasta, then place a lid on the Instant Pot and lock it into place to seal. Pressure Cook on High Pressure for 4 minutes. Use Quick Pressure Release.

Add coconut cream and mozzarella cheese.

Nutrition:

Calories 327, Total Fat 8. 9g, Saturated Fat 4. 4g, Cholesterol 67mg. Sodium 931mg, Total Carbohydrate 49g, Dietary Fiber 4. 7g, Total Sugars 5. 7g, Protein 13. 5g

48.   Creamy Mushroom Herb Pasta

Preparation Time:05 minutes | **Cooking Time:** 10 minutes | **Servings:** 2

Ingredients:

¼ cup of coconut oil	½ cup mushrooms
½ teaspoon garlic powder	1 1/2 tablespoon butter
1 1/2 tablespoon coconut flour	1 cup vegetable broth
1 sprig fresh thyme	½ teaspoon basil
Salt and pepper to taste	

Directions:

Add the coconut oil to the Instant Pot, hit "Sauté", add butter, when the butter melts add garlic powder, add the sliced mushrooms and continue to cook until the mushrooms have turned dark brown and all of the moisture they release has evaporated.

Add the flour, Whisk the vegetable broth into the Instant Pot with the flour and mushrooms. Add the thyme, basil, and some freshly cracked pepper.

Then add pasta, place the lid on the pot and lock it into place to seal. Pressure Cook on High Pressure for 4 minutes. Use Quick Pressure Release.

Serve and enjoy.

Nutrition:

Calories 107, Total Fat 7. 5g, Saturated Fat 4. 8g, Cholesterol 15mg, Sodium 439mg, Total Carbohydrate 5. 7g, Dietary Fiber 2. 8g, Total Sugars 1. 3g, Protein 4. 2g

49.   Cabbage and Noodles

Preparation Time:05 minutes | **Cooking Time:** 05 minutes | **Servings:** 2

Ingredients:

1 cup wide egg noodles	1 1/2 tablespoon butter
1 small onion	1/2 head green cabbage, shredded
Salt and pepper to taste	

Directions:

Add egg noodles, butter, water, onion, green cabbage, pepper, and salt to Instant Pot. Place lid on Instant Pot and lock into place to seal. Pressure Cook on High Pressure for 4 minutes. Use Quick Pressure Release.

Serve and enjoy.

Nutrition:

Calories183, Total Fat 6. 8g, Saturated Fat 3. 9g, Cholesterol 31mg, Sodium 78mg, Total Carbohydrate 27. 2g, Dietary Fiber 5. 9g, Total Sugars 7. 6g, Protein 5. 4g

50.   Lemon Garlic Broccoli Macaroni

Preparation Time:05 minutes | **Cooking Time:** 10 minutes | **Servings:** 2

Ingredients:

1 cup macaroni	½ cup broccoli
1 tablespoon butter	½ teaspoon garlic powder
1 lemon	Salt and pepper to taste
Enough water	

Directions:

Add macaroni, butter, water, broccoli, lemon, garlic powder, and salt to Instant Pot. Place the lid on the pot and lock it into place to seal. Pressure Cook on High Pressure for 4 minutes. Use Quick Pressure Release.

Nutrition:
Calories 254, Total Fat 7. 4g, Saturated Fat 3. 9g, Cholesterol 62mg, Sodium 66mg, Total Carbohydrate 39. 8g, Dietary Fiber 1. 5g, Total Sugars 1. 3g, Protein 8. 4g

51. Basil Spaghetti Pasta

Preparation Time:05 minutes | **Cooking Time:** 05 minutes | **Servings:** 2

Ingredients:

½ teaspoon garlic powder	1 cup spaghetti
2 large eggs	¼ cup grated Parmesan cheese
Freshly cracked pepper	Salt and pepper to taste
Handful fresh basil	Enough water

Directions:
In a medium bowl, whisk together the eggs, 1/2 cup of the Parmesan cheese, and a generous dose of freshly cracked pepper.

Add spaghetti, water, basil, garlic powder, pepper, and salt to Instant Pot. Place lid on Instant Pot and lock into place to seal. Pressure Cook on High Pressure for 4 minutes. Use Quick Pressure Release.

Pour the eggs and Parmesan mixture over the hot pasta.

Nutrition:
Calories216, Total Fat 2. 3g, Saturated Fat 0. 7g, Cholesterol 49mg, Sodium 160mg, Total Carbohydrate 36g, Dietary Fiber 0. 1g, Total Sugars 0. 4g, Protein 12. 2g

52. Parsley Hummus Pasta

Preparation Time:05 minutes | **Cooking Time:** 05 minutes | **Servings:** 2

Ingredients:

½ cup chickpeas	1/8 cup coconut oil
½ fresh lemon	1/8 cup tahini
½ teaspoon garlic powder	1/8 teaspoon cumin
1/4 teaspoon salt	
1/8 bunch fresh parsley, or to taste	1 green onion
	1 cup pasta
Enough water	

Directions:
Drain the chickpeas and add them to a food processor along with the coconut oil, juice from the lemon, tahini, garlic powder, cumin, and salt. Pulse the ingredients, adding a small amount of water if needed to keep it moving, until the hummus is smooth.

Slice the green onion (both white and green ends) and pull the parsley leaves from the stems. Add the green onion and parsley to the hummus in the food processor and process again until only small flecks of green remain. Taste the hummus and adjust the salt, lemon, or garlic if needed.

Add pasta, water into Instant Pot. Place the lid on the pot and lock it into place to seal. Pressure Cook on High Pressure for 4 minutes. Use Quick Pressure Release.

In Sauté mode add hummus to pasta. When it mixes, turn off the switch of Instant Pot.

Serve and enjoy.

Nutrition:
Calories 582, Total Fat 26. 3g, Saturated Fat 13. 5g, Cholesterol 47mg, Sodium 338mg, Total Carbohydrate 71g, Dietary Fiber 10. 8g, Total Sugars 6. 1g, Protein 19. 9g

53. Creamy Spinach Artichoke Pasta

Preparation Time:05 minutes | **Cooking Time:** 05 minutes | **Servings:** 2

Ingredients:

1 tablespoon butter	¼ teaspoon garlic powder
1 cup vegetable broth	1 cup of coconut milk
¼ teaspoon salt	Freshly cracked pepper
½ cup pasta	1/4 cup fresh baby spinach
½ cup quartered artichoke hearts	1/8 cup grated Parmesan cheese

Directions:
In the Instant Pot, hit "Sauté", add butter when it melts, add garlic powder just until it's tender and fragrant.

Add the vegetable broth, coconut milk, salt, some freshly cracked pepper, and pasta. Place the lid on the pot and lock it into place to seal.

Pressure Cook on High Pressure for 4 minutes. Use Quick Pressure Release.

Add the spinach, a handful at a time, to the hot pasta and toss it in the pasta until it wilts into Instant Pot in Sauté mode. Stir the chopped artichoke hearts into the pasta. Sprinkle grated Parmesan over the pasta, then stir slightly to incorporate the Parmesan. Top with an additional Parmesan then serve.

Nutrition:
Calories 457, Total Fat 36. 2g, Saturated Fat 29. 6g, Cholesterol 40mg, Sodium 779mg, Total Carbohydrate 27. 6g, Dietary Fiber 4g, Total Sugars 4. 7g, Protein 10. 3g

54. Easy Spinach Ricotta Pasta

Preparation Time:05 minutes | **Cooking Time:**10 minutes | **Servings:** 2

Ingredients:

½ cup pasta	1 cup vegetable broth
1/2 lb. uncooked tagliatelle	1 tablespoon coconut oil
½ teaspoon garlic powder	¼ cup almond milk
½ cup whole milk ricotta	1/8 teaspoon salt
Freshly cracked pepper	¼ cup chopped spinach

Directions:
Add the vegetable broth, tagliatelle, spinach, salt, some freshly cracked pepper, and the pasta. Place lid on Instant Pot and lock into place to seal. Pressure Cook on High Pressure for 4 minutes. Use Quick Pressure Release.

Prepare the ricotta sauce. Mince the garlic and add it to a large skillet with coconut oil. Cook over Medium-Low heat for 1-2 minutes, or just until soft and fragrant (but not browned). Add the almond milk and ricotta, then stir until relatively smooth (the ricotta may be slightly grainy). Allow the sauce to heat through and come to a low simmer. The sauce will thicken slightly as it simmers. Once it's thick enough to coat the spoon (3-5 minutes), season with salt and pepper.

Add the cooked and drained pasta to the sauce and toss to coat. If the sauce becomes too thick

or dry, add a small amount of the reserved pasta cooking water. Serve warm.

Nutrition:
Calories277, Total Fat 18. 9g, Saturated Fat 15. 2g, Cholesterol 16mg, Sodium 191mg, Total Carbohydrate 23. 8g, Dietary Fiber 1. 2g, Total Sugars 1. 4g, Protein 5. 1g

55. Roasted Red Pepper Pasta

Preparation Time:05 minutes | **Cooking Time:** 05 minutes | **Servings:** 2

Ingredients:

2 cups vegetable broth	½ cup spaghetti
1 small onion	½ teaspoon garlic minced
½ cup roasted red peppers	½ cup roasted diced tomatoes
¼ tablespoon dried mint	1/8 teaspoon crushed red pepper
Freshly cracked black pepper	½ cup goat cheese

Directions:
In an Instant Pot, combine the vegetable broth, onion, garlic, red pepper slices, diced tomatoes, mint, crushed red pepper, and some freshly cracked black pepper. Stir these ingredients to combine. Add spaghetti to the Instant Pot.

Place lid on Instant Pot and lock into place to seal. Pressure Cook on High Pressure for 4 minutes. Use Quick Pressure Release.

Divide the goat cheese into tablespoon-sized pieces, then add them to the Instant Pot. Stir the pasta until the cheese melts in and creates a smooth sauce. Serve hot.

Nutrition:
Calories198, Total Fat 4. 9g, Saturated Fat 2. 2g, Cholesterol 31mg, Sodium 909mg, Total Carbohydrate 26. 8g, Dietary Fiber 1. 9g, Total Sugars 5. 6g, Protein 11. 9g

56. Cheese Beetroot Greens Macaroni

Preparation Time:05 minutes | **Cooking Time:** 05 minutes | **Servings:** 2

Ingredients:

1 tablespoon butter	1 clove garlic minced

1 cup button mushrooms

½ bunch beetroot greens

½ cup vegetable broth

½ cup macaroni

¼ teaspoon salt

½ cup grated Parmesan cheese

Freshly cracked pepper

Directions:

In the Instant Pot, hit "Sauté", add butter, garlic and slice the mushrooms. Add the beetroot greens to the pot along with 1/2 cup vegetable broth. Stir the beetroot greens as it cooks until it is fully wilted.

Add vegetable broth, macaroni, salt, and pepper. Place lid on Instant Pot and lock into place to seal. Pressure Cook on High Pressure for 4 minutes. Use Quick Pressure Release. Add grated Parmesan cheese.

Nutrition:

Calories 147, Total Fat 8g, Saturated Fat 4. 8g, Cholesterol 23mg, Sodium 590mg, Total Carbohydrate 12. 7g, Dietary Fiber 1g, Total Sugars 1. 5g, Protein 6. 5g

57.   Pastalaya

Preparation Time:05 minutes | **Cooking Time:** 05 minutes | **Servings:** 2

Ingredients:

½ tablespoon avocado oil

½ teaspoon garlic powder

1 diced tomato

¼ teaspoon dried basil

¼ teaspoon smoked paprika

¼ teaspoon dried rosemary

Freshly cracked pepper

1 cup vegetable broth

½ cup of water

1 cup orzo pasta

1 tablespoon coconut cream

½ bunch fresh coriander

Directions:

In the Instant Pot, place the garlic powder and avocado oil, sauté for 15 seconds, or until the garlic is fragrant. Add diced tomatoes, basil, smoked paprika, rosemary, freshly cracked pepper, and orzo pasta to the Instant Pot. Finally, add the vegetable broth and ½ cup of water, and stir until everything is evenly combined.

Place the lid on the Instant Pot, and bring the toggle switch into the "Sealing" position. Press Manual or Pressure Cook and adjust the time for 5 minutes.

When the five minutes are up, do a Natural-release for 5 minutes and then move the toggle switch to "Venting" to release the rest of the pressure in the pot.

Remove the lid. If the mixture looks watery, press "Sauté" and bring the mixture up to a boil and let it boil for a few minutes. It will thicken as it boils. Add the coconut cream and leek to the Instant Pot, stir and let warm through for a few minutes.

Serve and garnish with coriander toast. Enjoy!

Nutrition:

Calories 351, Total Fat 6. 8g, Saturated Fat 3. 5g, Cholesterol 56mg. Sodium 869mg, Total Carbohydrate 45. 5g, Dietary Fiber 1. 5g, Total Sugars 2. 9g, Protein 26. 3g

58.   Pasta with Peppers

Preparation Time:5 minutes | **Cooking Time:** 15 minutes | **Servings:** 2

Ingredients:

1 1/2 cups spaghetti sauce

1 cup vegetable broth

½ tablespoon dried Italian seasoning blend

1 cup bell pepper strips

1 cup dried pasta

1 cup shredded Romano cheese

Directions:

Press the button Sauté. Set it for High, and set the time for 10 minutes.

Mix the sauce, broth, and seasoning blend in an Instant Pot. Cook, turn off the Sauté function; stir in the bell pepper strips and pasta. Lock the lid onto the pot.

Press Pressure Cook on Max Pressure for 5 minutes with the Keep Warm setting off.

Use the Quick Release method to bring the pot pressure back to normal. Unlatch the lid and open the cooker. Stir in the shredded Romano cheese. Set the lid askew over the pot and set aside for 5 minutes to melt the cheese and let the pasta continue to absorb excess liquid. Serve by the big spoon.

Nutrition:
Calories 291, Total Fat 6. 2g, Saturated Fat 2. 9g, Cholesterol 61mg, Sodium 994mg, Total Carbohydrate 43. 7g, Dietary Fiber 1g, Total Sugars 3. 5g, Protein 15. 1g

59.   Fresh Tomato Mint Pasta

Preparation Time:05 minutes | **Cooking Time:** 10 minutes | **Servings:** 2

Ingredients:

1 cup pasta	1 tablespoon coconut oil
½ teaspoon garlic powder	1 tomato
½ tablespoon butter	¼ cup fresh mint
¼ cup of coconut milk Enough water	Salt & pepper to taste

Directions:
Add the coconut oil to the Instant Pot hit "Sauté", add in the garlic, and stir. Add the tomatoes and a pinch of salt. Then add mint and pepper.
Next, add coconut milk, butter, and water. Stir well, lastly, add in the pasta.
Secure the lid and hit "Keep Warm/Cancel" and then hit "Manual" or "Pressure Cook" High Pressure for 6 minutes. Quick-release when done.
Enjoy.

Nutrition:
Calories 350, Total Fat 18. 5g, Saturated Fat 14. 3g, Cholesterol 54mg, Sodium 47mg, Total Carbohydrate 39. 4g, Dietary Fiber 1. 9g, Total Sugars 2g, Protein 8. 7g

60.   Corn and Chiles Fusilli

Preparation Time:05 minutes | **Cooking Time:** 05 minutes | **Servings:** 2

Ingredients:

½ tablespoon butter	1 tablespoon garlic minced
Salt and pepper to taste	2 oz. can green chills
½ cup frozen corn kernels	¼ teaspoon cumin
1/8 teaspoon paprika	1 cup fusilli
1 cup vegetable broth	¼ cup coconut cream
2 leeks, sliced	1/8 bunch parsley

1 oz. shredded mozzarella cheese

Directions:
In the Instant Pot, add butter when butter melt, place the minced garlic, salt, and pepper, then press Sauté   on the Instant Pot. Add the can of green chills (with juices), frozen corn kernels, cumin, and paprika.
Add the uncooked fusilli and vegetable broth to the Instant Pot.
Place the lid on the Instant Pot, and bring the toggle switch into the "Sealing" position. Press Manual or Pressure Cook and adjust the time for 5 minutes.
When the five minutes are up, do a Natural-release for 5 minutes and then move the toggle switch to "Venting" to release the rest of the pressure in the pot.
Remove the lid. If the mixture looks watery, press "Sauté", and bring the mixture up to a boil and let it boil for a few minutes. Then add the coconut cream and stir until it has fully coated the pasta. Stir in most of the sliced leek and parsley, reserving a little to sprinkle over top, mozzarella on top of the pasta.

Nutrition:
Calories 399, Total Fat 14. 4g, Saturated Fat 10g, Cholesterol 15mg, Sodium 531mg, Total Carbohydrate 56. 2g, Dietary Fiber 4. 9g, Total Sugars 7. 2g, Protein 15. 4g

61.   Creamy Penne with Vegetables

Preparation Time:05 minutes | **Cooking Time:** 10 minutes | **Servings:** 2

Ingredients:

½ tablespoon butter	1 cup penne
1 small onion	½ teaspoon garlic powder
1 carrot	½ red bell pepper
½ pumpkin	2 cups vegetable broth
2 oz. coconut cream	1/8 cup grated Parmesan cheese
1/8 teaspoon salt and pepper to taste	Dash hot sauce, optional
¼ cup cauliflower florets	

Directions:

Set Instant Pot to Sauté. Add the butter and allow it to melt. Add the onion and garlic powder and cook for 2 minutes. Stir regularly. Add the carrot, red pepper and pumpkin, and cauliflower to the pot.

Add penne, vegetable broth, coconut cream, salt, and pepper then add hot sauce.

Lock the lid and make sure the vent is closed. Set Instant Pot to Manual or Pressure Cook on High Pressure for 10 minutes. When cooking time ends, release pressure and wait for steam to completely stop before opening the lid.

Stir in cheese, sprinkle a bit on top of the pasta when you serve it.

Nutrition:

Calories 381, Total Fat 13. 2g, Saturated Fat 8. 7g, Cholesterol 56mg, Sodium 1006mg, Total Carbohydrate 52. 3g, Dietary Fiber 4. 7g, Total Sugars 8. 6g, Protein 15. 3g

62. Pasta with Eggplant Sauce

Preparation Time:05 minutes | **Cooking Time:** 10 minutes | **Servings:** 2

Ingredients:

1 tablespoon coconut oil	2 cloves garlic
1 small onion	1 medium eggplant
1 cup diced tomatoes	1 tablespoon tomato sauce
¼ teaspoon dried thyme	½ teaspoon honey
Pinch paprika	Freshly cracked pepper
¼ salt and pepper, or to taste	6 oz. spaghetti
2 cups vegetable broth	Handful fresh coriander, chopped

Directions:

Set Instant Pot to Sauté. Add the coconut oil and allow it to melt. Add the onion and garlic and cook for 2 minutes or until the onion is soft and transparent.

Add eggplant, diced tomatoes, tomato sauce, thyme, honey, paprika, and freshly cracked pepper. Stir them well to combine, Add spaghetti, and vegetable broth, salt, and pepper.

Lock the lid and make sure the vent is closed. Set Instant Pot to Manual or Pressure Cook on High Pressure for 10 minutes. When cooking time ends, release pressure and wait for steam to completely stop before opening the lid.

Top each serving with grated goat and a sprinkle of fresh coriander.

Nutrition:

Calories 306, Total Fat 18g, Saturated Fat 12. 9g, Cholesterol 30mg, Sodium 188mg, Total Carbohydrate 27g, Dietary Fiber 12. 6g 45%, Total Sugars 13. 9g, Protein 14. 2g

63. Creamy Pesto Pasta With Tofu & Broccoli

Preparation Time:05 minutes | **Cooking Time:** 10 minutes | **Servings:** 2

Ingredients:

4 oz. Farfalle pasta	4 oz. frozen broccoli florets
½ tablespoon coconut oil	½ cup tofu
¼ cup basil pesto	¼ cup vegetable broth
2 oz. heavy cream	

Directions:

In the Instant Pot, add Farfalline pasta, broccoli, coconut oil, tofu, basil pesto, vegetable broth. Cover the Instant Pot and lock it in.

Set the Manual or Pressure Cook timer for 10 minutes. Make sure the timer is set to "Sealing". Once the timer reaches zero, quickly release the pressure. Add heavy cream.

Enjoy.

Nutrition:

Calories 383, Total Fat 17. 8g, Saturated Fat 10. 1g, Cholesterol 39mg, Sodium 129mg, Total Carbohydrate 44g, Dietary Fiber 2. 4g, Total Sugars 3. 2g, Protein 13. 6g

64. Chili Cheese Cottage Cheese Mac

Preparation Time:05 minutes | **Cooking Time:** 12 minutes | **Servings:** 2

Ingredients:

½ tablespoon butter	1 cup cottage cheese

½ teaspoon garlic powder

1 tablespoon coconut flour

¼ teaspoon smoked paprika

1 cup tomato paste

1 cup dry macaroni

1 small onion

½ tablespoon chili powder

¼ teaspoon dried basil

2 cups vegetable broth

½ cup shredded sharp cheddar

Directions:

Set the Instant Pot to Sauté. Add butter and wait one minute to heat up.

Add the cottage cheese, sauté for one minute. Stir often. Add coconut flour, onion, and garlic powder.

Add the chili powder, smoked paprika, basil, tomato paste, and 2 cups of vegetable broth. Add the dry macaroni and cottage cheese. Stir well. Cover the Instant Pot and lock it in.

Set the Manual or Pressure Cook timer for 10 minutes. Make sure the timer is set to "Sealing". Once the timer reaches zero, quickly release the pressure.

Add shredded sharp cheddar cheese and enjoy.

Nutrition:

Calories 509, Total Fat 11. 3g, Saturated Fat 6. 4g, Cholesterol 23mg, Sodium 1454mg, Total Carbohydrate 70. 3g, Dietary Fiber 10. 8g, Total Sugars 20. 5g, Protein 34. 8g

65.   Spicy Cauliflower Pasta

Preparation Time:05 minutes | **Cooking Time:** 10 minutes | **Servings:** 2

Ingredients:

1 tablespoon coconut oil

¼ teaspoon paprika

½ cup broccoli florets

Salt & pepper to taste

1 teaspoon garlic powder

½ cup cauliflower florets

1 cup bow tie pasta

1 cup vegetable broth

Directions:

In the Instant Pot, set the Sauté button and add coconut oil when oil is hot, place garlic powder, paprika, cauliflower florets, broccoli florets, salt, and pepper.

Sauté the mixture until it's cooked thoroughly.

Add the vegetable broth, and dry bow tie pasta.

Mix very well and place the lid on the Instant Pot, and bring the toggle switch into the "Sealing" position.

Press Manual or Pressure Cook and adjust the time for 5 minutes.

When the five minutes are up, do a Natural-release for 5 minutes and then move the toggle switch to "Venting" to release the rest of the pressure in the pot.

Remove the lid. If the mixture looks watery, press "Sauté", and bring the mixture up to a boil and let it boil for a few minutes. It will thicken as it boils.

Serve and enjoy!

Nutrition:

Calories298, Total Fat 10. 4g, Saturated Fat 7. 2g, Cholesterol 50mg, Sodium 426mg, Total Carbohydrate 39. 6g, Dietary Fiber 1. 5g, Total Sugars 1. 8g, Protein 12. 2g

66.   Tasty Mac and Cheese

Preparation Time:05 minutes | **Cooking Time:** 10 minutes | **Servings:** 2

Ingredients:

½ cup of soy milk

Enough water

¼ teaspoon salt

1/8 teaspoon red chili powder

1 cup dry macaroni

½ cup shredded mozzarella cheese

¼ teaspoon Dijon mustard

Directions:

Add macaroni, soy milk, water, and salt, chili powder, Dijon mustard to the Instant Pot. Place lid on Instant Pot and lock into place to seal. Pressure Cook on High Pressure for 4 minutes. Use Quick Pressure Release. Stir cheese into macaroni and then stir in the cheeses until melted and combined.

Nutrition:

Calories 210, Total Fat 3g, Saturated Fat 1g, Cholesterol 4mg, Sodium 374mg, Total Carbohydrate 35. 7g, Dietary Fiber 1. 8g, Total Sugars 3. 6g, Protein 9. 6g

67. Jackfruit and Red Pepper Pasta

Preparation Time: 05 minutes | **Cooking Time:** 17 minutes | **Servings:** 2

Ingredients:

½ cup gnocchi	1/8 cup avocado oil
½ tablespoon garlic powder	1/2 teaspoon crushed red pepper
½ bunch fresh mint	½ cup jackfruit
Salt to taste	Enough water

Directions:

Set Instant Pot to Sauté. Add the avocado oil and allow it to sizzle. Add the garlic powder and cook for 2 minutes. Stir regularly.

Add jackfruit and cook until about 4 - 5 minutes. Add gnocchi, water, fresh mint, salt, and red pepper into Instant Pot.

Lock the lid and make sure the vent is closed. Set Instant Pot to Manual or Pressure Cook on High PRESSURE for 10 minutes. When cooking time ends, release pressure and wait for steam to completely stop before opening the lid.

Enjoy.

Nutrition:

Calories 110, Total Fat 2. 3g, Saturated Fat 0. 4g, Cholesterol 0mg, Sodium 168mg, Total Carbohydrate 21. 5g, Dietary Fiber 2. 5g, Total Sugars 0. 6g, Protein 2. 3g

68. Creamy Mushroom Pasta with Broccoli

Preparation Time: 05 minutes | **Cooking Time:** 12 minutes | **Servings:** 2

Ingredients:

1 tablespoon coconut oil	1 small onion
½ teaspoon garlic powder	1 cup mushrooms
1 tablespoon coconut flour	1 cup of water
¼ cup red wine	1/8 cup coconut cream
¼ teaspoon dried basil	Salt and pepper to taste
1/8 bunch fresh cilantro	½ cup mozzarella cheese

4 oz. pasta	½ cup broccoli

Directions:

Set Instant Pot to Sauté. Add the coconut oil and allow it to sizzle. Add coconut flour and mushrooms, sauté for 2 minutes. Stir regularly. It will coat the mushrooms and will begin to turn golden in color. Just make sure to keep stirring so that the flour does not burn.

Combine water along with the red wine, basil, salt, and pepper. Whisk until no flour lumps remain.

Add pasta, broccoli, cilantro, onion, and garlic powder. Lock the lid and make sure the vent is closed. Set Instant Pot to Manual or Pressure Cook on High Pressure for 10 minutes. When cooking time ends, release pressure and wait for steam to completely stop before opening the lid. Stir in cheese and coconut cream.

Serve hot and enjoy.

Nutrition:

Calories 363, Total Fat 14. 2g, Saturated Fat 11g, Cholesterol 45mg, Sodium 91mg, Total Carbohydrate 43. 4g, Dietary Fiber 4. 6g, Total Sugars 3. 9g, Protein 12. 1g

69. Peanut Noodles Stir Fry

Preparation Time: 05 minutes | **Cooking Time:** 17 minutes | **Servings:** 2

Ingredients:

½ teaspoon ginger powder	¼ cup natural peanut butter
¼ cup hoisin sauce	1 cup hot water
¼ teaspoon sriracha hot sauce	1 tablespoon vegetable oil
½ teaspoon garlic powder	1 cup frozen stir fry vegetables
2 oz. soba noodles	2 sliced leek, optional

Directions:

Prepare the sauce first. Add ginger powder into a bowl. Add the peanut butter, hoisin sauce, sriracha hot sauce, and ¼ cup of hot water. Stir or whisk until smooth. Set the sauce aside until it is needed.

Set the Instant Pot to Sauté. Add the vegetable oil and allow it to sizzle. Add garlic powder and ginger powder and cook for 2 minutes. Add the bag of frozen vegetables and cook for 5 minutes. Add the remaining water and soba noodles.

Lock the lid and make sure the vent is closed. Set Instant Pot to Manual or Pressure Cook on High Pressure for 10 minutes. When cooking time ends, release pressure and wait for steam to completely stop before opening the lid.

Stir until everything is combined and coated with sauce. Garnish with sliced leek if desired.

Nutrition:
Calories 501, Total Fat 24. 4g, Saturated Fat 4. 6g, Cholesterol 1mg, Sodium 788mg, Total Carbohydrate 58. 1g, Dietary Fiber 6g, Total Sugars 15. 8g, Protein 17. 3g

70.   Cauliflower Shells Cheese

Preparation Time:05 minutes | **Cooking Time:** 15 minutes | **Servings:** 2

Ingredients:

4 oz. macaroni	1 cup vegetable broth
½ cup cauliflower florets	1/2 small onion
1 1/2 tablespoons butter	1 1/2 tablespoons coconut flour
1 1/2 cups coconut milk	1 cup sharp cheddar, shredded
Salt and pepper to taste	

Directions:
Set the Instant Pot to Sauté, add the coconut flour, butter, and onion. The flour and butter will form a paste, whisk for 1-2 minutes more taking care not to let it scorch. This slightly cooks the flour preventing the cheese sauce from having an overly strong flour flavor or paste-like flavor.

Whisk the milk into the roux until no lumps remain. Add some freshly cracked pepper to the sauce. Bring the mixture up to a simmer, stirring often. Set aside.

Add macaroni and vegetable broth into Instant Pot. Lock the lid and make sure the vent is closed. Add cauliflower and set Instant Pot to Manual or Pressure Cook on High Pressure for 10 minutes. When cooking time ends, release pressure and wait for steam to completely stop before opening the lid.

Add cheddar and stir sauce mix well with macaroni.

Nutrition:
Calories 643, Total Fat 53. 6g, Saturated Fat 42. 1g, Cholesterol 75mg, Sodium 443mg, Total Carbohydrate 26. 2g, Dietary Fiber 6. 6g, Total Sugars 6. 2g, Protein 18. 4g

71.   Lemon Mozzarella Pasta

Preparation Time:05 minutes | **Cooking Time:** 10 minutes | **Servings:** 2

Ingredients:

4 oz. macaroni	¼ cup peas
½ cup mozzarella cheese	½ tablespoon olive oil
1 lemon	Salt and pepper

Directions:
Set Instant Pot to Sauté. Add the olive oil and allow it to sizzle. Add macaroni, peas, lemon, salt, and pepper.

Lock the lid and make sure the vent is closed. Set Instant Pot to Manual or Pressure Cook on High Pressure for 10 minutes. When cooking time ends, release pressure and wait for steam to completely stop before opening the lid.

Add mozzarella cheese and Stir until everything is combined and coated with sauce.

Enjoy.

Nutrition:
Calories 273, Total Fat 5. 9g, Saturated Fat 1. 3g, Cholesterol 4mg, Sodium 44mg, Total Carbohydrate 46. 6g, Dietary Fiber 3. 7g, Total Sugars 2. 8g, Protein 10. 3g

72.   Kale Lasagna Roll-Ups

Preparation Time:10 minutes | **Cooking Time:** 15 minutes | **Servings:** 2

Ingredients:

½ cup Lasagna noodles	½ cup goat cheese
½ cup mozzarella, shredded	1 large egg
¼ cup kale	½ cup marinara sauce
Salt and pepper to taste	Enough water

Directions:

Set Instant Pot to Sauté. Add the kale with goat cheese, mozzarella, egg, pepper, and salt. Stir regularly.

Add marinara sauce, water, noodles. Mix well. Stir to make sure noodles are covered with the liquid.

Lock the lid and make sure the vent is closed. Set Instant Pot to Manual or Pressure Cook on High Pressure for 15 minutes. When cooking time ends, release pressure and wait for steam to completely stop before opening the lid.

if you would like to sprinkle a bit on top of the Lasagna when you serve it.

Nutrition:

Calories 343, Total Fat 23. 6g, Saturated Fat 22. 1g, Cholesterol 17. 5mg, Sodium 243mg, Total Carbohydrate 16. 2g, Dietary Fiber 3. 6g, Total Sugars 2. 2g, Protein 16. 4g

73.   Zucchini Noodles

Preparation Time: 10 minutes | **Cooking Time:** 15 minutes | **Servings:** 2

Ingredients:

2 zucchini, peeled	Marinara sauce of your choice
Any other seasonings you wish to use	

Directions:

Peel & spiralizer your zucchini into noodles.

Add some of your favorite sauce to Instant Pot, hit "Sauté" and "Adjust" so it's on the "More" or "High" setting.

Once the sauce is bubbling, add the noodles to the pot, toss them in the sauce, and allow them to heat up and soften for a few minutes for about 2-5 minutes.

Serve in bowls and top with some grated parmesan, if desired.

Enjoy!

Nutrition:

Calories 86, Total Fat 2g, Saturated Fat 0. 5g, Cholesterol 1mg, Sodium 276mg, Total Carbohydrate 15. 2g, Dietary Fiber 3. 8g, Total Sugars 8. 9g, Protein 3. 5g

74.   Lemon Parsley Pasta

Preparation Time: 10 minutes | **Cooking Time:** 15 minutes | **Servings:** 2

Ingredients:

1 cup ziti pasta	½ cup fresh parsley, finely chopped
1 lemon zest	1 teaspoon garlic powder
1 1/2 tablespoon coconut oil	½ tablespoon butter
2 tablespoon parmesan cheese	Salt and fresh black pepper
Enough water	

Directions:

Add butter to the Instant Pot, hit "Sauté" and once the butter is melted and sizzled, Add parsley, lemon zest, garlic powder, coconut oil, salt, and black pepper.

Lock the lid and make sure the vent is closed. Add water and ziti pasta. Set Instant Pot to Manual or Pressure Cook on High PRESSURE for 10 minutes. When cooking time ends, release pressure and wait for steam to completely stop before opening the lid.

Stir in cheese. Serve and enjoy.

Nutrition:

Calories 377, Total Fat 17. 4g, Saturated Fat 11. 9g, Cholesterol 74mg, Sodium 306mg, Total Carbohydrate 40. 7g, Dietary Fiber 1. 5g, Total Sugars 1. 2g, Protein 17. 3g

75.   Creamy Tofu Marsala Pasta

Preparation Time: 10 minutes | **Cooking Time:** 15 minutes | **Servings:** 2

Ingredients:

¼ cup butter	1 tablespoon coconut oil
1 small onion, diced	2 cup mushrooms, sliced
½ cup tofu, diced into chunks	½ teaspoon garlic powder
1 1/2 cups of vegetable broth	1 cup of white wine
½ cup sun-dried tomatoes	1 cup fusilli
1/4 cup coconut cream	½ cup grated goat cheese

Directions:

Add the butter to the Instant Pot. Hit "Sauté". Add the onion and mushrooms and cook for 3-5 minutes, until the mushrooms have softened and browned a bit.

Then, add the tofu and the coconut oil from the sun-dried tomatoes and cook for another 2-3 minutes until the tofu is slightly white.

Toss in the garlic powder and cook for 1 more minute and then add in the white wine and let it simmer for 1 minute more.

Add in the vegetable broth and stir together well. Pour in the fusilli so it's laying on top of the broth, gently smoothing and pushing it down with a spatula so it's submerged, but do not stir it with the rest of the broth.

Secure the lid and hit "Manual" or "Pressure Cook" High Pressure for 6 minutes. Quick-release when done and give it all a good stir.

Stir in the coconut cream and goat cheese. Let it sit for about 5 minutes, stirring occasionally and it will thicken up into an incredible sauce, coating all the pasta perfectly.

Transfer to a serving bowl, plate it up, and sprinkle any extra goat cheese if desired.

Enjoy!

Nutrition:

Calories 510, Total Fat 20. 6g, Saturated Fat 14. 8g, Cholesterol 7mg, Sodium 432mg, Total Carbohydrate 45. 9g, Dietary Fiber 4. 8g, Total Sugars 7. 8g, Protein 19. 1g

76.   Classic Goulash

Preparation Time:10 minutes | **Cooking Time:** 15 minutes | **Servings:** 2

Ingredients:

1 cup crumbled tofu	2 onions, chopped
1 teaspoon garlic powder	2 cups of water
1 cup tomato paste	1cup diced tomatoes
1 1/2 tablespoons soy sauce	½ tablespoon dried basil
1 bay leaf	¼ tablespoon seasoned salt, or to taste
1 cup uncooked elbow macaroni	

Directions:

Set Instant Pot to Sauté. Add crumbled tofu. Add the onions and garlic powder and cook for 2 minutes. Stir regularly.

Stir water, tomato paste, diced tomatoes, soy sauce, dried basil, bay leaf, and seasoned salt into the tofu mixture.

Stir macaroni into the mixture, Secure the lid, and hit "Manual" or "Pressure Cook" High Pressure for 6 minutes. Quick-release when done.

Enjoy.

Nutrition:

Calories 425, Total Fat 7. 5g, Saturated Fat 1. 2g, Cholesterol 0mg, Sodium 647mg, Total Carbohydrate 73. 5g, Dietary Fiber 10. 7g, Total Sugars 24. 3g, Protein 23. 8g

77.   Penne with Spicy Vodka Tomato Cream Sauce

Preparation Time:10 minutes | **Cooking Time:** 15 minutes | **Servings:** 2

Ingredients:

½ cup uncooked penne pasta	1/8 cup coconut oil
Enough water	1 teaspoon garlic powder
¼ teaspoon paprika	½ cup crushed tomatoes
½ teaspoon salt	1 tablespoon vodka
½ cup coconut cream	1/8 cup chopped fresh cilantro

Directions:

Add penne pasta, coconut oil, water, paprika, crushed tomatoes, vodka, garlic powder, and salt to Instant Pot.

Place the lid on the pot and lock it into place to seal. Pressure Cook on High Pressure for 4 minutes. Use Quick Pressure Release. Stir coconut cream into penne pasta and then stir in the fresh cilantro and combine.

Nutrition:

Calories 394, Total Fat 28. 7g, Saturated Fat 24. 6g, Cholesterol 23mg, Sodium 720mg, Total Carbohydrate 27g, Dietary Fiber 3. 6g, Total Sugars 5. 9g, Protein 6. 8g

78. Creamy Pesto Tofu

Preparation Time: 10 minutes | **Cooking Time:** 15 minutes | **Servings:** 2

Ingredients:

½ cup vermicelli pasta	¼ cup butter
1/2 teaspoon ground black pepper	¼ cup grated mozzarella cheese
¼ cup basil pesto	½ cup tofu, peeled
Enough water	

Directions:

Set the Instant Pot to Sauté. Add butter and wait one minute to heat up.

Add the tofu, basil pesto sauté for one minute. Stir often.

Add water, vermicelli pasta, and pepper. Place the lid on the pot and lock it into place to seal. Pressure Cook on High Pressure for 4 minutes. Use Quick Pressure Release.

Stir mozzarella cheese. Serve and enjoy.

Nutrition:

Calories 711, Total Fat 62. 3g, Saturated Fat 52. 7g, Cholesterol 15mg, Sodium 77mg, Total Carbohydrate 32. 5g, Dietary Fiber 6. 8g, Total Sugars 8. 8g, Protein 15. 6g

79. Garlic Lasagna

Preparation Time: 10 minutes | **Cooking Time:** 20min | **Servings:** 2

Ingredients:

½ tablespoon butter	½ tablespoon coconut oil
1 small onion chopped	1 tablespoon garlic powder
½ cup ground cauliflower	½ cup pasta sauce
2 cups vegetable broth	1/8 cup white wine
1 cup of water	1teaspoon Italian seasoning
1 cup uncooked Lasagna noodles	½ cup shredded goat cheese divided
1/4 cup Parmesan cheese	

Directions:

Set Instant Pot to Sauté. Add the coconut oil and butter and allow it to sizzle. Add the onions and garlic powder and cook for 2 minutes. Stir regularly.

Add ground cauliflower and cook until about 4 - 5 minutes into Instant Pot.

Add pasta sauce, vegetable broth, white wine, water, and Italian seasonings. Mix well.

Add Lasagna noodles. Stir to make sure noodles are covered with the liquid.

Lock the lid and make sure the vent is closed. Set Instant Pot to Manual or Pressure Cook on high pressure for 10 minutes. When cooking time ends, release pressure and wait for steam to completely stop before opening the lid.

Stir in goat cheese and Parmesan cheese, but reserve about 1/8 cup Parmesan cheese if you would like to sprinkle a bit on top of the Lasagna when you serve it.

Nutrition:

Calories 325, Total Fat 13. 4g, Saturated Fat 7. 5g, Cholesterol 31mg, Sodium 1117mg, Total Carbohydrate 34. 5g, Dietary Fiber 3. 4g, Total Sugars 9. 7g, Protein 14g

80. Tomato Sauce with Pumpkin

Preparation Time: 10 minutes | **Cooking Time:** 15 minutes | **Servings:** 2

Ingredients:

½ cup avocado oil	1 small onion diced
1 teaspoon garlic minced	1 cup pumpkin
1/8 cup fresh coriander washed and chopped	1 cup crushed tomatoes
1 tablespoon tomato paste	½ tablespoon dried basil
1/2 teaspoon salt and pepper	

Directions:

Set the Instant Pot to Sauté. Add avocado oil and wait one minute to heat up.

Add the onion and garlic, sauté for one minute. Stir often.

Add the pumpkin, coriander, and sauté for one minute. Stir often.

Add the crushed tomatoes, tomato paste, dried basil, salt, and pepper. Stir well. Cover the Instant Pot and lock it in.

Set the Manual or Pressure Cook timer for 10 minutes. Make sure the timer is set to "Sealing". Once the timer reaches zero, quickly release the pressure.
Enjoy!

Nutrition:
Calories191, Total Fat 7. 6g, Saturated Fat 1. 7g, Cholesterol 0mg, Sodium 840mg, Total Carbohydrate 28. 9g, Dietary Fiber 11. 4g, Total Sugars, Protein 6g

81. Eggplant Fettuccine Pasta

Preparation Time:05 minutes | **Cooking Time:** 25 minutes | **Servings:** 2

Ingredients:

1 tablespoon coconut oil	1 onion finely diced
1 medium zucchini chopped	2 cloves garlic minced
1 tablespoon tomato paste	1/2 cup vegetable broth
1 teaspoon dried thyme	1 teaspoon dried oregano
1 teaspoon kosher salt	¼ teaspoon pepper
½ cup diced tomatoes	1 cup eggplant, diced
1 tablespoon corn-starch	1 cup juice
Shredded goat cheese for garnish	

Directions:
Add coconut oil to the Instant Pot. Using the display panel select the Sauté function.
When oil gets hot, add onion to the Instant Pot and sauté for 3 minutes. Add zucchini and cook for 3 minutes more. Add garlic and tomato paste and cook for 1-2 minutes more.
Add vegetable broth and seasonings to the Instant pot and deglaze by using a wooden spoon to scrape the brown bits from the bottom of the pot.
Add tomatoes to the Instant Pot and stir. Add eggplant to the Instant Pot, turning once to coat. Turn the Instant pot off by selecting Cancel, then secure the lid, making sure the vent is closed.
Using the display panel select the Manual or Pressure Cook function. Use the + /- keys and program the Instant Pot for 20 minutes.

When the time is up, let the pressure naturally release for 15 minutes, then quickly release the remaining pressure.
In a small bowl, mix 1/4 cup of Instant pot juices and corn-starch. Stir into the pot until thickened. Serve hot topped with shredded cheese.

Nutrition:
Calories 405, Total Fat 14. 2g, Saturated Fat 9. 8g, Cholesterol 62mg, Sodium 1443mg, Total Carbohydrate 56. 1g, Dietary Fiber 5. 2g, Total Sugars 8g, Protein 16. 1g

82. Pasta Puttanesca

Preparation Time:05 minutes | **Cooking Time:** 25 minutes | **Servings:** 2

Ingredients:

1 teaspoon garlic powder	½ cup pasta sauce
2 cups of water	2 cups dried rigatoni
1/8 teaspoon crushed red pepper flakes	1/2 cup pitted Kalamata olives sliced
½ teaspoon fine sea salt	1/4 teaspoon ground black pepper
1 teaspoon grated lemon zest	½ cup broccoli

Directions:
Combine all of the ingredients in the inner cooking pot and stir to coat the pasta.
Lock the lid into place and turn the valve to "Sealing. " Select Manual or Pressure Cook and adjust the pressure to High. Set the time for 5 minutes. When cooking ends, carefully turn the valve to "Venting" to quickly release the pressure. Unlock and remove the lid.
Serve hot.

Nutrition:
Calories 383, Total Fat 4. 2g, Saturated Fat 0. 9g, Cholesterol 1mg, Sodium 1269mg, Total Carbohydrate 73. 8g, Dietary Fiber 5g, Total Sugars 9g, Protein 12. 4g

83. Basil-Coconut Peas and Broccoli

Preparation Time:05 minutes | **Cooking Time:** 25 minutes | **Servings:** 2

Ingredients:

1 cup of coconut milk	1 cup basil
1 bell pepper seeded and cut into chunks	1 leek green part only, cut into chunks
1 teaspoon garlic powder	¼ teaspoon salt
½ cup of water	1 cup noodles
1 cup green peas	½ cup broccoli florets

Directions:

In a blender add the coconut milk, basil, bell pepper, leek, garlic powder, and salt. Blend until smooth.

Pour the sauce into the inner pot and add the water. Select Sauté and adjust to High heat. Bring just to a simmer, then turn the Instant Pot off.

Break up the noodles into 3 or 4 pieces and place them in the pot in a single layer as much as possible. Layer the broccoli over the noodles.

Lock the lid into place. Select Pressure Cook or Manual, and adjust the pressure to Low and the time to 25 minutes. After cooking, quickly release the pressure.

Unlock the lid. Gently stir the mixture until the broccoli and peas are coated with sauce. Ladle into bowls and serve immediately.

Nutrition:

Calories 499, Total Fat 31g, Saturated Fat 25. 8g, Cholesterol 23mg, Sodium 337mg, Total Carbohydrate 49. 2g, Dietary Fiber 10g, Total Sugars 12. 4g, Protein 12. 8g

84. Spaghetti Squash with Mushroom Sauce Pasta

Preparation Time:05 minutes | **Cooking Time:** 25 minutes | **Servings:** 2

Ingredients:

½ tablespoon avocado oil	1 cup mushrooms
1 cloves garlic minced	1/8 cup finely chopped onion
¼ cup crushed tomatoes	1 teaspoon Italian seasoning blend
1 teaspoon garlic powder	½ teaspoon dried basil
½ teaspoon of sea salt	½ teaspoon ground black pepper
1/4 cup vegetable broth	1 bay leaf
1 cup spaghetti squash washed and dried	1 tablespoon tomato paste
1 tablespoon grated Parmesan cheese	1 tablespoon fresh parsley

Directions:

Select Sauté (Normal), once the pot is hot, add the avocado oil, mushrooms, garlic, and onions. Sauté, stirring continuously, for about 5 minutes or until the mushrooms are browned.

Add the crushed tomatoes, Italian seasoning, garlic powder, basil, sea salt, black pepper, and vegetable broth to the pot. Using a wooden spoon, stir and scrape the bottom of the pot to loosen any browned bits. Add the bay leaf.

Using a paring knife, pierce the spaghetti squash 4 or 5 times on each side to create holes for venting the steam. Place the squash in the pot and on top of the sauce.

Cover, lock the lid and flip the steam release handle to the sealing position. Select Manual or Pressure Cook (High) and set the cooking time to 8 minutes. When the cooking time is complete, allow the pressure to release naturally for 20 minutes and then quickly release the remaining pressure.

Open the lid. Using a slotted spoon, carefully transfer the squash to a cutting board and set aside to cool.

Add the tomato paste to the pot and stir. Select Sauté (Less or Low), replace the lid, and let the sauce simmer for 6 minutes.

While the sauce is simmering, slice the cooled squash in half and use a spoon to scoop out the seeds. Using a fork, scrape the flesh to create the noodles.

Transfer the noodles to a colander to drain, pressing down on the noodles with paper towels to expel any excess moisture. Transfer the noodles to a serving platter.

Remove and discard the bay leaf. Ladle the sauce over top of the noodles and garnish with the Parmesan and parsley. Serve warm.

Nutrition:
Calories 115, Total Fat 4. 1g, Saturated Fat 2. 2g, Cholesterol 10mg, Sodium 893mg, Total Carbohydrate 13. 9, Dietary Fiber 3. 6g 13%, Total Sugars 6. 1g, Protein 8. 5g

85. Smoked Tofu and Cherry Tomatoes

Preparation Time:05 minutes | **Cooking Time:** 25 minutes | **Servings:** 2

Ingredients:

1 tablespoon coconut oil	1 small onion finely diced
1/2 cup dry red wine	3 cups vegetable broth
1 1/4 cups coconut cream	1 /2 teaspoon salt
1 tablespoon fresh dill	1 cup fettuccine pasta, broken in half
1 cup cherry or grape tomatoes halved	2 cups smoked tofu sliced and cut into bite-sized pieces
Freshly ground pepper	

Directions:
Add coconut oil to the Instant Pot. Using the display panel select the Sauté function.

Add onion and red wine to the pot and deglaze by using a wooden spoon to scrape any brown bits from the bottom of the pot.

Add vegetable broth, coconut cream, salt, and herbs to the pot and stir to combine.

Carefully fan the pasta in the pot and ensure it is completely submerged.

Add the halved cherry tomatoes in a single layer, do not stir.

Turn the pot off by selecting Cancel, then secure the lid, making sure the vent is closed.

Using the display panel select the Manual or Pressure Cook function. Use the + /- keys and program the Instant Pot for 5 minutes.

When the time is up, let the pressure naturally release for 5 minutes, then quickly release the remaining pressure.

Gently stir the pasta, breaking up any clumps.

Fold in smoked tofu pieces and serve immediately garnished with freshly ground pepper and additional herbs.

Nutrition:
Calories 501, Total Fat 31g, Saturated Fat 25. 6g, Cholesterol 31mg, Sodium 1182mg, Total Carbohydrate 40g, Dietary Fiber 3. 7g, Total Sugars 9. 7g, Protein 13g

86. Cheesy Creamy Farfalle

Preparation Time:05 minutes | **Cooking Time:** 25 minutes | **Servings:** 2

Ingredients:

1 cup vegetable broth	¼ cup coconut cream
1 teaspoon garlic powder	½ teaspoon salt
¼ teaspoon pepper	1 cup dried Farfalle pasta
1 cup pasta sauce	¼ cup goat cheese shredded
1 cup mozzarella cheese shredded	½ cups fresh kale finely chopped

Directions:
Layer vegetable broth, coconut cream, garlic powder, salt, pepper, and Farfalle pasta in that order in the pot--do not stir. Ensure all pasta is submerged.

Secure the lid, making sure the vent is closed.

Using the display panel select the Manual or Pressure Cook function. Use the + /- keys and program the Instant Pot for 6 minutes.

When the time is up, let the pressure naturally release for 6 minutes, then quickly release the remaining pressure.

Stir in the pasta sauce and kale.

Add the cheeses, 1/3 cup at a time, stirring until fully melted and incorporated.

Serve hot garnished with finely chopped kale

Nutrition:
Calories 365, Total Fat 15g, Saturated Fat 9. 4g, Cholesterol 12mg, Sodium 1586mg, Total Carbohydrate 44. 3g, Dietary Fiber 5. 4g, Total Sugars 14. 3g, Protein 13. 8g

87. Basil Pesto Mushrooms Pasta

Preparation Time:10 minutes | **Cooking Time:** 22 minutes | **Servings:** 2

Ingredients:

1 tablespoon coconut oil	½ teaspoon garlic powder

½ cup mushrooms
½ cup cherry tomatoes
1 cup pasta
½ cup basil pesto
1/8 bunch fresh mint
Salt and pepper to taste
Enough water

Directions:

Set Instant Pot to Sauté. Add coconut oil when it gets hot then add garlic powder. Stir regularly.

Add mushrooms and cook until about 4 - 5 minutes, cherry tomatoes, basil pesto, fresh mint, salt, and pepper.

Add water and pasta. Lock the lid and make sure the vent is closed. Set Instant Pot to Manual or Pressure Cook on High Pressure for 15 minutes. When cooking time ends, release pressure and wait for steam to completely stop before opening the lid.

Nutrition:

Calories 259, Total Fat 8. 5g, Saturated Fat 6. 1g, Cholesterol 47mg, Sodium 21mg, Total Carbohydrate 38. 1g, Dietary Fiber 1g, Total Sugars 1. 7g, Protein 8. 5g

88.   Instant Pot Spaghetti

Preparation Time:20 minutes | **Cooking Time:** 15 minutes | **Servings:** 2

Ingredients:

1 tablespoon coconut oil
½ cup tofu
½ onion, diced
½ teaspoon garlic powder
¼ teaspoon dried thyme
¼ teaspoon dried basil
¼ teaspoon salt
Freshly ground black pepper
½ cup jarred spaghetti sauce
2 tablespoons tomato paste
1 cups vegetable broth
2 tablespoon goat cheese, plus extra for serving
6 ounces of spaghetti noodles

Directions:

Press Sauté   on your Instant Pot. Add the coconut oil and tofu to the Instant Pot.

Cook for about 3 minutes, stirring and breaking up with a spoon occasionally.

Add the chopped onion. Stir, and cook for about 4 minutes.

Stir in the garlic powder, thyme, basil, salt, pepper, spaghetti sauce, tomato paste, broth, and goat cheese. Stir very well.

Turn off the Instant Pot.

Break the noodles in half, and layer them in the tomato mixture, ensuring they are covered by the liquid. Press Pressure Cook and set the timer for 8 minutes.

Place the lid on the Instant Pot, and turn the valve to Sealing.

When the timer goes off, very carefully do a forced pressure release, cover your hand with a kitchen towel, and gently release the steam. When you hear the float valve drop down, all of the pressure is released.

Open the lid to the Instant Pot. It may look like there is a bit too much liquid, but just stir until it all comes together.

If it's still too much liquid for you, press Sauté and cook to reduce for 2 minutes.

Divide into bowls, and serve topped with more goat cheese.

Nutrition:

Calories 522, Total Fat 22. 3g, Saturated Fat 13. 9g, Cholesterol 92mg, Sodium 817mg, Total Carbohydrate 54. 9g, Dietary Fiber 2g 7%, Total Sugars 4. 6g, Protein 27g

89.   Mushrooms Creamed Noodles

Preparation Time:5 minutes | **Cooking Time:** 20 minutes | **Servings:** 2

Ingredients:

½ cup heavy cream
2 cups vegetable broth
½ teaspoon dried oregano
½ teaspoon garlic minced
½ teaspoon red pepper flakes
1 cup noodles
1 cup mushrooms

Directions:

Put ¼ cup of the heavy cream in an Instant Pot. Stir in the broth, oregano, garlic, and red pepper flakes until smooth. Stir in the noodles, then set the block of mushrooms right on top. Lock the lid onto the Instant Pot.

Press Pressure Cook on Max Pressure for 3 minutes with the Keep Warm setting off.

When the Instant Pot has finished cooking, turn it off and let its pressure return to normal naturally for 1 minute. Then use the Quick-release method to get rid of any residual pressure in the pot.

Unlatch the lid and open the cooker. Stir in the remaining 1/4 cup heavy cream. Set the lid askew over the pot and let sit for a couple of minutes so the noodles continue to absorb some of the liquid. Serve hot.

Nutrition:
Calories182, Total Fat 5. 3g, Saturated Fat 1. 6g, Cholesterol 31mg, Sodium 850mg, Total Carbohydrate 23. 9g, Dietary Fiber 1. 9g, Total Sugars 2g, Protein 10. 2g

90. Singapore Noodles with Garlic

Preparation Time:15 minutes | **Cooking Time:** 20 minutes | **Servings:** 2

Ingredients:

1 cup vermicelli noodles	¼ tablespoon hot curry powder
½ teaspoon garlic powder	½ teaspoon ginger powder
1 tablespoon olive oil	½ bunch spinach
1 medium carrot	½ cup green cabbage
½ green onions	1/8 cup soy sauce
1 teaspoon sesame oil	1 teaspoon chili garlic sauce, optional

Directions:
Place the dry vermicelli noodles in a bowl and cover with room temperature water. Let it soak for 15 minutes. Drain in a colander after they have soaked and are softened. Return the noodles to the bowl, cut the noodles into pieces (approximately 6 inches in length) to facilitate stir-frying later. Sprinkle the noodles with curry powder and toss to coat. Set noodles aside.

In the Instant Pot inner pot, place the heated olive oil. add the garlic powder and ginger powder. Stir fry very briefly (1 minute or less) then add all of the vegetables. Stir fry the vegetables until they just begin to soften.

Add sesame oil, water noodles, soy sauce, salt, pepper, and chili garlic sauce.

Lock the lid and make sure the vent is closed. Set Instant Pot to Manual or Pressure Cook on High

Pressure for 15 minutes. When cooking time ends, release pressure and wait for steam to completely stop before opening the lid.
Serve.

Nutrition:
Calories 244, Total Fat 11. 5g, Saturated Fat 1. 7g, Cholesterol 23mg, Sodium 1036mg, Total Carbohydrate 30. 2g, Dietary Fiber 4. 8g, Total Sugars 3. 3g, Protein 7. 9g

91. Garlic Noodles

Preparation Time:10 minutes | **Cooking Time:** 15 minutes | **Servings:** 2

Ingredients:

½ cup spaghetti	1 cup of coconut milk
1 tablespoon goat cheese	2 tablespoon butter
1 teaspoon soy sauce	1 tablespoon honey
1 tablespoon oyster sauce	1 teaspoon olive oil
Enough water	Salt to taste

Directions:
Add the oyster sauce, honey, soy sauce, and olive oil to a bowl and stir until combined.

Add spaghetti, water, and salt to Instant Pot. Place the lid on the pot and lock it into place to seal. Pressure Cook on High Pressure for 4 minutes. Use Quick Pressure Release. Stir milk into Spaghetti and then stir in the cheeses until melted and combined.

Add sauce mix well.

Nutrition:
Calories 239, Total Fat 11. 2g, Saturated Fat 6. 1g, Cholesterol 58mg, Sodium 199mg, Total Carbohydrate 29. 5g, Dietary Fiber 0. 1g, Total Sugars 3. 6g, Protein 5. 6g

92. Green Goddess Pasta

Preparation Time:10 minutes | **Cooking Time:** 15 minutes | **Servings:** 2

Ingredients:

1 tablespoon butter	1 cup mushrooms, sliced
½ tablespoon garlic powder	1 cup pasta vegetable
2 cups vegetable broth	½ cup baby kale

½ cup peas

½ cup coconut cream, cubed

¼ cup pesto sauce

¼ cup grated goat cheese

Directions:

Add butter to the Instant Pot, hit "Sauté" and once the butter is melted and sizzled, add in the mushrooms and cook for 2-3 minutes until they begin lightly brown. Then, add the garlic powder and stir for another 2 minutes.

Next, add in the pasta vegetable and broth.

Top off with the kale and secure the lid and hit "Keep Warm/Cancel" and then hit "Manual" or "Pressure Cook" High Pressure for 6 minutes. Quick-release when done.

Stir in the peas. Then, add in the coconut cream and pesto, and goat cheese and stir for about 2 minutes more until the cheese is completely melted into the sauce. Transfer to a serving dish and top with grated goat cheese.

Enjoy!

Nutrition:

Calories 677, Total Fat 43. 4g, Saturated Fat 20. 4g, Cholesterol 137mg, Sodium 1203mg, Total Carbohydrate 48. 6g, Dietary Fiber 3. 2g, Total Sugars 6. 1g, Protein 24. 4g

93.   Simply Kale Lasagna

Preparation Time:15 minutes | **Cooking Time:** 45 minutes | **Servings:** 2

Ingredients:

1 cup pasta sauce

1/8 cup water

1 large egg

2-1/2 cups shredded Italian cheese blend divided

1 cup ricotta cheese

½ cup kale

1 cup oven-ready (no-boil) lasagna noodles

Directions:

Add 1/2 cup sauce into a pan. Transfer the remaining sauce to a bowl and stir in water.

In a large bowl, whisk the egg. Stir in 1-3/4 cups Italian cheese and ricotta blend them.

Layer one-quarter of the noodles on top of the sauce in the pan, breaking noodles as needed to evenly cover the sauce. Top with one-third of the cheese mixture with kale, then one-quarter of the sauce. Continue with two more layers

each of noodles, cheese mixture, and sauce, gently pressing down on the noodles between each layer. Finish with a layer of noodles and a layer of sauce.

Add 1 1/2 cups water and the steam rack to the Instant Pot. Place the baking pan on the rack.

Close and lock the lid and turn the steam release handle to Sealing. Set your Instant Pot to Pressure Cook on High for 14 minutes.

When the cooking time is done, press Cancel and turn the steam release handle to Venting. When the float valve drops down, remove the lid. Sprinkle with the remaining Italian cheese blend. Close and lock the lid and let it stand for 10 minutes or until the cheese is melted.

Using the handles of the rack, carefully remove the rack and pan. Let Lasagna stand for 10 minutes. Cut into wedges.

Nutrition:

Calories 491, Total Fat 22. 4g, Saturated Fat 11. 3g, Cholesterol 156mg, Sodium 898mg, Total Carbohydrate 43. 8g, Dietary Fiber 4. 3g, Total Sugars 12. 1g, Protein 29. 5g

94.   Mozzarella Lemon Pasta

Preparation Time:05 minutes | **Cooking Time:** 45 minutes | **Servings:** 2

Ingredients:

½ tablespoon olive oil

½ teaspoon garlic powder

2 cups vegetable broth

Zest of one lemon

1 tablespoon lemon juice divided

1 cup ziti noodles

½ cup grated/shredded mozzarella cheese

½ cup coconut cream

Salt and pepper to taste

½ tablespoon cornstarch

1 tablespoon cold water

1 tablespoon finely chopped parsley for serving

Additional mozzarella for serving

Directions:

Add olive oil to the Instant Pot. Using the display panel select the Sauté function.

Add garlic powder, vegetable broth, lemon zest, and lemon juice to the pot and deglaze by using a wooden spoon to scrape any brown bits from the bottom of the pot.

Break noodles in half and fan across the bottom of the pot, making sure all noodles are submerged.

Turn the pot off by selecting Cancel, then secure the lid, making sure the vent is closed.

Using the display panel select the Manual or Pressure Cook function. Use the + /- keys and program the Instant Pot for 3 minutes.

When the time is up, let the pressure naturally release for 10 minutes, then quickly release the remaining pressure.

Stir, breaking up any pasta clumps, and allow to cool slightly.

Add mozzarella cheese, coconut cream, and remaining lemon juice. Add salt and pepper to taste.

In a small bowl, mix cornstarch and cold water. Stir into the pot until thickened, returning to Sauté mode as needed.

Serve warm topped finely chopped parsley and additional mozzarella.

Nutrition:
Calories 331, Total Fat 21g, Saturated Fat 14. 4g, Cholesterol 4mg, Sodium 895mg, Total Carbohydrate 26. 3g, Dietary Fiber 2. 5g, Total Sugars 4g, Protein 12g

95.   Grilled Tempeh With Green Beans

Preparation Time: 15-30 minutes | **Cooking Time:** 15 minutes | **Servings:** 4

Ingredients:

1 tbsp plant butter, melted	1 lb tempeh, sliced into 4 pieces
1 lb green beans, trimmed	Salt and black pepper to taste
2 sprigs thyme	2 tbsp olive oil
1 tbsp pure corn syrup	1 lemon, juiced

Directions:
Preheat a grill pan over medium heat and brush with the plant butter.

Season the tempeh and green beans with salt, black pepper, and place the thyme in the pan. Grill the tempeh and green beans on both sides until golden brown and tender, 10 minutes.

Transfer to serving plates.

In a small bowl, whisk the olive oil, corn syrup, lemon juice, and drizzle all over the food.

Serve warm.

Nutrition:
Calories 352 Fats 22. 5g Carbs 21. 8g Protein 22. 6g

96.   Creamy Fettuccine With Peas

Preparation Time: 15-30 minutes | **Cooking Time:** 25 minutes | **Servings:** 4

Ingredients:

16 oz whole-wheat fettuccine	Salt and black pepper to taste
¾ cup flax milk	½ cup cashew butter, room temperature
1 tbsp olive oil	2 garlic cloves, minced
1 ½ cups frozen peas	½ cup chopped fresh basil

Directions:
Add the fettuccine and 10 cups of water to a large pot, and cook over medium heat until al dente, 10 minutes. Drain the pasta through a colander and set aside. In a bowl, whisk the flax milk, cashew butter, and salt until smooth. Set aside.

Heat the olive oil in a large skillet and sauté the garlic until fragrant, 30 seconds. Mix in the peas, fettuccine, and basil. Toss well until the pasta is well-coated in the sauce and season with some black pepper. Dish the food and serve warm.

Nutrition:
Calories 654 Fats 23. 7g Carbs 101. 9g Protein 18. 2g

97.   Buckwheat Cabbage Rolls

Preparation Time: 15-30 minutes | **Cooking Time:** 30 minutes | **Servings:** 4

Ingredients:

2 tbsp plant butter	2 cups extra-firm tofu, pressed and crumbled
½ medium sweet onion, finely chopped	2 garlic cloves, minced
Salt and black pepper to taste	1 cup buckwheat groats
1 ¾ cups vegetable stock	1 bay leaf

2 tbsp chopped fresh cilantro + more for garnishing
1 (23 oz) canned chopped tomatoes

1 head Savoy cabbage, leaves separated (scraps kept)

Directions:

Melt the plant butter in a large bowl and cook the tofu until golden brown, 8 minutes. Stir in the onion and garlic until softened and fragrant, 3 minutes. Season with salt, black pepper, and mix in the buckwheat, bay leaf, and vegetable stock.

Close the lid, allow boiling, and then simmer until all the liquid is absorbed. Open the lid; remove the bay leaf, adjust the taste with salt, black pepper, and mix in the cilantro.

Lay the cabbage leaves on a flat surface and add 3 to 4 tablespoons of the cooked buckwheat onto each leaf. Roll the leaves to firmly secure the filling.

Pour the tomatoes with juices into a medium pot, season with a little salt, black pepper, and lay the cabbage rolls in the sauce. Cook over medium heat until the cabbage softens, 5 to 8 minutes. Turn the heat off and dish the food onto serving plates. Garnish with more cilantro and serve warm.

Nutrition:

Calories 1147 Fats 112. 9g Carbs 25. 6g Protein 23. 8g

98.   Bbq Black Bean Burgers

Preparation Time: 15-30 minutes | **Cooking Time:** 20 minutes | **Servings:** 4

Ingredients:

3 (15 oz) cans black beans, drained and rinsed
2 tbsp quick-cooking oats
2 tbsp pure barbecue sauce
Salt and black pepper to taste
For topping:
Tomato slices
Additional barbecue sauce

2 tbsp whole-wheat flour
¼ cup chopped fresh basil
1 garlic clove, minced
4 whole-grain hamburger buns, split
Red onion slices
Fresh basil leaves

Directions:

In a medium bowl, mash the black beans and mix in the flour, oats, basil, barbecue sauce, garlic salt, and black pepper until well combined. Mold 4 patties out of the mixture and set aside. Heat a grill pan to medium heat and lightly grease with cooking spray.

Cook the bean patties on both sides until light brown and cooked through, 10 minutes.

Place the patties between the burger buns and top with the onions, tomatoes, basil, and some barbecue sauce.

Serve warm.

Nutrition:

Calories 589 Fats 17. 7g Carbs 80. 9g Protein 27. 9g

99.   Paprika & Tomato Pasta Primavera

Preparation Time: 15-30 minutes | **Cooking Time:** 25 minutes | **Servings:** 4

Ingredients:

2 tbsp olive oil
½ tsp paprika
2 garlic cloves, minced
Salt and black pepper to taste
3 tbsp plant butter, cut into ½-in cubes
1 cup packed fresh basil leaves

8 oz whole-wheat fedelini
1 small red onion, sliced
1 cup dry white wine
2 cups cherry tomatoes, halved
1 lemon, zested and juiced

Directions:

Heat the olive oil in a large pot and mix in the fedelini, paprika, onion, garlic, and stir-fry for 2-3 minutes.

Mix in the white wine, salt, and black pepper. Cover with water. Cook until the water absorbs and the fedelini al dente, 5 minutes. Mix in the cherry tomatoes, plant butter, lemon zest, lemon juice, and basil leaves.

Dish the food and serve warm.

Nutrition:

Calories 380 kcal Fats 24. 1g Carbs 33. 7g Protein 11. 2g

100. Green Lentil Stew With Brown Rice

Preparation Time: 15-30 minutes | **Cooking Time:** 50 minutes | **Servings:** 4

Ingredients:

For the stew:	2 tbsp olive oil
1 lb tempeh, cut into cubes	Salt and black pepper to taste
1 tsp chili powder	1 tsp onion powder
1 tsp cumin powder	1 tsp garlic powder
1 yellow onion, chopped	2 celery stalks, chopped
2 carrots diced	4 garlic cloves, minced
2 cups vegetable broth	1 tsp oregano
1 cup green lentils, rinsed	¼ cup chopped tomatoes
1 lime, juiced	For the brown rice:
1 cup of brown rice	1 cup of water
Salt to taste	

Directions:

Heat the olive oil in a large pot, season the tempeh with salt, black pepper, and cook in the oil until brown, 10 minutes.

Stir in the chili powder, onion powder, cumin powder, garlic powder, and cook until fragrant, 1 minute. Mix in the onion, celery, carrots, garlic, and cook until softened. Pour in the vegetable broth, oregano, green lentils, tomatoes, and green chilies.

Cover the pot and cook until the tomatoes soften and the stew reduces by half, 10 to 15 minutes. Open the lid, adjust the taste with salt, black pepper, and mix in the lime juice. Dish the stew and serve warm with the brown rice.

Meanwhile, as the stew cooks, add the brown rice, water, and salt to a medium pot. Cook over medium heat until the rice is tender and the water is absorbed for about 15 to 25 minutes.

Nutrition:

Calories 1305 kcal Fats 130. 9g Carbs 25. 1g Protein 24. 3g

101. Nutty Tofu Loaf

Preparation Time: 15-30 minutes | **Cooking Time:** 65 minutes | **Servings:** 4

Ingredients:

2 tbsp olive oil + extra for brushing	2 white onions, finely chopped
4 garlic cloves, minced	1 lb firm tofu, pressed and crumbled
2 tbsp soy sauce	¾ cup chopped mixed nuts
¼ cup flaxseed meal	1 tbsp sesame seeds
1 cup chopped mixed bell peppers	Salt and black pepper to taste
1 tbsp Italian seasoning	½ tsp pure date syrup
½ cup tomato sauce	

Directions:

Preheat the oven to 350 F and grease an 8 x 4-inch loaf pan with olive oil.

Heat 1 tbsp of olive oil in a small skillet and sauté the onion and garlic until softened and fragrant, 2 minutes.

Pour the onion mixture into a large bowl and mix with the tofu, soy sauce, nuts, flaxseed meal, sesame seeds, bell peppers, salt, black pepper, Italian seasoning, and date syrup until well combined.

Spoon the mixture into the loaf pan, press to fit, and spread the tomato sauce on top.

Bake the tofu loaf in the oven for 45 minutes to 1 hour or until well compacted.

Remove the loaf pan from the oven, invert the tofu loaf onto a chopping board, and cool for 5 minutes. Slice and serve warm.

Nutrition:

Calories 544 Fats 39. 2g Carbs 30. 4g Protein 25g

102. Taco Rice Bowls

Preparation Time: 15-30 minutes | **Cooking Time:** 50 minutes | **Servings:** 4

Ingredients:

2 tbsp olive oil	2 cups chopped soy chorizo
1 tsp taco seasoning	2 green bell peppers, deseeded and sliced
1 cup of brown rice	2 cups vegetable broth
Salt to taste	¼ cup of salsa

1 lemon, zested and juiced

1 (7 oz) can sweet corn kernels, drained

2 tbsp freshly chopped parsley

1 (8 oz) can pinto beans, drained and rinsed

2 green onions, chopped

Directions:

Heat the olive oil in a medium pot and cook the soy chorizo until golden brown, 5 minutes.

Season with the taco seasoning and stir in the bell peppers; cook until the peppers slightly soften, 3 minutes.

Stir in the brown rice, vegetable broth, salt, salsa, and lemon zest.

Close the lid and cook the food until the rice is tender and all the liquid is absorbed for about 15 to 25 minutes.

Mix in the lemon juice, pinto beans, corn kernels, and green onions. Allow warming for 3 to 5 minutes and dish the food.

Garnish with the parsley and serve warm.

Nutrition:

Calories 253 Fats 8. 4g Carbs 32. 7g Protein 15. 5g

103. Red Sauce Mushroom Pizza

Preparation Time: 15-30 minutes | **Cooking Time:** 40 minutes | **Servings:** 4

Ingredients:

For the crust:

2 tbsp flax seed powder + 6 tbsp water

¾ cup whole-wheat flour

½ tsp salt

½ cup tofu mayonnaise

1 tsp baking powder

For the topping:

1 cup sliced mixed mushrooms

1 tbsp basil pesto

½ cup red pizza sauce

2 tbsp olive oil

Salt and black pepper

¾ cup shredded plant-based Parmesan cheese

Directions:

Preheat the oven to 350 F.

In a medium bowl, mix the flax seed powder with water and allow thickening for 5 minutes to make the flax egg. Mix in the tofu mayonnaise,

whole-wheat flour, baking powder, and salt until dough forms. Spread the dough on a pizza pan and bake in the oven for 10 minutes or until the dough sets.

In a medium bowl, mix the mushrooms, olive oil, basil pesto, salt, and black pepper.

Remove the pizza crust and spread the pizza sauce on top. Scatter mushroom mixture on the crust and top with plant-based Parmesan cheese. Bake further until the cheese melts and the mushrooms soften, 10 to 15 minutes. Remove the pizza, slice, and serve.

Nutrition:

Calories 515 Fats 35g Carbs 35. 9g Protein 16. 2g

104. Sweet Quinoa Veggie Burger

Preparation Time: 15-30 minutes | **Cooking Time:** 35 minutes | **Servings:** 4

Ingredients:

1 cup quick-cooking quinoa

1 shallot, chopped

1 garlic clove, minced

2 tbsp whole-wheat flour

2 tbsp pure maple syrup

4 whole-grain hamburger buns, split

½ cup tofu mayonnaise for topping

1 tbsp olive oil

2 tbsp chopped fresh celery

1 (15 oz) can pinto beans, drained and rinsed

¼ cup chopped fresh basil

Salt and black pepper to taste

4 small lettuce leaves for topping

Directions:

Cook the quinoa with 2 cups of water in a medium pot until the liquid is absorbed for about 10 to 15 minutes.

Meanwhile, heat the olive oil in a medium skillet over medium heat and sauté the shallot, celery, and garlic until softened and fragrant, 3 minutes.

Transfer the quinoa and shallot mixture to a medium bowl and add the pinto beans, flour, basil, maple syrup, salt, and black pepper. Mash and mold 4 patties out of the mixture and set aside.

Heat a grill pan to medium heat and lightly grease with cooking spray. Cook the patties on both sides until light brown, compacted, and cooked through, 10 minutes. Place the patties between the burger buns and top with the lettuce and tofu mayonnaise. Serve warm.

Nutrition:
Calories 290 Fats 6. 2g Carbs 50. 2g Protein 12g

105. Cheesy Broccoli Casserole

Preparation Time: 15-30 minutes | **Cooking Time:** 50 minutes | **Servings:** 4

Ingredients:

1 tbsp olive oil	2 cups broccoli florets
1 (10 oz) can cream of mushroom soup	1 cup tofu mayonnaise
Salt and black pepper to taste	3 tbsp coconut cream
1 medium red onion, chopped	2 cups grated plant-based cheddar cheese
¾ cup whole-wheat bread crumbs	3 tbsp plant butter, melted

Directions:
Preheat the oven to 350 F.
Heat the olive oil in a medium skillet and sauté the broccoli florets until softened, 8 minutes.
Turn the heat off and mix in the mushroom soup, mayonnaise, salt, black pepper, coconut cream, and onion. Spread the mixture into the baking sheet.
In a small bowl, mix the breadcrumbs with the plant butter and evenly distribute the mixture on top. Add the cheddar cheese and bake the casserole in the oven until golden on top and the cheese melts.
Remove the casserole from the oven, allow cooling for 5 minutes, dish, and serve warm.

Nutrition:
Calories 412 Fats 38. 14g Carbs 13. 19g Protein 6. 57g

106. Hummus & Vegetable Pizza

Preparation Time: 15-30 minutes | **Cooking Time:** 30 minutes | **Servings:** 4

Ingredients:

For the pizza crust:	3 ½ cups whole-wheat flour
1 tsp yeast	1 tsp salt
1 pinch sugar	3 tbsp olive oil
1 cup of warm water	For the topping:
1 cup hummus	10 cremini mushrooms, sliced
½ cup fresh baby spinach	½ cup cherry tomatoes halved
½ cup sliced Kalamata olives	½ medium onion, sliced
2 tsp dried oregano	

Directions:
Preheat the oven the 350 F and lightly grease a pizza pan with cooking spray.
In a medium bowl, mix the flour, nutritional yeast, salt, sugar, olive oil, and warm water until smooth dough forms. Allow rising for an hour or until the dough doubles in size.
Spread the dough on the pizza pan and apply the hummus on the dough. Add the mushrooms, spinach, tomatoes, olives, onion, and top with the oregano. Bake the pizza for 20 minutes or until the mushrooms soften.
Remove from the oven, cool for 5 minutes, slice, and serve.

Nutrition:
Calories 592 Fats 19. 9g Carbs 92. 5g Protein 18g

107. Chickpea Burgers With Guacamole

Preparation Time: 15-30 minutes | **Cooking Time:** 20 minutes | **Servings:** 4

Ingredients:

For the guacamole:	1 large avocado, pitted and peeled
1 tomato, chopped	1 small red onion, chopped
For the burgers:	3 (15 oz) cans chickpeas, drained and rinsed
2 tbsp almond flour	2 tbsp quick-cooking oats

¼ cup chopped fresh parsley	1 tbsp hot sauce
1 garlic clove, minced	¼ tsp garlic salt
1/8 tsp black pepper	4 whole-grain hamburger buns, split

Directions:

In a medium bowl, mash avocados and mix in the tomato, onion, and parsley. Set aside.

In a medium bowl, mash the chickpeas and mix in the almond flour, oats, parsley, hot sauce, garlic, garlic salt, and black pepper. Mold 4 patties out of the mixture and set aside.

Heat a grill pan to medium heat and lightly grease with cooking spray. Cook the bean patties on both sides until light brown and cooked through, 10 minutes. Place each patty between each burger bun and top with the guacamole.

Nutrition:

Calories 369 kcal Fats 12. 7g Carbs 52. 7g Protein 15. 6g

108.   Chili Seitan Stew With Brown Rice

Preparation Time: 15-30 minutes | **Cooking Time:** 50 minutes | **Servings:** 4

Ingredients:

For the stew:

2 tbsp olive oil	1 lb seitan, cut into cubes
Salt and black pepper to taste	1 tsp chili powder
1 tsp onion powder	1 tsp cumin powder
1 tsp garlic powder	1 yellow onion, chopped
2 celery stalks, chopped	2 carrots diced
4-5 cloves garlic	1 cup vegetable broth
1 cup of water	1 tsp oregano
1 cup chopped tomatoes	3 green chilies, deseeded and chopped
1 lime, juiced	

For the brown rice:

| 1 cup of brown rice | 1 cup of water |
| Salt to taste | |

Directions:

Heat the olive oil in a large pot, season the seitan with salt, black pepper, and cook in the oil until brown, 10 minutes.

Stir in the chili powder, onion powder, cumin powder, garlic powder, and cook until fragrant, 1 minute. Mix in the onion, celery, carrots, garlic, and cook until softened. Pour in the vegetable broth, water, oregano, tomatoes, and green chilies.

Cover the pot and cook until the tomatoes soften and the stew reduces by half, 10 to 15 minutes. Open the lid, adjust the taste with salt, black pepper, and mix in the lime juice. Dish the stew and serve warm with the brown rice.

Meanwhile, as the stew cooks, add the brown rice, water, and salt to a medium pot. Cook over medium heat until the rice is tender and the water absorbs 15 to 20 minutes.

Nutrition:

Calories 1290 Fats 131. 8g Carbs 15. 2g Protein 24. 4g

109.   Potato And Pea Stir-Fry

Preparation Time: 15-30 minutes | **Cooking Time:** 21 minutes | **Servings:** 4

Ingredients:

4 medium potatoes, peeled and diced	2 tbsp olive oil
1 medium onion, chopped	1 tsp red chili powder
1 tsp fresh ginger-garlic paste	1 tsp cumin powder
¼ tsp turmeric powder	Salt and black pepper to taste
1 cup fresh green peas	

Directions:

Steam potatoes in a safe microwave bowl for 8-10 minutes or until softened. Heat the olive oil in a wok and sauté the onion until softened, 3 minutes.

Mix in the chili powder, ginger-garlic paste, cumin powder, turmeric powder, salt, and black pepper. Cook until the fragrant releases, 1 minute. Stir in the green peas, potatoes, and cook until softened, 2 to 3 minutes. Serve warm.

Nutrition:

Calories 394 kcal Fats 7. 7g Carbs 73. 9g Protein 10. 2g

110. Mongolian Seitan

Preparation Time: 15-30 minutes | **Cooking Time:** 20 minutes | **Servings:** 4

Ingredients:
For the sauce:

2 tsp olive oil	½ tsp freshly grated ginger
3 garlic cloves, minced	1/3 tsp red chili flakes
1/3 tsp allspice	1/2 cup low-sodium soy sauce
½ cup + 2 tbsp pure date sugar	2 tsp cornstarch
2 tbsp cold water	

For the crisped seitan:

1 ½ tbsp olive oil	1 lb seitan, cut into 1-inch pieces
For topping:	1 tbsp toasted sesame seeds
1 tbsp sliced scallions	

Directions:
Heat the olive oil in a wok and sauté the ginger and garlic until fragrant, 30 seconds.

Mix in the red chili flakes, Chinese allspice, soy sauce, and date sugar. Allow the sugar to melt and set aside.

In a small bowl, mix the cornstarch and water. Stir the cornstarch mixture into the sauce and allow thickening for 1 minute. Turn the heat off. Heat the olive oil in a medium skillet over medium heat and fry the seitan on both sides until crispy, 10 minutes,

Mix the seitan into the sauce and warm over low heat. Dish the food, garnish with the sesame seeds and scallions. Serve warm with brown rice.

Nutrition:
Calories 354 kcal Fats 20. 8g Carbs 17. 7g Protein 25. 2g

111. Alfredo Pasta With Cherry Tomatoes

Preparation Time: 15-30 minutes | **Cooking Time:** 20 minutes | **Servings:** 4

Ingredients:

2 cups almond milk	1 ½ cups vegetable broth
3 tbsp plant butter	1 large garlic clove, minced
16 oz whole-wheat fettuccine	½ cup coconut cream
¼ cup halved cherry tomatoes	¾ cup grated plant-based Parmesan cheese
Salt and black pepper to taste	Chopped fresh parsley to garnish

Directions:
Bring almond milk, vegetable broth, butter, and garlic to a boil in a large pot, 5 minutes. Mix in the fettuccine and cook until tender, while frequently tossing around 10 minutes.

Mix in coconut cream, tomatoes, plant Parmesan cheese, salt, and pepper. Cook for 3 minutes or until the cheese melts. Garnish with some parsley and serve warm.

Nutrition:
Calories 698 kcal Fats 26. 1g Carbs 101. 8g Protein 22. 6g

112. Tempeh Tetrazzini With Garden Peas

Preparation Time: 15-30 minutes | **Cooking Time:** 50 minutes | **Servings:** 4

Ingredients:

16 oz whole-wheat bow-tie pasta	2 tbsp olive oil, divided
2/3 lb tempeh, cut into 1-inch cubes	Salt and black pepper to taste
1 medium yellow onion, chopped	½ cup sliced white mushrooms
2 tbsp whole-wheat flour	¼ cup white wine
¾ cup vegetable stock	¼ cup oats milk
2 tsp chopped fresh thyme	¼ cup chopped cauliflower
½ cup grated plant-based Parmesan cheese	3 tbsp whole-wheat breadcrumbs

Directions:
Cook the pasta in 8 cups of slightly salted water for 10 minutes or until al dente. Drain and set aside.

Preheat the oven to 375 F.

Heat the 1 tbsp of olive oil in a skillet over medium heat, season the tempeh with salt, pepper, and cook until golden brown all around. Mix in onion, mushrooms, and cook until softened, 5 minutes. Stir in flour and cook for 1 more minute. Mix in wine and add two-thirds of the vegetable stock. Cook for 2 minutes while occasionally stirring and then add milk; continue cooking until the sauce thickens, 4 minutes.

Season with the thyme, salt, black pepper, and half of the Parmesan cheese. Once the cheese melts, turn the heat off and allow cooling.

Add the rest of the vegetable stock and cauliflower to a food processor and blend until smooth. Pour the mixture into a bowl, pour in the sauce, and mix in pasta until combined.

Grease a 2 quarts glass baking dish with cooking spray and spread the mixture in the baking dish. Drizzle the remaining olive oil on top, breadcrumbs, some more thyme, and the remaining cheese. Bake until the cheese melts and is golden brown on top, 30 minutes. Remove the dish from the oven, allow cooling for 3 minutes, and serve.

Nutrition:
Calories 799 kcal Fats 57. 7g Carbs 54. 3g Protein 27g

113. Tomato, Kale, and White Bean Skillet

Preparation Time: 10 minutes | **Cooking Time:** 10 minutes | **Servings:** 4

Ingredients:

30 ounces cooked cannellini beans	3. 5 ounces sun-dried tomatoes, packed in oil, chopped
6 ounces kale, chopped	1 teaspoon minced garlic
1/4 teaspoon ground black pepper	1/4 teaspoon salt
1/2 tablespoon dried basil	1/8 teaspoon red pepper flakes
1 tablespoon apple cider vinegar	1 tablespoon olive oil
2 tablespoons oil from sun-dried tomatoes	

Directions:
Prepare the dressing and for this, place basil, black pepper, salt, vinegar, and red pepper flakes in a small bowl, add oil from sun-dried tomatoes and whisk until combined.

Take a skillet pan, place it over medium heat, add olive oil and when hot, add garlic and cook for 1 minute until fragrant.

Add kale, splash with some water and cook for 3 minutes until kale leaves have wilted.

Add tomatoes and beans, stir well and cook for 3 minutes until heated.

Remove pan from heat, drizzle with the prepared dressing, toss until mixed and serve.

Nutrition:
Calories: 264 Cal Fat: 12 g Carbs: 38 g Protein: 9 g Fiber: 13 g

114. Chard Wraps With Millet

Preparation Time: 25 minutes | **Cooking Time:** 0 minute | **Servings:** 4

Ingredients:

1 carrot, cut into ribbons	1/2 cup millet, cooked
1/2 of a large cucumber, cut into ribbons	1/2 cup chickpeas, cooked
1 cup sliced cabbage Mint leaves as needed for topping Hemp seeds as needed for topping 1 bunch of Swiss rainbow chard	1/3 cup hummus

Directions:
Spread hummus on one side of the chard, place some millet, vegetables, and chickpeas on it, sprinkle with some mint leaves and hemp seeds and wrap it like a burrito.

Serve straight away.

Nutrition:
Calories: 152 Cal Fat: 4. 5 g Carbs: 25 g Protein: 3. 5 g Fiber: 2. 4 g

115. Quinoa Meatballs

Preparation Time: 10 minutes | **Cooking Time:** 35 minutes | **Servings:** 4

Ingredients:

1 cup quinoa, cooked	1 tablespoon flax meal
1 cup diced white onion	1 ½ teaspoon minced garlic

1/2 teaspoon salt

1 teaspoon lemon zest

1 teaspoon dried basil

2 tablespoons olive oil

1 teaspoon dried oregano

1 teaspoon paprika

3 tablespoons water

1 cup grated vegan mozzarella cheese

Marinara sauce as needed for serving

Directions:

Place flax meal in a bowl, stir in water, and set aside until required.

Take a large skillet pan, place it over medium heat, add 1 tablespoon oil and when hot, add onion and cook for 2 minutes.

Stir in all the spices and herbs, then stir in quinoa until combined and cook for 2 minutes.

Transfer quinoa mixture in a bowl, add flax meal mixture, lemon zest, and cheese, stir until well mixed and then shape the mixture into twelve 1 ½ inch balls.

Arrange balls on a baking sheet lined with parchment paper, refrigerate the balls for 30 minutes and then bake for 20 minutes at 400 degrees F.

Serve balls with marinara sauce.

Nutrition:

Calories: 100 Cal Fat: 100 g Carbs: 100 g Protein: 100 g Fiber: 100 g

116. Rice Stuffed Jalapeños

Preparation Time: 5 minutes | **Cooking Time:** 15 minutes | **Servings:** 6

Ingredients:

3 medium-sized potatoes, peeled, cubed, boiled

3 tablespoons water

1 teaspoons salt

1/4 teaspoon garlic powder

3 tablespoons water

3 jalapeños pepper, halved

½ cup vegetable broth

2 large carrots, peeled, chopped, boiled

1/4 teaspoon onion powder

1/2 cup nutritional yeast

1 lime, juiced

Cooked rice as needed

1 red bell pepper, sliced, for garnish

Directions:

Place boiled vegetables in a food processor, pour in the broth, and pulse until smooth.

Add garlic powder, onion powder, salt, water, and lime juice, pulse until combined, then add yeast and blend until smooth.

Tip the mixture in a bowl, add rice, and stir until incorporated.

Cut each jalapeno into half lengthwise, brush them with oil, season them with some salt, stuff them with rice mixture and bake them for 20 minutes at 400 degrees F until done.

Serve straight away.

Nutrition:

Calories: 148 Cal Fat: 3. 7 g Carbs: 12. 2 g Protein: 2 g Fiber: 2 g

117. Pineapple Fried Rice

Preparation Time: 5 minutes | **Cooking Time:** 12 minutes | **Servings:** 2

Ingredients:

2 cups brown rice, cooked

2/3 cup green peas

1 large red bell pepper, cored, diced

2/3 cup pineapple chunks with juice

1 bunch of green onions, sliced

4 tablespoons soy sauce

1/2 teaspoon sesame oil

1/2 cup sunflower seeds, toasted

1 teaspoon minced garlic

1 tablespoon grated ginger

2 tablespoons coconut oil

For the Sauce:

1/2 cup pineapple juice

1/2 a lime, juiced

Directions:

Take a skillet pan, place it over medium-high heat, add oil, and when hot, add red bell pepper, pineapple pieces, and two-third of onion, cook for 5 minutes, then stir in ginger and garlic and cook for 1 minute.

Switch heat to the high level, add rice to the pan, stir until combined, and cook for 5 minutes.

When done, fold in sunflower seeds and peas and set aside until required.

Prepare the sauce and for this, place sesame oil in a small bowl, add soy sauce and pineapple juice and whisk until combined.

Drizzle sauce over rice, drizzle with lime juice and serve straight away.

Nutrition:
Calories: 179 Cal Fat: 5. 5 g Carbs: 30 g Protein: 3. 3 g Fiber: 2 g

118. Portobello Kale Florentine

Preparation Time: 15-30 minutes | **Cooking Time:** 25 minutes | **Servings:** 4

Ingredients:

4 large portobello mushrooms, stems removed	1/8 tsp black pepper
1/8 tsp garlic salt	½ tsp olive oil
1 small onion, chopped	1 cup chopped fresh kale
¼ cup crumbled tofu cheese	1 tbsp chopped fresh basil

Directions:
Preheat the oven to 350 F and grease a baking sheet with cooking spray.

Lightly oil the mushrooms with some cooking spray and season with the black pepper and garlic salt. Arrange the mushrooms on the baking sheet and bake in the oven until tender, 10 to 15 minutes.

Heat the olive oil in a medium skillet over medium heat and sauté the onion until tender, 3 minutes. Stir in the kale until wilted, 3 minutes. Turn the heat off. Spoon the mixture into the mushrooms and top with the tofu cheese and basil. Serve.

Nutrition:
Calories 65 kcal Fats 1. 6g Carbs 10. 1g Protein 4. 9g

119. Tempeh Oat Balls With Maple Asparagus

Preparation Time: 15-30 minutes | **Cooking Time:** 40 minutes | **Servings:** 4

Ingredients:
For tempeh balls:

1 tbsp flax seed powder + 3 tbsp water	1 lb tempeh, crumbled
¼ cup chopped red bell pepper	Salt and black pepper to taste
1 tbsp almond flour	1 tsp garlic powder
1 tsp onion powder	1 tsp tofu mayonnaise
Olive oil for brushing	

For maple asparagus:

2 tbsp plant butter	1 lb asparagus, hard part trimmed
2 tbsp pure maple syrup	1 tbsp freshly squeezed lemon juice

Directions:
Preheat the oven to 400 F and line a baking sheet with parchment paper.

In a medium bowl, mix the flax seed powder with water and allow thickening for 5 minutes. Add the tempeh, bell pepper, salt, black pepper, almond flour, garlic powder, onion powder, and tofu mayonnaise. Mix well and form 1-inch balls from the mixture.

Arrange on the baking sheet, brush with cooking spray, and bake in the oven for 15 to 20 minutes or until brown and compacted. Remove from the oven and set aside for serving.

Melt the butter in a large skillet and sauté the asparagus until softened with some crunch, 7 minutes. Mix in the maple syrup and lemon juice. Cook for 2 minutes and plate the asparagus. Serve warm with the tempeh balls.

Nutrition:
Calories 365 kcal Fats 22. 1g Carbs 24. 5g Protein 24. 2g

120. Chili Mushroom Spaghetti With Watercress

Preparation Time: 15-30 minutes | **Cooking Time:** 30 minutes | **Servings:** 4

Ingredients:

1 lb whole-wheat spaghetti	3 tbsp plant butter
2 tbsp olive oil	2 shallots, finely chopped
2 garlic cloves, minced	½ lb chopped white button mushrooms
1 tbsp sake	3 tbsp soy sauce
1 tsp hot sauce	A handful of fresh watercress
¼ cup chopped fresh parsley	Black pepper to taste

Directions:
Cook the spaghetti in slightly salted water in a large pot over medium heat until al dente, 10 minutes. Drain the spaghetti and set aside.

Heat the butter and olive oil in a large skillet over medium heat and sauté the shallots, garlic, and mushrooms until softened, 5 minutes.

Stir in the sake, soy sauce, and hot sauce. Cook further for 1 minute.

Toss the spaghetti in the sauce along with the watercress and parsley. Cook for 1 minute and season with the black pepper. Dish the food and serve warm.

Nutrition:
Calories 393 kcal Fats 22. 2g Carbs 42. 9g Protein 9. 3g

121. Zucchini Rolls In Tomato Sauce

Preparation Time: 15-30 minutes | **Cooking Time:** 60 minutes | **Servings:** 4

Ingredients:

3 large zucchinis, sliced lengthwise into strips	Salt and black pepper to taste
1 tbsp olive oil	¾ lb crumbled tempeh
1 cup crumbled tofu cheese	1/3 cup grated plant-based Parmesan cheese
¼ cup chopped fresh basil leaves	2 garlic cloves, minced
1 ½ cups marinara sauce, divided	2 cups shredded plant-based mozzarella, divided

Directions:
Line a baking sheet with paper towels and lay the zucchini slices in a single layer on the sheet. Sprinkle each side with some salt and allow the release of liquid for 15 minutes.

Heat the olive oil in a large skillet over medium heat and cook the tempeh until browned, 10 minutes. Set aside.

In a medium bowl, mix the tempeh, tofu cheese, plant Parmesan cheese, basil, and garlic; season with salt and black pepper.

Preheat the oven to 400 F.

Spread 1 cup of marinara sauce onto the bottom of a 10-inch oven-proof skillet and set aside.

Spread 1 tbsp of the cheese mixture evenly along with each zucchini slice; sprinkle with 1 tbsp of plant mozzarella cheese. Roll up the zucchini slices over the filling and arrange them in the skillet. Top with the remaining ½ cup of marinara sauce and sprinkle with the remaining plant mozzarella.

Bake in the oven for 25-30 minutes or until the zucchini rolls are heated through and the cheese begins to brown. Serve immediately.

Nutrition:
Calories 428 kcal Fats 14. 5g Carbs 31. 3g Protein 40. 3g

122. Cannellini Beans Bow Ties

Preparation Time: 15-30 minutes | **Cooking Time:** 35 minutes | **Servings:** 4

Ingredients:

2 ½ cups whole-wheat bow tie pasta	1 tbsp olive oil
1 medium zucchini, sliced	2 garlic cloves, minced
2 large tomatoes, chopped	1 (15 oz) can cannellini beans, rinsed and drained
1 (2 ¼ oz) can pitted green olives, sliced	½ cup crumbled tofu cheese

Directions:
Cook the pasta in 8 cups of slightly salted water in a medium pot over medium heat until al dente, 10 minutes. Drain the pasta and set aside. Heat olive oil in a skillet and sauté zucchini and garlic for 4 minutes. Stir in tomatoes, beans, and olives. Cook until the tomatoes soften, 10 minutes. Mix in pasta. Allow warming for 1 minute. Stir in tofu cheese and serve warm.

Nutrition:
Calories 206 kcal Fats 5. 1g Carbs 35. 8g Protein 7. 6g

123. Crispy Tofu Burgers

Preparation Time: 15-30 minutes | **Cooking Time:** 20 minutes | **Servings:** 4

Ingredients:

1 tbsp flax seed powder + 3 tbsp water	2/3 lb crumble tofu
1 tbsp quick-cooking oats	1 tbsp toasted almond flour
½ tsp garlic powder	½ tsp onion powder

Salt and black pepper to taste

3 tbsp whole-grain breadcrumbs

¼ tsp curry powder

4 whole-wheat burger buns, halved

Directions:

In a small bowl, mix the flax seed powder with water and allow thickening for 5 minutes to make the flax egg. Set aside.

In a medium bowl, mix the tofu, oats, almond flour, garlic powder, onion powder, salt, black pepper, and curry powder. Mold 4 patties out of the mixture and lightly brush both sides with the flax egg.

Pour the breadcrumbs onto a plate and coat the patties in the crumbs until well covered.

Heat a pan to medium heat and grease well with cooking spray.

Cook the patties on both sides until crispy, golden brown, and cooked through, 10 minutes. Place each patty between each burger bun and top with the guacamole.

Serve immediately.

Nutrition:

Calories 238 kcal Fats 15. 8g Carbs 14. 8g Protein 14. 1g

124. Green Bean And Mushroom Biryani

Preparation Time: 15-30 minutes | **Cooking Time:** 50 minutes | **Servings:** 4

Ingredients:

1 cup of brown rice	2 cups of water
Salt to taste	3 tbsp plant butter
3 medium white onions, chopped	6 garlic cloves, minced
1 tsp ginger puree	1 tbsp turmeric powder + more for dusting
¼ tsp cinnamon powder	2 tsp garam masala
½ tsp cardamom powder	½ tsp cayenne powder
½ tsp cumin powder	1 tsp smoked paprika
3 large tomatoes, diced	2 green chilies, deseeded and minced
1 tbsp tomato puree	1 cup chopped cremini mushrooms

1 cup chopped mustard greens

1 cup plant-based yogurt for topping

Directions:

Melt the butter in a large pot and sauté the onions until softened, 3 minutes. Mix in the garlic, ginger, turmeric, cardamom powder, garam masala, cardamom powder, cayenne pepper, cumin powder, paprika, and salt. Stir-fry while cooking until fragrant, 1 to 2 minutes. Stir in the tomatoes, green chili, tomato puree, and mushrooms. Once boiling, mix in the rice and cover with water. Cover the pot and cook over medium heat until the liquid absorbs and the rice is tender, 15-20 minutes.

Open the lid and fluff in the mustard greens and half of the parsley. Dish the food, top with the coconut yogurt, garnish with the remaining parsley and serve warm.

Nutrition:

Calories 255 Fats 16. 8g Carbs 25. 6g Protein 5. 8g

125. Cabbage & Bell Pepper Skillet

Preparation Time: 15-30 minutes | **Cooking Time:** 30 minutes | **Servings:** 4

Ingredients:

1 can (28 oz) whole plum tomatoes, undrained	1 lb crumbled tempeh
1 large yellow onion, chopped	1 can (8 oz) tomato sauce
2 tbsp plain vinegar	1 tbsp pure date sugar
1 tsp dried mixed herbs	3 large tomatoes, chopped
½ tsp black pepper	1 small head cabbage, thinly sliced
1 medium green bell pepper, deseeded and cut into thin strips	

Directions:

Drain the tomatoes and reserve their liquid. Chop the tomatoes and set them aside.

Add the tempeh to a large skillet and cook until brown, 10 minutes. Mix in the onion, tomato sauce, vinegar, date sugar, mixed herbs, and chopped tomatoes. Close the lid and cook until the liquid reduces and the tomato softens for about 10 minutes.

Stir in the cabbage and bell pepper; cook until softened, 5 minutes.

Dish the food and serve it with cooked brown rice.

Nutrition:

Calories 403 Fats 16. 9g Carbs 44. 1g Protein 27. 3g

126. Mixed Bean Burgers With Cashew Cheese

Preparation Time: 15-30 minutes | **Cooking Time:** 30 minutes | **Servings:** 4

Ingredients:

1 (15 oz) can chickpea, drained and rinsed	1 (15 oz) can pinto beans, drained and rinsed
1 (15 oz) can red kidney beans, drained and rinsed	2 tbsp whole-wheat flour
¼ cup dried mixed herbs	¼ tsp hot sauce
½ tsp garlic powder	Salt and black pepper to taste
4 slices cashew cheese	4 whole-grain hamburger buns, split
4 small lettuce leaves for topping	

Directions:

In a medium bowl, mash the chickpea, pinto beans, kidney beans and mix in the flour, mixed herbs, hot sauce, garlic powder, salt, and black pepper. Mold 4 patties out of the mixture and set aside.

Heat a grill pan to medium heat and lightly grease with cooking spray.

Cook the bean patties on both sides until light brown and cooked through, 10 minutes.

Lay a cashew cheese slice on each and allow slight melting, 2 minutes.

Remove the patties between the burger buns and top with the lettuce and serve warm.

Nutrition:

Calories 456 Fats 16. 8g Carbs 56. 1g Protein 24g

127. Cheesy Bean & Rice Burritos

Preparation Time: 15-30 minutes | **Cooking Time:** 50 minutes | **Servings:** 4

Ingredients:

1 cups brown rice	Salt and black pepper to taste
1 tbsp olive oil	1 medium red onion, chopped
1 medium green bell pepper, deseeded and diced	2 garlic cloves, minced
1 tbsp chili powder	1 tsp cumin powder
1/8 tsp red chili flakes	1 (15 oz) can black beans, rinsed and drained
4 (8-inch) whole-wheat flour tortillas, warmed	1 cup of salsa
1 cup coconut cream for topping	1 cup grated plant-based cheddar cheese for topping

Directions:

Add 2 cups of water and brown rice to a medium pot, season with some salt, and cook over medium heat until the water absorbs and the rice is tender, 15 to 20 minutes.

Heat the olive oil in a medium skillet over medium heat and sauté the onion, bell pepper, and garlic until softened and fragrant, 3 minutes.

Mix in the chili powder, cumin powder, red chili flakes, and season with salt and black pepper. Cook for 1 minute or until the food releases fragrance. Stir in the brown rice, black beans, and allow warming through, 3 minutes.

Lay the tortillas on a clean, flat surface and divide the rice mixture in the center of each. Top with the salsa, coconut cream, and plant cheddar cheese. Fold the sides and ends of the tortillas over the filling to secure. Serve immediately.

Nutrition:

Calories 421 Fats 29. 1g Carbs 37g Protein 9. 3g

128. Avocado and Cauliflower Hummus

Preparation Time: 5 minutes | **Cooking Time:** 25 minutes | **Servings:** 2

Ingredients:

1 medium cauliflower, stem removed and chopped	1 large Hass avocado, peeled, pitted, and chopped
¼ cup extra virgin olive oil	2 garlic cloves
½ tbsp. lemon juice	½ tsp. onion powder
Sea salt and ground black pepper to taste	2 large carrots
¼ cup fresh cilantro, chopped	

Directions:

Preheat the oven to 450°F, and line a baking tray with aluminum foil.

Put the chopped cauliflower on the baking tray and drizzle with 2 tablespoons of olive oil.

Roast the chopped cauliflower in the oven for 20-25 minutes, until lightly brown.

Remove the tray from the oven and allow the cauliflower to cool down.

Add all the ingredients—except the carrots and optional fresh cilantro—to a food processor or blender, and blend the ingredients into a smooth hummus.

Transfer the hummus to a medium-sized bowl, cover, and put it in the fridge for at least 30 minutes.

Take the hummus out of the fridge and, if desired, top it with the optional chopped cilantro and more salt and pepper to taste; serve with the carrot fries, and enjoy!

Nutrition:

Calories 416 Carbohydrates 8. 4 g Fats 40. 3 g Protein 3. 3 g

129. Raw Zoodles with Avocado and Nuts

Preparation Time: 10 minutes | **Cooking Time:** 3-30 minutes | **Servings:** 2

Ingredients:

1 medium zucchini	1½ cups basil
1/3 cup water	5 tbsp. pine nuts
2 tbsp. lemon juice	1 medium avocado, peeled, pitted, sliced
Optional: 2 tbsp. olive oil	6 yellow cherry tomatoes, halved
Optional: 6 red cherry tomatoes, halved	Sea salt and black pepper to taste

Directions:

Add the basil, water, nuts, lemon juice, avocado slices, optional olive oil (if desired), salt, and pepper to a blender.

Blend the ingredients into a smooth mixture. Add more salt and pepper to taste and blend again. Divide the sauce and the zucchini noodles between two medium-sized bowls for serving, and combine in each.

Top the mixtures with the halved yellow cherry tomatoes, and the optional red cherry tomatoes (if desired); serve and enjoy!

Nutrition:

Calories 317 Carbohydrates 7. 4 g Fats 28. 1 g Protein 7. 2 g

130. Cauliflower Sushi

Preparation Time: 30 minutes | **Cooking Time:** 3-30 minutes | **Servings:** 4

Ingredients:

Sushi Base:	6 cups cauliflower florets
½ cup vegan cheese	1 medium spring onion, diced
4 nori sheets	Sea salt and pepper to taste
1 tbsp. rice vinegar or sushi vinegar	1 medium garlic clove, minced
Filling:	1 medium Hass avocado, peeled, sliced
½ medium cucumber, skinned, sliced	4 asparagus spears
A handful of enoki mushrooms	

Directions:

Put the cauliflower florets in a food processor or blender. Pulse the florets into a rice-like substance. When using ready-made cauliflower rice, add this to the blender.

Add the vegan cheese, spring onions, and vinegar to the food processor or blender. Top these ingredients with salt and pepper to taste, and pulse everything into a chunky mixture. Make sure not to turn the ingredients into a puree by pulsing too long.

Taste and add more vinegar, salt, or pepper to taste. Add the optional minced garlic clove to the blender and pulse again for a few seconds.

Lay the nori sheets and spread the cauliflower rice mixture out evenly between the sheets. Make sure to leave at least 2 inches of the top and bottom edges empty.

Place one or more combinations of multiple filling ingredients along the center of the spread-out rice mixture. Experiment with different ingredients per nori sheet for the best flavor.

Roll up each nori sheet tightly. (Using a sushi mat will make this easier.)

Either serve the sushi as a nori roll or, slice each roll up into sushi pieces.

Serve right away with a small amount of wasabi, pickled ginger, and soy sauce!

Nutrition:
Calories 189 Carbohydrates 7. 6 g Fats 14. 4 g Protein 6. 1 g

131. Pinwheel Greens

Preparation Time: 5 minutes | **Cooking Time:** 1 minute | **Servings:** 16

Ingredients:

½ cup of water	4 tablespoons white vinegar
3 tablespoons lemon juice	3 tablespoons tahini paste
1 clove garlic, minced	Salt and pepper to taste
Canned artichokes, drained, thinly sliced	Cherry tomatoes, thinly sliced
Olives, thinly sliced	Lettuce or baby spinach
Tortillas	

Directions:
In a bowl, combine the water, vinegar, lemon juice, and Tahini paste; whisk together until smooth.

Add the garlic, salt, and pepper to taste; whisk to combine. Set the bowl aside.

Lay a tortilla on a flat surface and spread with one tablespoon of the sauce.

Lay some lettuce or spinach slices on top, then scatter some artichoke, tomato, and olive slices on top.

Tightly roll the tortilla and fold in the sides. Cut the ends off and then slice into four or five pinwheels.

Nutrition:
Calories 322 Carbohydrates 5 g Fats 4 g Protein 30 g

132. Guacamole Rice and Bean Burritos

Preparation Time: 10 minutes | **Cooking Time:** 15 minutes | **Servings:** 8

Ingredients:

2 16-ounce cans fat-free refried beans	6 tortillas
2 cups cooked rice	½ cup of salsa
1 tablespoon olive oil	1 bunch green onions, chopped
2 bell peppers, finely chopped	Guacamole

Directions:
Preheat the oven to 375°F.

Dump the refried beans into a saucepan and place over medium heat to warm.

Heat the tortillas and lay them out on a flat surface.

Spoon the beans in a long mound that runs across the tortilla, just a little off from the center.

Spoon some rice and salsa over the beans; add the green pepper and onions to taste, along with any other finely chopped vegetables you like.

Fold over the shortest edge of the plain tortilla and roll it up, folding in the sides as you go.

Place each burrito, seam side down, on a baking sheet sprayed with a non-stick spray.

Brush with olive oil and bake for 15 minutes. Serve with guacamole.

Nutrition:
Calories 290 Carbohydrates 49 g Fats 6 g Protein 9 g

133. Ricotta Basil Pinwheels

Preparation Time: 10 minutes | **Cooking Time:** 3-30 minutes | **Servings:** 4

Ingredients:

½ cup unsalted cashews	Water
7 ounces firm tofu, cut into pieces	¼ cup almond milk
1 teaspoon white wine vinegar	1 clove garlic, smashed
20 to 25 fresh basil leaves	Salt and pepper to taste
8 tortillas	7 ounces fresh spinach
½ cup black olives, sliced	2 to 3 tomatoes, cut into small pieces

Directions:

Soak the cashews for 30 minutes in enough water to cover them. Drain them well and pat them dry with paper towels.

Place the cashews in a blender along with the tofu, almond milk, vinegar, garlic, basil leaves, salt, and pepper to taste. Blend until smooth and creamy.

Spread the resulting mixture on the eight tortillas, dividing it equally.

Top with spinach leaves, olives, and tomatoes.

Tightly roll each loaded tortilla.

Cut off the ends with a sharp knife and slice into four or five pinwheels.

Nutrition:

Calories 236 Carbohydrates 6. 1 g Fats 21. 6 g Protein 4. 2 g

134. Delicious Sloppy Joes With No Meat

Preparation Time: 6 minutes | **Cooking Time:** 5 minutes | **Servings:** 4

Ingredients:

5 tablespoons vegetable stock	2 stalks celery, diced
1 small onion, diced	1 small red bell pepper, diced
1 teaspoon garlic powder	1 teaspoon chili powder
1 teaspoon ground cumin	1 teaspoon salt

1 cup cooked bulgur wheat	1 cup red lentils
1 15-ounce can tomato sauce	4 tablespoons tomato paste
3½ cups water	2 teaspoons balsamic vinegar
1 tablespoon Hoisin sauce	

Directions:

In a Dutch oven, heat the vegetable stock and add the celery, onion, and bell pepper. Sauté until vegetables are soft, about five minutes.

Add the garlic powder, chili powder, cumin, and salt and mix in.

Add the bulgur wheat, lentils, tomato sauce, tomato paste, water, vinegar, and Hoisin sauce. Stir and bring to a boil.

Turn the heat down to a simmer and cook uncovered for 30 minutes. Stir occasionally to prevent sticking and scorching.

Taste to see if the lentils are tender.

When the lentils are done, serve on buns.

Nutrition:

Calories 451 Fats 10 g Carbohydrates 61 g Protein 27 g

135. Coconut Curry Lentils

Preparation Time: 10 minutes | **Cooking Time:** 40 minutes | **Servings:** 4

Ingredients:

1 cup brown lentils	1 small white onion, peeled, chopped
1 teaspoon minced garlic	1 teaspoon grated ginger
3 cups baby spinach	1 tablespoon curry powder
2 tablespoons olive oil	13 ounces coconut milk, unsweetened
2 cups vegetable broth	

For Servings:

4 cups cooked rice	1/4 cup chopped cilantro

Directions:

Place a large pot over medium heat, add oil and when hot, add ginger and garlic and cook for 1 minute until fragrant.

Add onion, cook for 5 minutes, stir in curry powder, cook for 1 minute until toasted, add lentils, and pour in broth.

Switch heat to medium-high level, bring the mixture to a boil, then switch heat to the low level and simmer for 20 minutes until tender and all the liquid is absorbed.

Pour in milk, stir until combined, turn heat to medium level, and simmer for 10 minutes until thickened.

Then remove the pot from heat, stir in spinach, let it stand for 5 minutes until its leaves wilts and then top with cilantro.

Serve lentils with rice.

Nutrition:
Calories: 184 Cal Fat: 3. 7 g Carbs: 30 g Protein: 11. 3 g Fiber: 10. 7 g

136. Cauliflower-Onion Patties

Preparation Time: 05 minutes | **Cooking Time:** 10 minutes | **Servings:** 4

Ingredients:

3 cups cauliflower florets	1/2 cup onion
2 large eggs	2 tablespoons all-purpose white flour
2 tablespoons olive oil	

Directions:
Dice cauliflower and chop onion.

Boil the diced cauliflower in a small amount of water for 5 minutes; drain.

Break eggs into a medium bowl and beat. Add the flour and mix well.

Add the cauliflower and onion and stir into the flour/egg mixture until well mixed.

Add olive oil to a frying pan and heat.

Drop the mixture by spoonful's into the hot oil, making 4 equal portions (or 8 portions smaller size are desired).

Using a spatula, flatten the latkes and fry until brown on both sides.

Drain on a paper towel to soak up extra oil.

Serve hot.

Nutrition:
Calories 134, Total Fat 9.6g, Saturated Fat 1.8g, Cholesterol 93mg, Sodium 58mg, Total Carbohydrate 8.5g, Dietary Fiber 2.3g, Total Sugars 2.6g, Protein 5.2g, Calcium 34mg, Iron 1mg, Potassium 286mg, Phosphorus 229 mg

137. Roasted Garlic Broccoli

Preparation Time: 15 minutes | **Cooking Time:** 25 minutes | **Servings:** 4

Ingredients:

2 tablespoons minced garlic	3 tablespoons olive oil
1 large head broccoli, separated into florets	1/3 cup grated Parmesan cheese
Salt and black pepper to taste	1 tablespoon chopped fresh basil

Directions:
Preheat the oven to 450 degrees F. Grease a large casserole dish.

Place the olive oil and garlic in a large resealable bag. Add broccoli, and shake to mix. Pour into the prepared casserole dish, and season with salt and pepper to taste.

Bake for 25 minutes, stirring halfway through. Top with Parmesan cheese and basil, and broil for 3 to 5 minutes, until golden brown.

Nutrition:
Calories 112, Total Fat 11.1g, Saturated Fat 1.8g, Cholesterol 2mg, Sodium 30mg, Total Carbohydrate 3g, Dietary Fiber 0.7g, Total Sugars 0.4g, Protein 1.7g, Calcium 40mg, Iron 0mg, Potassium 91mg Phosphorus 89 mg

138. Carrot Casserole

Preparation Time: 15 minutes | **Cooking Time:** 15 minutes | **Servings:** 4

Ingredients:

½ pound carrots	½ cup graham crackers
1 tablespoon olive oil	1 tablespoon onion
1/8 teaspoon black pepper	1/6 cup shredded cheddar cheese
Salt	

Directions:
Preheat the oven to 350º F.

Peel carrots and slice into 1/4-inch rounds. Place carrots in a large saucepan over medium-high heat and boil until soft enough to mash. Drain and reserve 1/3-cup liquid.

Mash carrots until they are smooth.

Crush graham crackers, heat oil, and minced onion. Stir crackers, onion, oil, salt, pepper, and reserved liquid into mashed carrots.

Place in a greased small casserole dish. Sprinkle shredded cheese on top and bake for 15 minutes. Serve hot.

Nutrition:

Calories 118, Total Fat 6.1g, Saturated Fat 1.7g, Cholesterol 5mg, Sodium 86mg, Total Carbohydrate 14g, Dietary Fiber 1.8g, Total Sugars 6.2g, Protein 2.4g, Calcium 56mg, Iron 1mg, Potassium 205mg, Phosphorus 189 mg

139. Carrot-Pineapple Casserole

Preparation Time: 10 minutes | **Cooking Time:** 50 minutes | **Servings:** 4

Ingredients:

3 large carrots	1 large pineapple
2 tablespoons all-purpose flour	1 tablespoon honey
½ teaspoon ground cinnamon	1 tablespoon olive oil
1/2 cup pineapple juice	

Directions:

Preheat the oven to 350 degrees F.

Peel and slice carrots and pineapples. Bring 1 quart of water to a boil in a medium-sized pot. Boil carrots for 5 minutes or until tender. Drain. Layer carrots and pineapples in a large casserole dish.

Using a fork, mix flour, honey, and cinnamon in a small bowl. Mix in olive oil to make a crumb topping.

Sprinkle flour mixture over carrots and pineapples then drizzle with juice.

Bake for 50 minutes or until pineapples and carrots are tender and the topping is golden brown.

Nutrition:

Calories 94, Total Fat 2.9g, Saturated Fat 0.4g, Cholesterol 0mg, Sodium 31mg, Total Carbohydrate 17.4g, Dietary Fiber 1.8g, Total Sugars 11.2g, Protein 0.9g, Calcium 23mg, Iron 0mg, Potassium 206mg, Phosphorus 27 mg

140. Broccoli with Garlic Butter and Almonds

Preparation Time: 10 minutes | **Cooking Time:** 50 minutes | **Servings:** 4

Ingredients:

1 pound fresh broccoli, cut into bite-size pieces	¼ cup olive oil
½ tablespoon honey	1-1/2 tablespoons soy sauce
¼ teaspoon ground black pepper	2 cloves garlic, minced
¼ cup chopped almonds	

Directions:

Place the broccoli into a large pot with about 1 inch of water in the bottom. Bring to a boil, and cook for 7 minutes, or until tender but still crisp. Drain, and arrange broccoli on a serving platter. While the broccoli is cooking, heat the oil in a small skillet over medium heat. Mix in the honey, soy sauce, pepper, and garlic. Bring to a boil, then remove from the heat. Mix in the almonds, and pour the sauce over the broccoli. Serve immediately.

Nutrition:

Calories 177, Total Fat 17.3g, Saturated Fat 2.1g, Cholesterol 0mg, Sodium 234mg, Total Carbohydrate 5.3g, Dietary Fiber 1.2g, Total Sugars 2.7g, Protein 2.9g, Calcium 20mg, Iron 1mg, Potassium 131mg, Phosphorus 67 mg

141. Roasted Vegetables

Preparation Time: 15 minutes | **Cooking Time:** 40 minutes | **Servings:** 4

Ingredients:

¼ summer squash, cubed	1 red bell peppers, seeded and diced
1 red onion, quartered	¼ cup green beans
1 tablespoon chopped fresh thyme	2 tablespoons chopped fresh rosemary
1/4 cup olive oil	½ tablespoon lemon juice
Salt and freshly ground black pepper	

Directions:
Preheat the oven to 475 degrees F.

In a large bowl, combine the squash, red bell peppers, and green beans. Separate the red onion quarters into pieces, and add them to the mixture. In a small bowl, stir together thyme, rosemary, olive oil, lemon juice, salt, and pepper. Toss with vegetables until they are coated. Spread evenly on a large roasting pan.

Roast for 35 to 40 minutes in the preheated oven, stirring every 10 minutes, or until vegetables are cooked through and browned.

Nutrition:
Calories 145, Total Fat 13.1g, Saturated Fat 2g, Cholesterol 0mg, Sodium 4mg, Total Carbohydrate 8g, Dietary Fiber 2.5g, Total Sugars 3.5g, Protein 1.3g, Calcium 47mg, Iron 2mg, Potassium 160mg, Phosphorus 110mg

142. Honey Roasted Cauliflower

Preparation Time: 10 minutes | **Cooking Time:** 35 minutes | **Servings:** 4

Ingredients:

2 cups cauliflower	2 tablespoons diced onion
2 tablespoons olive oil	1 tablespoon honey
1 teaspoon dry mustard	1 pinch salt
1 pinch ground black pepper	

Directions:
Preheat the oven to 375 degrees F. Lightly coat an 11x7 inch baking dish with non-stick cooking spray.

Place cauliflower in a single layer in a prepared dish, and top with onion. In a small bowl, combine olive oil, honey, mustard, salt, and pepper; drizzle over cauliflower and onion.

Bake in the preheated 375 degrees F oven for 35 minutes or until tender, stirring halfway through the cooking time.

Nutrition:
Calories 88, Total Fat 7.3g, Saturated Fat 1g, Cholesterol 0mg, Sodium 47mg, Total Carbohydrate 6.4g, Dietary Fiber 0.9g, Total Sugars 5.2g, Protein 0.8g, Calcium 11mg, Iron 0mg, Potassium 92mg, Phosphorus 70mg

143. Broccoli Steaks

Preparation Time: 10 minutes | **Cooking Time:** 25 minutes | **Servings:** 4

Ingredients:

1 medium head broccoli	3 tablespoons unsalted butter
¼ teaspoon garlic powder	¼ teaspoon onion powder
1/8 teaspoon salt	¼ teaspoon pepper

Directions:
Preheat the oven to 400 degrees F. Please parchment paper on a roasting pan.

Trim the leaves off the broccoli and cut off the bottom of the stem. Cut the broccoli head in half. Cut each half into 1 to 3/4-inch slices, leaving the core in place. Cut off the smaller ends of the broccoli and save for another recipe. There should be 4 broccoli steaks.

Mix butter, garlic powder, onion powder, salt, and pepper.

Lay the broccoli on the parchment-lined baking sheet. Using half of the butter mixture, brush onto the steaks. Place in the preheated oven for 20 minutes. Remove from the oven and flip the steaks over. Brush steaks with remaining butter and roast for about 20 more minutes, until they are golden brown on the edges.

Nutrition:
Calories 86, Total Fat 8.7g, Saturated Fat 5.5g, Cholesterol 23mg, Sodium 143mg, Total Carbohydrate 1.9g, Dietary Fiber 0.7g, Total Sugars 0.5g, Protein 0.8g, Calcium 15mg, Iron 0mg, Potassium 80mg, Phosphorus 61 mg

144. Roasted Garlic Lemon Cauliflower

Preparation Time: 10 minutes | **Cooking Time:** 15 minutes | **Servings:** 4

Ingredients:

2 heads cauliflower, separated into florets	2 teaspoons olive oil
½ teaspoon ground black pepper	1 clove garlic, minced
½ teaspoon lemon juice	

Directions:
Preheat the oven to 400 degrees F.

In a large bowl, toss broccoli florets with olive oil, pepper, and garlic. Spread the broccoli out in an even layer on a baking sheet.

Bake in the preheated oven until florets are tender enough to pierce the stems with a fork, 15 to 20 minutes. Remove and transfer to a serving platter. Squeeze lemon juice liberally over the broccoli before serving for a refreshing, tangy finish.

Nutrition:
Calories 37, Total Fat 1.7g, Saturated Fat 0.2g, Cholesterol 0mg, Sodium 27mg, Total Carbohydrate 5g, Dietary Fiber 2.3g, Total Sugars 2.1g, Protein 1.8g, Calcium 21mg, Iron 0mg, Potassium 272mg, Phosphorus 161 mg

145. Broccoli with Garlic Sauce

Preparation Time: 10 minutes | **Cooking Time:** 15 minutes | **Servings:** 4

Ingredients:

2 cups broccoli florets	1 garlic cloves
½ tablespoon butter	2 teaspoons honey
1-1/2 tablespoons apple cider vinegar	1 tablespoon fresh parsley

Directions:
In a large saucepan with a steamer rack, steam broccoli over boiling water for 8 to 10 minutes or until crisp-tender (cover with a lid while steaming).

In a small saucepan, cook minced garlic in butter for 30 seconds then remove the pan from heat.

Stir in honey, apple cider vinegar, and chopped parsley. Return the saucepan to heat until the sauce is heated.

Transfer steamed broccoli to a serving dish.

Pour sauce over hot broccoli and toss to coat.

Nutrition:
Calories 41, Total Fat 1.6g, Saturated Fat 0.9g, Cholesterol 4mg, Sodium 26mg, Total Carbohydrate 6.2g, Dietary Fiber 1.2g, Total Sugars 3.7g, Protein 1.4g, Calcium 25mg, Iron 0mg, Potassium 157mg, Phosphorus 100 mg

146. Cranberry Cabbage

Preparation Time: 10 minutes | **Cooking Time:** 15 minutes | **Servings:** 4

Ingredients:

8 ounces canned whole-berry cranberry sauce	1 tablespoon fresh lemon juice
1/4 teaspoon ground cloves	1 medium head red cabbage

Directions:
In a large pan heat cranberry sauce, lemon juice, and cloves together and bring to a simmer.

Stir cabbage into melted cranberry sauce, mixing well. Bring mixture to a boil; reduce heat to simmer. Continue cooking until cabbage is tender, stirring occasionally.

Serve hot.

Nutrition:
Calories 38, Total Fat 0.1g, Saturated Fat 0g, Cholesterol 0mg, Sodium 20mg, Total Carbohydrate 7.9g, Dietary Fiber 2.6g, Total Sugars 3.8g, Protein 1g, Calcium 37mg, Iron 1mg, Potassium 224mg, Phosphorus 120 mg

147. Deviled Green Beans

Preparation Time: 10 minutes | **Cooking Time:** 15 minutes | **Servings:** 4

Ingredients:

2 cups frozen green beans	5 teaspoons unsalted butter
2 teaspoons mustard	1/2 teaspoon black pepper
1 teaspoon Worcestershire sauce	1 tablespoon graham crackers crumbs

Directions:
Prepare green beans as directed on the package.

Make a sauce by mixing 2 teaspoons melted butter, mustard, and pepper, and Worcestershire sauce. Heat in the microwave for 30 seconds.

Toss sauce with hot cooked green beans.

Mix remaining butter (melted with graham crackers crumbs. Sprinkle on top of the beans and serve.

Nutrition:
Calories 75, Total Fat 5.4g, Saturated Fat 0.8g, Cholesterol 0mg, Sodium 84mg, Total Carbohydrate 6.1g, Dietary Fiber 2.3g, Total Sugars 1.4g, Protein 1.6g, Calcium 32mg, Iron 1mg, Potassium 132mg, Phosphorus 80 mg

148. Lemon Green Beans with Almonds

Preparation Time: 15 minutes | **Cooking Time:** 15 minutes | **Servings:** 4

Ingredients:

1/2 cup chopped almonds	1 pound green beans, trimmed and cut into 2 inch pieces
2 1/2 tablespoons olive oil	1 lemon, juiced and zest
Salt and pepper to taste	

Directions:
Preheat the oven to 375 degrees F. Arrange nuts in a single layer on a baking sheet. Toast in the preheated oven until lightly browned, approximately 5 to 10 minutes.
Place green beans in a steamer over 1 inch of boiling water, and cover. Steam for 8 to 10 minutes, or until tender, but still bright green.
Place cooked beans in a large bowl, and toss with olive oil, lemon juice, and lemon zest. Season with salt and pepper. Transfer beans to a serving dish, and sprinkle with toasted almonds. Serve immediately.

Nutrition:
Calories 211, Total Fat 18.2g, Saturated Fat 1.8g, Cholesterol 0mg, Sodium 7mg, Total Carbohydrate 11g, Dietary Fiber 5.3g, Total Sugars 2.1g, Protein 6g, Calcium 55mg, Iron 2mg, Potassium 339mg, Phosphorus 180 mg

149. Eggplant Casserole

Preparation Time: 15 minutes | **Cooking Time:** 20 minutes | **Servings:** 4

Ingredients:

3 cups eggplant	3 large eggs
1/8 teaspoon salt	½ teaspoon pepper
¼ teaspoon sage	½ cup white bread crumbs

1 tablespoon olive oil

Directions:
Preheat the oven to 350 degrees F.
Peel and cut up eggplant. Place eggplant pieces in a pan, cover with water, and boil until tender. Drain and mash.
Combine beaten eggs, salt, pepper, and sage with mashed eggplant. Place in a greased casserole dish.
Mix olive oil with white bread crumbs.
Top the casserole with breadcrumbs and bake for 20 minutes or until the top begins to brown.

Nutrition:
Calories 153, Total Fat 8.1g, Saturated Fat 1.8g, Cholesterol 140mg, Sodium 226mg, Total Carbohydrate 13.8g, Dietary Fiber 2.9g, Total Sugars 3g, Protein 7.2g, Calcium 52mg, Iron 2mg, Potassium 221mg, Phosphorus 115mg

150. Garlic Green Beans

Preparation Time: 10 minutes | **Cooking Time:** 15 minutes | **Servings:** 4

Ingredients:

1 tablespoon butter	3 tablespoons olive oil
1 medium head garlic - peeled and sliced	2 (14.5 ounces) cans green beans, drained
Salt and pepper to taste	¼ cup grated Parmesan cheese
1 teaspoon dried basil	

Directions:
In a large skillet over medium heat, melt butter with olive oil; add garlic, and cook until lightly browned, stirring frequently. Stir in green beans, and season with salt and pepper. Cook until beans are tender, about 10 minutes. Remove from heat, and sprinkle with Parmesan cheese and basil.

Nutrition:
Calories 96, Total Fat 9.2g, Saturated Fat 2.4g, Cholesterol 6mg, Sodium 27mg, Total Carbohydrate 3.6g, Dietary Fiber 1.3g, Total Sugars 0.5g, Protein 1.3g, Calcium 30mg, Iron 0mg, Potassium 89mg, Phosphorus 71mg

151. Ginger Veggie Stir-Fry

Preparation Time: 10 minutes | **Cooking Time:** 15 minutes | **Servings:** 4

Ingredients:

1 tablespoon corn-starch	1 1/2 cloves garlic, crushed
2 teaspoons chopped fresh ginger root, divided	1/4 cup olive oil, divided
1 small head broccoli, cut into florets	3/4 cup julienned carrots
1/2 cup halved green beans	½ tablespoon soy sauce
2 1/2 tablespoons water	1/4 cup chopped onion

Directions:

In a large bowl, blend corn-starch, garlic, 1 teaspoon ginger, and 2 tablespoons olive oil until corn-starch is dissolved. Mix in broccoli, carrots, and green beans, tossing to lightly coat. Heat the remaining 2 tablespoons oil in a large skillet or wok over medium heat. Cook vegetables in oil for 2 minutes, stirring constantly to prevent burning. Stir in soy sauce and water. Mix in onion and remaining 1 teaspoon ginger. Cook until vegetables are tender but still crisp.

Nutrition:

Calories 102, Total Fat 8.5g, Saturated Fat 1.2g, Cholesterol 0mg, Sodium 91mg, Total Carbohydrate 6.5g, Dietary Fiber 1.6g, Total Sugars 1.9g, Protein 1.4g, Calcium 25mg, Iron 1mg, Potassium 154mg, Phosphorus 101mg

152. Roasted Green Beans

Preparation Time: 10 minutes | **Cooking Time:** 25 minutes | **Servings:** 4

Ingredients:

2 pounds fresh green beans, trimmed	1 tablespoon olive oil, or as needed
Salt to taste	1/2 teaspoon freshly ground black pepper

Directions:

Preheat the oven to 400 degrees F.
Pat green beans dry with paper towels if necessary; spread onto a jelly roll pan. Drizzle with olive oil and sprinkle with salt and pepper. Use your fingers to coat beans evenly with olive oil and spread them out so they don't overlap. Roast in the preheated oven until beans are slightly shriveled and have brown spots, 20 to 25 minutes.

Nutrition:

Calories 48, Total Fat 3.6g, Saturated Fat 0.5g, Cholesterol 0mg, Sodium 585mg, Total Carbohydrate 4.1g, Dietary Fiber 1.9g, Total Sugars 0.8g, Protein 1g, Calcium 22mg, Iron 1mg, Potassium 118mg, Phosphorus 91mg

153. French Fries Made with Zucchini

Preparation Time: 10 minutes | **Cooking Time:** 25 minutes | **Servings:** 4

Ingredients:

2 medium zucchini	1 cup of soy milk
2 large eggs	3/4 cup corn-starch
3/4 cup dry unseasoned bread crumbs	3 teaspoons dried basil
½ cup olive oil	

Directions:

Peel and slice zucchini into 3/4-inch sticks, 4-inch long. Rinse zucchini and pat dry.
In a medium bowl, mix milk and eggs until well blended. In a wide, shallow bowl, combine corn-starch, bread crumbs, and basil.
Heat oil in a frying pan on high heat.
Dip zucchini sticks into the egg mixture and then roll each piece in bread crumb mixture.
Place in oil, flipping regularly, and fry for 3 minutes or until golden brown.
Drain on paper towels and serve immediately.

Nutrition:

Calories 129, Total Fat 11.7g, Saturated Fat 1.8g, Cholesterol 37mg, Sodium 44mg, Total Carbohydrate 4.6g, Dietary Fiber 0.5g, Total Sugars 1.6g, Protein 2.6g, Calcium 19mg, Iron 1mg, Potassium 109mg, Phosphorus 80mg

154. Garlicky Ginger Eggplant

Preparation Time: 10 minutes | **Cooking Time:** 00 minutes | **Servings:** 4

Ingredients:

2 cups eggplant	2 teaspoons minced ginger
2 garlic cloves	1/4 cup fresh Parsley
2 tablespoons olive oil	1/2 cup fresh mushroom pieces
1/4 teaspoon red chili pepper flakes	

Directions:

Slice eggplant into 1-1/2-inch long pieces. Mince garlic cloves. Chop parsley.

Heat olive oil in a large skillet. Add eggplant, ginger, garlic, and mushrooms. Stir-fry over medium-high heat until eggplant begins to soften, 4-6 minutes.

Add parsley, chili pepper flakes to eggplant. Continue cooking for 1-2 minutes. Remove from heat and serve.

Nutrition:

Calories 78, Total Fat 7.2g, Saturated Fat 1g, Cholesterol 0mg, Sodium 2mg, Total Carbohydrate 3.9g, Dietary Fiber 1.7g, Total Sugars 1.4g, Protein 0.9g, Calcium 10mg, Iron 1mg, Potassium 145mg, Phosphorus 48mg

155. Garlic Kale Buckwheat

Preparation Time: 10 minutes | **Cooking Time:** 25 minutes | **Servings:** 4

Ingredients:

2/3 cup water	1/3 cup buckwheat
1 tablespoon olive oil	1 cup chopped kale
1 clove garlic, minced	Salt and ground black pepper to taste

Directions:

Bring 2/3 cup water and buckwheat to a boil in a saucepan. Reduce heat to medium-low, cover, and simmer until buckwheat is tender and water has been absorbed, 15 to 20 minutes.

Heat olive oil in a skillet over medium heat; sauté kale and garlic in the hot oil until kale is wilted, about 5 minutes. Season with salt and pepper.

Stir buckwheat into kale mixture; cook until flavors blend, about 5 more minutes. Add 1 tablespoon of water to the mixture to keep it from sticking.

Nutrition:

Calories 88, Total Fat 4g, Saturated Fat 0.6g, Cholesterol 0mg, Sodium 9mg, Total Carbohydrate 12.1g, Dietary Fiber 1.7g, Total Sugars 0g, Protein 2.4g, Calcium 28mg, Iron 1mg, Potassium 151mg, Phosphorus 104mg

156. Glazed Zucchini

Preparation Time: 05 minutes | **Cooking Time:** 10 minutes | **Servings:** 4

Ingredients:

2 cups Zucchini	1 tablespoon honey
1 teaspoon corn-starch	1/8 teaspoon salt
1/4 teaspoon ground ginger	1/4 cup apple juice
2 tablespoons unsalted butter	

Directions:

Slice zucchini into -inch thick slices. Place zucchinis and 1/4 cup water in a pot. Cover and cook until slightly tender.

Mix honey, corn-starch, salt, ginger, apple juice, and melted butter. Pour mixture over zucchini and water.

Cook, stirring occasionally, for 10 minutes or until mixture thickens.

Nutrition:

Calories 86, Total Fat 5.9g, Saturated Fat 3.7g, Cholesterol 15mg, Sodium 121mg, Total Carbohydrate 8.8g, Dietary Fiber 0.7g, Total Sugars 6.8g, Protein 0.8g, Calcium 12mg, Iron 0mg, Potassium 170mg, Phosphorus 56 Mg

157. Grilled Summer Squash

Preparation Time: 05 minutes | **Cooking Time:** 10 minutes | **Servings:** 4

Ingredients:

2 medium summer squash	Non-stick cooking spray
1/4 teaspoon garlic powder	1/4 teaspoon black pepper

Directions:

Wash summer squash with mild soap and water; rinse well.

Cut each squash into four pieces; cut both vertically and horizontally.

Place on a cookie sheet or large platter and spray with non-stick cooking spray.

Sprinkle with garlic powder and black pepper, to taste (both optional).

Cook on either a gas grill. Cook for approximately three to five minutes, flipping once. The squash should be tender but not mushy. If cooking on a gas grill, place the flat surface down on a sheet of aluminum foil sprayed with non-stick cooking spray.

Cook approximately 5 to 7 minutes over a medium flame, watching carefully. Flip and cook for approximately 2 more minutes on the "round" side.

Nutrition:

Calories 17, Total Fat 0.2g, Saturated Fat 0.1g, Cholesterol 0mg, Sodium 2mg, Total Carbohydrate 3.4g, Dietary Fiber 0.9g, Total Sugars 3g, Protein 0.9g, Calcium 18mg, Iron 0mg, Potassium 190mg, Phosphorus100mg

158. Pineapple and Pepper Curry

Preparation Time: 05 minutes | **Cooking Time:** 15 minutes | **Servings:** 4

Ingredients:

2 cups green bell pepper	1/2 cup red onion
1 tablespoon cilantro	1 tablespoon ginger root
2 tablespoons olive oil	1/2 cup pineapple juice
1 teaspoon curry powder	1/2 tablespoon lemon juice

Directions:

Chop bell pepper, onion, and cilantro. Shred ginger root.

Heat oil and when hot add ginger and red onion. Cook until the onion is transparent.

Microwave peppers on high for 6 minutes. Add the peppers to the onion mixture. Close the lid of the pan and cook on low for 10 minutes, stirring to avoid burning peppers.

Add pineapple juice and simmer for 2 minutes. Add curry powder and cilantro. Turn the vegetables once and let simmer on low for 2 minutes.

Garnish lemon juice before serving.

Nutrition:

Calories 107, Total Fat 6g, Saturated Fat 0.8g, Cholesterol 0mg, Sodium 4mg, Total Carbohydrate 12.5g, Dietary Fiber 2.6g, Total Sugars 7.1g, Protein 2.3g, Calcium 20mg, Iron 1mg, Potassium 222mg, Phosphorus150mg

159. Stuffed Mushrooms

Preparation Time: 25 minutes | **Cooking Time:** 20 minutes | **Servings:** 4

Ingredients:

8 whole fresh mushrooms	½ tablespoon olive oil
½ tablespoon minced garlic	1 (8 ounces) package cream cheese, softened
1/8 cup grated Parmesan cheese	1/8 teaspoon ground black pepper
1/8 teaspoon onion powder	1/8 teaspoon ground cayenne pepper

Directions:

Preheat the oven to 350 degrees F. Spray a baking sheet with cooking spray. Clean mushrooms with a damp paper towel. Carefully break off stems. Chop stems extremely fine, discarding the tough end of stems.

Heat oil in a large skillet over medium heat. Add garlic and chopped mushroom stems to the skillet. Fry until any moisture has disappeared, taking care not to burn the garlic. Set aside to cool.

When garlic and mushroom mixture is no longer hot, stir in cream cheese, Parmesan cheese, black pepper, onion powder, and cayenne pepper. The mixture should be very thick. Using a little spoon, fill each mushroom cap with a generous amount of stuffing. Arrange the mushroom caps on the prepared cookie sheet.

Bake for 20 minutes in the preheated oven, or until the mushrooms are piping hot and liquid starts to form under caps.

Nutrition:
Calories 150, Total Fat 14.5g, Saturated Fat 8.6g, Cholesterol 42mg, Sodium 171mg, Total Carbohydrate 2g, Dietary Fiber 0.4g, Total Sugars 0.3g, Protein 3.6g, Calcium 37mg, Iron 1mg, Potassium 50mg, Phosphorus10mg

160. Sautéed Mushrooms

Preparation Time: 10 minutes | **Cooking Time:** 15 minutes | **Servings:** 4

Ingredients:

3 tablespoons olive oil	3 tablespoons unsalted butter
1 pound button mushrooms, sliced	1 clove garlic, thinly sliced
1/8 teaspoon salt, or to taste	Freshly ground black pepper to taste

Directions:
Heat olive oil and unsalted butter in a large saucepan over medium heat. Cook and stir mushrooms, garlic, salt, and black pepper in the hot oil and butter until mushrooms are lightly browned, about 5 minutes. Reduce heat to low and simmer until mushrooms are tender, 5 to 8 more minutes.

Nutrition:
Calories 171, Total Fat 19.2g, Saturated Fat 7g, Cholesterol 23mg, Sodium 62mg, Total Carbohydrate 0.9g, Dietary Fiber 0.2g, Total Sugars 0.3g, Protein 0.7g, Calcium 4mg, Iron 1mg, Potassium 62mg, Phosphorus 50mg

161. Mushroom Rice

Preparation Time: 05 minutes | **Cooking Time:** 25 minutes | **Servings:** 4

Ingredients:

2 teaspoons olive oil	6 mushrooms, coarsely chopped
1 clove garlic, minced	1 green onion, finely chopped
1 cup uncooked white rice	1/2 teaspoon chopped fresh parsley
Salt and pepper to taste	1-1/2 cups water

Directions:
Heat olive oil in a saucepan over medium heat. Cook mushrooms, garlic, and green onion until mushrooms are cooked and liquid has evaporated. Stir in water and rice. Season with parsley, salt, and pepper. Reduce heat, cover, and simmer for 20 minutes.

Nutrition:
Calories 197, Total Fat 2.7g, Saturated Fat 0.4g, Cholesterol 0mg, Sodium 5mg, Total Carbohydrate 38.4g, Dietary Fiber 1g, Total Sugars 0.6g, Protein 4.3g, Calcium 17mg, Iron 3mg, Potassium 154mg, Phosphorus 110mg

162. Roasted Asparagus and Mushrooms

Preparation Time: 10 minutes | **Cooking Time:** 15 minutes | **Servings:** 4

Ingredients:

1 bunch fresh asparagus, trimmed	1/2 pound fresh mushrooms, quartered
2 sprigs fresh rosemary, minced	2 teaspoons olive oil
Freshly ground black pepper to taste	

Directions:
Preheat the oven to 450 degrees F. Lightly spray a cookie sheet with vegetable cooking spray. Place the asparagus and mushrooms in a bowl. Drizzle with the olive oil, then season with rosemary and pepper; toss well. Lay the asparagus and mushrooms out on the prepared pan in an even layer. Roast in the preheated oven until the asparagus is tender, about 15 minutes.

Nutrition:
Calories 31, Total Fat 2.5g, Saturated Fat 0.4g, Cholesterol 0mg, Sodium 1mg, Total Carbohydrate 2g, Dietary Fiber 1.1g, Total Sugars 0.8g, Protein 1g, Calcium 16mg, Iron 1mg, Potassium 102mg, Phosphorus 70mg

163. Buckwheat Bake

Preparation Time: 10 minutes | **Cooking Time:** 1hr.15 minutes | **Servings:** 4

Ingredients:

1/4 cup olive oil	1 medium onion, diced
1 cup uncooked buckwheat	2 green onions, thinly sliced
1/2 cup sliced fresh mushrooms	1/2 cup chopped fresh parsley
1/8 teaspoon salt	1/8 teaspoon pepper
2 water	

Directions:
Preheat the oven to 350 degrees F.
Melt olive oil in a skillet over medium-high heat. Stir in onion, buckwheat. Cook and stir until buckwheat is lightly browned. Mix in green onions, mushrooms, and parsley. Season with salt and pepper. Transfer the mixture to a 2-quart casserole dish, and stir in the water.
Bake 1 hour and 15 minutes in the preheated oven, or until liquid has been absorbed and buckwheat is tender.

Nutrition:
Calories 181, Total Fat 9.5g, Saturated Fat 1.4g, Cholesterol 0mg, Sodium 102mg, Total Carbohydrate 22.9g, Dietary Fiber 3.6g, Total Sugars 1g, Protein 4.4g, Calcium 20mg, Iron 1mg, Potassium 218mg, Phosphorus 170mg

164. Stir-Fry Vegetables

Preparation Time: 10 minutes | **Cooking Time:** 20 minutes | **Servings:** 4

Ingredients:

2 cups green pepper	2 cups red pepper
1 cup fresh sliced mushrooms	1 cup celery
¼ cup onion	1 garlic clove
½ teaspoon honey	½ teaspoon dried oregano
1/8 teaspoon salt	1/8 teaspoon pepper
1 tablespoon olive oil	

Directions:
Cut green and red peppers. Slice celery and chop onion. Crush garlic.

In a large skillet, heat oil. Add green pepper, red pepper, mushrooms, celery, onion, garlic, honey, oregano, salt, and pepper.
Stir-fry over medium-high heat until peppers are crisp-tender.
Serve hot.

Nutrition:
Calories 36, Total Fat 1.6g, Saturated Fat 0.2g, Cholesterol 0mg, Sodium 69mg, Total Carbohydrate 5.4g, Dietary Fiber 1.2g, Total Sugars 2.6g, Protein 0.9g, Calcium 13mg, Iron 1mg, Potassium 162mg, Phosphorus 120mg

165. Roasted Apples and Cabbage

Preparation Time: 15 minutes | **Cooking Time:** 20 minutes | **Servings:** 4

Ingredients:

1 cup chopped cabbage	2 apples - peeled, cored, and cut into 3/4-inch chunks
2 tablespoons olive oil, or as needed	Salt and ground black pepper to taste
1 pinch garlic powder to taste	Zest from 1 lemon
Juice from 1 lemon	

Directions:
Preheat the oven to 425 degrees F.
Arrange cabbage in a single layer on a rimmed baking sheet; sprinkle apple pieces evenly around the baking sheet. Drizzle the cabbage, apples with olive oil; sprinkle with salt, black pepper, and garlic powder. Toss the mixture gently to coat.
Roast in the preheated oven until the cabbage is hot and fragrant, about 20 minutes. Sprinkle with lemon zest, and squeeze juice from zested lemon over the cabbage to serve.

Nutrition:
Calories 127, Total Fat 7.3g, Saturated Fat 1g, Cholesterol 0mg, Sodium 4mg, Total Carbohydrate 17.8g, Dietary Fiber 3.6g, Total Sugars 12.5g, Protein 0.7g, Calcium 11mg, Iron 1mg, Potassium 170mg, Phosphorus 80mg

166. Cabbage Bake

Preparation Time: 15 minutes | **Cooking Time:** 30 minutes | **Servings:** 4

Ingredients:

1 cup of water	1 cup cabbage
½ tablespoon olive oil	1 egg, beaten
½ cup shredded Cheddar cheese	½ cup graham crackers

Directions:

Preheat the oven to 350 degrees F.

Bring water to boil in a medium saucepan. Place chopped cabbage in the water, and return to boil. Reduce heat, and simmer 2 minutes, until tender; drain.

In a medium bowl, mix cabbage with oil, egg, Cheddar cheese, and 1/3 cup graham crackers. Transfer to a medium baking dish and top with remaining graham crackers.

Cover, and bake for 25 minutes in the preheated oven, until bubbly. Uncover, and continue baking 5 minutes, until lightly browned.

Nutrition:

Calories 91, Total Fat 5.7g, Saturated Fat 2.5g, Cholesterol 37mg, Sodium 114mg, Total Carbohydrate 6.2g, Dietary Fiber 0.5g, Total Sugars 2.7g, Protein 3.9g, Calcium 79mg, Iron 1mg, Potassium 49mg, Phosphorus 20mg

167. Zippy Zucchini

Preparation Time: 10 minutes | | **Cooking Time:** 15 minutes | **Servings:** 4

Ingredients:

2 cups zucchini	½ medium onion
2 large eggs	¼ cup shredded cheddar cheese
1/8 teaspoon salt	1/8 teaspoon black pepper

Directions:

Cut zucchini into chunks. Thinly slice the onion. Place zucchini and onion in a 10" x 6" x 2" dish. Cover with plastic wrap, turning one edge back slightly to vent. Microwave on high for 7 minutes. Drain liquid.

In a large bowl, mix beaten eggs, cheese, salt, and pepper. Add zucchini and onions, stirring well.

Grease dish in which vegetables were microwaved.

Pour mixture into a dish and cover with a paper towel. Microwave on medium-high for 4 minutes. Remove the paper towel and stir.

Continue to microwave uncovered for 4 to 6 minutes until the center is set.

Nutrition:

Calories 80, Total Fat 5g, Saturated Fat 2.3g, Cholesterol 100mg, Sodium 159mg, Total Carbohydrate 3.7g, Dietary Fiber 1g, Total Sugars 1.9g, Protein 5.8g, Calcium 77mg, Iron 1mg, Potassium 224mg, Phosphorus 124mg

168. Barley with Beans

Preparation Time: 10 minutes | | **Cooking Time:** 20 minutes | **Servings:** 4

Ingredients:

1 tablespoon olive oil	1 cup uncooked barley
2 cups of water	1/4 cup chopped onion
1 clove garlic, minced	1 teaspoon chopped fresh basil
1/2 teaspoon black pepper	3/4 cup green beans
1/2 cup grated parmesan cheese, divided	2 tablespoons chopped fresh parsley

Directions:

Heat the oil in a saucepan over medium heat. Stir in the barley, and cook for 2 minutes until toasted. Pour in the water, onion, garlic, basil, and black pepper. Cover, and let come to a boil. Once boiling, stir in the green beans. Recover, reduce heat to medium-low, and continue simmering until the barley is tender and has absorbed the water, 15 to 20 minutes.

Stir in half of the parmesan cheese and the parsley until evenly mixed. Scoop the barley into a serving dish, and sprinkle with the remaining parmesan cheese to serve.

Nutrition:

Calories 155, Total Fat 3.6g, Saturated Fat 0.8g, Cholesterol 2mg, Sodium 43mg, Total Carbohydrate 26.3g, Dietary Fiber 6.6g, Total Sugars 1.4g, Protein 5.8g, Calcium 43mg, Iron 2mg, Potassium 180mg, Phosphorus 120mg

169. Zucchini Stir-Fry

Preparation Time: 10 minutes | **Cooking Time:** 05 minutes | **Servings:** 4

Ingredients:

1 tablespoon olive oil	1 teaspoon cumin
2 cups zucchini	1/2 cup red onion
1 teaspoon black pepper	1 tablespoon lemon juice
1/4 cup fresh parsley	

Directions:

Peel and slice zucchini and onion. Chop parsley. Heat olive oil in a non-stick skillet over medium heat.

Sauté cumin to brown.

Add zucchini and onion and sprinkle with black pepper. Stir a few times to mix.

Cover and cook for approximately 5 minutes to medium tenderness, stirring a few times.

Add lemon juice and chopped parsley. Mix, cook another minute, and serve.

Nutrition:

Calories 51, Total Fat 3.8g, Saturated Fat 0.6g, Cholesterol 0mg, Sodium 11mg, Total Carbohydrate 4.3g, Dietary Fiber 1.3g, Total Sugars 1.8g, Protein 1.2g, Calcium 25mg, Iron 1mg, Potassium 225mg, Phosphorus 108mg

170. Couscous Primavera

Preparation Time: 15 minutes | **Cooking Time:** 20 minutes | **Servings:** 4

Ingredients:

1 cup dry couscous	½ cup broccoli
1/2 cup chopped green onions	2 tablespoons olive oil
1/2 teaspoon ground cumin	1 pinch ground black pepper
2 cups of water	1 bunch asparagus, trimmed and cut into 1/4-inch pieces
1 cup shelled fresh or thawed frozen beans Salt and freshly ground black pepper to taste	2 tablespoons chopped fresh basil

Directions:

Combine couscous, green onion, broccoli, olive oil, cumin, and black pepper in a large bowl; stir until the olive oil is completely incorporated.

Bring water, asparagus, and beans to a boil in a saucepan over high heat.

Pour water, asparagus, and peas over couscous mixture; shake the bowl to settle couscous into liquid. Cover and let stand for 10 minutes. Fluff with a fork, then stir in basil and season with salt and pepper to taste.

Nutrition:

Calories 174, Total Fat 5g, Saturated Fat 0.7g, Cholesterol 0mg, Sodium 57mg, Total Carbohydrate 26.9g, Dietary Fiber 3.2g, Total Sugars 1.6g, Protein 5.6g, Calcium 24mg, Iron 1mg, Potassium 124mg, Phosphorus 108mg

171. Lemon Pepper Beans

Preparation Time: 01 minutes | **Cooking Time:** 05 minutes | **Servings:** 4

Ingredients:

1 cup frozen green beans, thawed	1 tablespoon water
2 tablespoons olive oil	1 pinch lemon pepper
1 pinch dried rosemary	

Directions:

Place the beans and water into a microwave-safe bowl. Cover loosely, and microwave for 3 to 4 minutes, or until beans are tender. Stir in oil, and sprinkle with lemon pepper and rosemary. Serve warm.

Nutrition:

Calories 90, Total Fat 7.2g, Saturated Fat 1g, Cholesterol 0mg, Sodium 2mg, Total Carbohydrate 5.3g, Dietary Fiber 1.9g, Total Sugars 2.1g, Protein 2g, Calcium 10mg, Iron 1mg, Potassium 89mg, Phosphorus 45 mg

172. Sweet Bean and Noodles

Preparation Time: 15 minutes | **Cooking Time:** 15 minutes | **Servings:** 4

Ingredients:

12 ounces egg noodle	1 cup green beans
1 onion, chopped	1/2 cup mayonnaise

1 dash black pepper

Directions:
In a large pot of boiling water, cook noodles until al dente, rinse under cold water and drain.
In a mixing bowl, combine the noodle, green beans, onions, mayonnaise, and a dash of black pepper. Mix well and chill before serving.

Nutrition:
Calories 265, Total Fat 11.7g, Saturated Fat 1.8g, Cholesterol 31mg, Sodium 106mg, Total Carbohydrate 35g, Dietary Fiber 3.4g, Total Sugars 5.4g, Protein 6.2g, Calcium 29mg, Iron 1mg, Potassium 81mg, Phosphorus 25 mg

173. Bean Rice

Preparation Time: 15 minutes | **Cooking Time:** 20 minutes | **Servings:** 4

Ingredients:

1 cup white rice	1 tablespoon olive oil
2 whole cloves	1 (2-inch) piece of cinnamon stick
1 bell pepper, chopped	1 teaspoon minced fresh ginger root
¼ cup green beans	¼ teaspoon honey
2 cups of water	

Directions:
Wash and drain the rice.
Heat a saucepan over medium heat. Add olive oil and let heat it. Stir in cloves, cinnamon, bell pepper, and ginger. Sauté briefly. Mix in rice and stir to coat it evenly. Stir in beans, honey. Pour in water and bring the water to a boil.
Reduce heat to simmer and let rice cook covered for 15 to 20 minutes; or until rice is tender.

Nutrition:
Calories 224, Total Fat 4.2g, Saturated Fat 0.7g, Cholesterol 0mg, Sodium 10mg, Total Carbohydrate 42.5g, Dietary Fiber 2.4g, Total Sugars 2.5g, Protein 4.2g, Calcium 40mg, Iron 2mg, Potassium 151mg, Phosphorus 125 mg

174. Fried Cabbage

Preparation Time: 05 minutes | **Cooking Time:** 45 minutes | **Servings:** 4

Ingredients:

2 teaspoons olive oil	1 cup of water
1 head cabbage, cored and coarsely chopped	1 pinch salt and pepper to taste

Directions:
Bring the oil and water to a boil in a large skillet. Reduce heat to low and add the cabbage. Cover and cook over low heat to steam the cabbage for about 45 minutes, stirring frequently, or until the cabbage is tender and sweet. Season with salt and pepper and serve.

Nutrition:
Calories 43, Total Fat 1.7g, Saturated Fat 0.3g, Cholesterol 0mg, Sodium 21mg, Total Carbohydrate 6.9g, Dietary Fiber 3g, Total Sugars 3.8g, Protein 1.5g, Calcium 48mg, Iron 1mg, Potassium 202mg, Phosphorus 100 mg

175. Roasted Cabbage

Preparation Time: 10 minutes | **Cooking Time:** 30 minutes | **Servings:** 4

Ingredients:

2 tablespoons butter	1/2 head green cabbage, cut into 4 wedges
1 pinch garlic powder, or to taste	1 pinch red pepper flakes, or to taste
Salt and ground black pepper to taste	2 lemons, halved

Directions:
Preheat the oven to 450 degrees F.
Brush both sides of each cabbage wedge with melted butter. Sprinkle garlic powder, red pepper flakes, salt, and pepper over each wedge. Arrange wedges on a baking sheet.
Roast in the preheated oven for 15 minutes; flip cabbage and continue roasting until browned and charred in some areas, about 15 minutes more. Squeeze lemon over each wedge.

Nutrition:
Calories 89, Total Fat 6g, Saturated Fat 3.7g, Cholesterol 15mg, Sodium 58mg, Total Carbohydrate 9.4g, Dietary Fiber 3.3g, Total Sugars 3.6g, Protein 1.8g, Calcium 48mg, Iron 1mg, Potassium 195mg, Phosphorus 90 mg

176. Okra Buckwheat

Preparation Time: 10 minutes | **Cooking Time:** 30 minutes | **Servings:** 4

Ingredients:

1 large onion, chopped	3 cups sliced fresh okra
1 cup of water	½ teaspoon olive oil
1 cup uncooked buckwheat	

Directions:

In the skillet, heat olive oil and sauté onion over medium-high heat until tender, about 3 minutes. Sliced okra, and water. Reduce heat and simmer until okra is tender and falling apart, about 15 minutes. Stir in buckwheat and water. Cover, and simmer for 20 minutes, or until fluffy.

Nutrition:

Calories 127, Total Fat 1.1g, Saturated Fat 0.2g, Cholesterol 0mg, Sodium 6mg, Total Carbohydrate 26.3g, Dietary Fiber 5g, Total Sugars 1.8g, Protein 5g, Calcium 53mg, Iron 1mg, Potassium 317mg, Phosphorus 190 mg

177. Black Beans, Corn, and Yellow Rice

Preparation Time: 10 minutes | **Cooking Time:** 25 minutes | **Servings:** 8

Ingredients:

8 ounces yellow rice mix	15.25 ounces cooked kernel corn
1 1/4 cups water	15 ounces cooked black beans
1 teaspoon ground cumin	2 teaspoons lime juice
2 tablespoons olive oil	

Directions:

Place a saucepan over high heat, add oil, water, and rice, bring the mixture to a bowl, and then switch heat to medium-low level.

Simmer for 25 minutes until rice is tender and all the liquid has been absorbed and then transfer the rice to a large bowl.

Add remaining ingredients into the rice, stir until mixed and serve straight away.

Nutrition:

Calories: 100 Cal Fat: 4.4 g Carbs: 15.1 g Protein: 2 g Fiber: 1.4 g

178. Okra Curry

Preparation Time: 05 minutes | **Cooking Time:** 10 minutes | **Servings:** 4

Ingredients:

1 pound okra, ends trimmed, cut into 1/4-inch rounds	1 tablespoon olive oil
1/2 teaspoon curry powder	1/2 teaspoon all-purpose flour
1/2 teaspoon black pepper	

Directions:

Microwave the okra on High for 3 minutes. Heat olive oil in a large skillet over medium heat. Gently mix in the curry powder, all-purpose flour, and black pepper; cook 2 minutes more. Serve immediately.

Nutrition:

Calories 45, Total Fat 3.7g, Saturated Fat 0.5g, Cholesterol 0mg, Sodium 3mg, Total Carbohydrate 2.7g, Dietary Fiber 1g, Total Sugars 0.4g, Protein 0.7g, Calcium 28mg, Iron 1mg, Potassium 92mg, Phosphorus 60 mg

179. Frying Pan Okra

Preparation Time: 05 minutes | **Cooking Time:** 10 minutes | **Servings:** 4

Ingredients:

1 tablespoon olive oil	2 onions, sliced
½ pound fresh okra, sliced into 1/8 inch pieces	½ teaspoon ground turmeric

Directions:

Heat olive oil in a medium saucepan over medium heat and sauté onion until translucent. Stir in okra and turmeric. Reduce heat to low and cook for 15 minutes, or until tender.

Nutrition:

Calories 32, Total Fat 1.8g, Saturated Fat 0.3g, Cholesterol 0mg, Sodium 2mg, Total Carbohydrate 3.6g, Dietary Fiber 1g, Total

Sugars 1.4g, Protein 0.6g, Calcium 17mg, Iron 0mg, Potassium 81mg, Phosphorus 50 mg

180. Lemony Grilled Okra

Preparation Time: 10min | **Cooking Time:** 10 minutes | **Servings:** 4

Ingredients:

1 pound okra, stems trimmed	1 tablespoon olive oil, or more as needed
1 pinch paprika, or to taste	1 pinch garlic powder, or to taste
Salt and freshly ground black pepper to taste	1 pinch cayenne pepper
1 lemon, juiced	1/4 teaspoon chopped fresh dill, or to taste
1/4 teaspoon chopped fresh basil, or to taste	

Directions:
Preheat an outdoor grill for high heat and lightly oil the grate.
Toss okra with olive oil, paprika, garlic powder, salt, pepper, and cayenne pepper in a bowl.
Grill okra on the preheated grill until 1 side is bright green with visible grill marks, about 5 minutes. Turn okra, cover grill, and cook until tender, about 5 minutes.
Transfer okra to a serving bowl; sprinkle with lemon juice, dill weed, and basil.

Nutrition:
Calories 45, Total Fat 3.6g, Saturated Fat 0.5g, Cholesterol 0mg, Sodium 2mg, Total Carbohydrate 3.4g, Dietary Fiber 1.3g, Total Sugars 0.8g, Protein 0.7g, Calcium 26mg, Iron 0mg, Potassium 101mg, Phosphorus 90 mg

181. Stuffed Okra

Preparation Time: 15min | **Cooking Time:** 05 minutes | **Servings:** 4

Ingredients:

1 teaspoon ground ginger	1 teaspoon ground cumin
1 teaspoon ground turmeric	1/2 teaspoon chili powder (optional)
1/8 teaspoon salt	1/2 teaspoon butter
1 pound large okra	1/4 cup all-purpose flour

Olive oil for frying

Directions:
Combine ginger, cumin, turmeric, chili powder, salt, and 1/2 teaspoon butter in a bowl; set aside for flavors to blend for 2 hours.
Heat olive oil in a deep-fryer or large saucepan to 350 degrees F.
Trim okra and make a slit lengthwise down the side of each okra, creating a pocket. Fill each pocket with the spice mixture.
Place all-purpose flour in a resealable plastic bag; add filled okra and shake to coat.
Fry okra in the hot oil until golden brown, 5 to 8 minutes. Transfer fried okra using a slotted spoon to a paper towel-lined plate.

Nutrition:
Calories 43, Total Fat 0.5g, Saturated Fat 0.2g, Cholesterol 1mg, Sodium 43mg, Total Carbohydrate 8g, Dietary Fiber 2.1g, Total Sugars 1.1g, Protein 1.6g, Calcium 51mg, Iron 1mg, Potassium 194mg, Phosphorus 80 mg

182. Mashed Turnip

Preparation Time: 10 minutes | **Cooking Time:** 50 minutes | **Servings:** 4

Ingredients:

1 large turnip, peeled and cubed	1 cup cauliflower
1/4 cup soy milk	1 tablespoon olive oil
1 teaspoon honey	1/8 teaspoon salt
1/4 teaspoon pepper	

Directions:
Preheat the oven to 375 degrees F.
Place turnip and cauliflower in a large pot with enough water to cover, and bring to a boil. Cook for 25 to 30 minutes, until tender. Remove from heat, and drain.
Mix soy milk, ¼ tablespoon olive oil, and honey with the turnip and cauliflower. Season with salt and pepper. Mash until slightly lumpy.
Transfer turnip mixture to a small baking dish. Dot with remaining olive oil. Cover loosely, and bake 15 minutes in the preheated oven. Remove cover, and continue baking for about 8 minutes, until lightly browned.

Nutrition:
Calories 42, Total Fat 2.6g, Saturated Fat 0.4g, Cholesterol 0mg, Sodium 321mg, Total Carbohydrate 4.5g, Dietary Fiber 1.1g, Total Sugars 2.9g, Protein 0.9g, Calcium 16mg, Iron 0mg, Potassium 123mg, Phosphorus 70 mg

183. Sautéed Zucchini and Leeks

Preparation Time: 15 minutes | **Cooking Time:** 20 minutes | **Servings:** 4

Ingredients:

2 leeks, finely chopped	2 zucchini, finely chopped
1/3 cup water	2 tablespoons olive oil
1 tablespoon honey	1/2 teaspoon dried basil
Pinch of salt	1/8 teaspoon ground black pepper

Directions:
Combine leeks, zucchinis, water, olive oil, honey, basil, salt, and pepper in a skillet; bring to a boil. Reduce heat and simmer until liquid evaporates for about 15 minutes. Cook and stir mixture until leeks and carrots are lightly browned, 2 to 3 minutes.

Nutrition:
Calories 79, Total Fat 4.9g, Saturated Fat 0.7g, Cholesterol 0mg, Sodium 40mg, Total Carbohydrate 9.3g, Dietary Fiber 1.3g, Total Sugars 5.2g, Protein 1.3g, Calcium 28mg, Iron 1mg, Potassium 227mg, Phosphorus 180 mg

184. Black Beans and Rice

Preparation Time: 10 minutes | **Cooking Time:** 30 minutes | **Servings:** 4

Ingredients:

3/4 cup white rice	1 medium white onion, peeled, chopped
3 1/2 cups cooked black beans	1 teaspoon minced garlic
1/4 teaspoon cayenne pepper	1 teaspoon ground cumin
1 teaspoon olive oil	1 1/2 cups vegetable broth

Directions:
Take a large pot over medium-high heat, add oil and when hot, add onion and garlic and cook for 4 minutes until saute.
Then stir in rice, cook for 2 minutes, pour in the broth, bring it to a boil, switch heat to the low level and cook for 20 minutes until tender.
Stir in remaining ingredients, cook for 2 minutes, and then serve straight away.

Nutrition:
Calories: 140 Cal Fat: 0.9 g Carbs: 27.1 g Protein: 6.3 g Fiber: 6.2 g

185. Brown Rice Pilaf

Preparation Time: 5 minutes | **Cooking Time:** 25 minutes | **Servings:** 4

Ingredients:

1 cup cooked chickpeas	3/4 cup brown rice, cooked
1/4 cup chopped cashews	2 cups sliced mushrooms
2 carrots, sliced	½ teaspoon minced garlic
1 1/2 cups chopped white onion	3 tablespoons vegan butter
½ teaspoon salt	¼ teaspoon ground black pepper
1/4 cup chopped parsley	

Directions:
Take a large skillet pan, place it over medium heat, add butter and when it melts, add onions and cook them for 5 minutes until softened.
Then add carrots and garlic, cook for 5 minutes, add mushrooms, cook for 10 minutes until browned, add chickpeas and cook for another minute.
When done, remove the pan from heat, add nuts, parsley, salt, and black pepper, toss until mixed, and garnish with parsley.
Serve straight away.

Nutrition:
Calories: 409 Cal Fat: 17.1 g Carbs: 54 g Protein: 12.5 g Fiber: 6.7 g

186. Barley and Mushrooms with Beans

Preparation Time: 5 minutes | **Cooking Time:** 15 minutes | **Servings:** 6

Ingredients:

1/2 cup uncooked barley	15.5 ounces white beans
1/2 cup chopped celery	3 cups sliced mushrooms
1 cup chopped white onion	1 teaspoon minced garlic
1 teaspoon olive oil	3 cups vegetable broth

Directions:

Take a saucepan, place it over medium heat, add oil and when hot, add vegetables and cook for 5 minutes until tender.

Pour in broth, stir in barley, bring the mixture to boil, and then simmer for 50 minutes until tender.

When done, add beans into the barley mixture, stir until mixed and continue cooking for 5 minutes until hot.

Serve straight away.

Nutrition:

Calories: 202 Cal Fat: 2.1 g Carbs: 39 g Protein: 9.1 g Fiber: 8.8 g

187. Vegan Curried Rice

Preparation Time: 5 minutes | **Cooking Time:** 25 minutes | **Servings:** 4

Ingredients:

1 cup white rice	1 tablespoon minced garlic
1 tablespoon ground curry powder	1/3 teaspoon ground black pepper
1 tablespoon red chili powder	1 tablespoon ground cumin
2 tablespoons olive oil	1 tablespoon soy sauce
1 cup vegetable broth	

Directions:

Take a saucepan, place it over low heat, add oil and when hot, add garlic and cook for 3 minutes. Then stir in all spices, cook for 1 minute until fragrant, pour in the broth, and switch heat to a high level.

Stir in soy sauce, bring the mixture to boil, add rice, stir until mixed, then switch heat to the low level and simmer for 20 minutes until rice is tender and all the liquid has absorbed.
Serve straight away.

Nutrition:

Calories: 262 Cal Fat: 8 g Carbs: 43 g Protein: 5 g Fiber: 2 g

188. Lentils and Rice with Fried Onions

Preparation Time: 5 minutes | **Cooking Time:** 7 minutes | **Servings:** 4

Ingredients:

3/4 cup long-grain white rice, cooked	1 large white onion, peeled, sliced
1 1/3 cups green lentils, cooked	½ teaspoon salt
1/4 cup vegan sour cream	¼ teaspoon ground black pepper
6 tablespoons olive oil	

Directions:

Take a large skillet pan, place it over medium heat, add oil, and when hot, add onions, and cook for 10 minutes until browned, set aside until required.

Take a saucepan, place it over medium heat, grease it with oil, add lentils and beans and cook for 3 minutes until warmed.

Season with salt and black pepper, cook for 2 minutes, then stir in half of the browned onions, and top with cream and remaining onions.
Serve straight away.

Nutrition:

Calories: 535 Cal Fat: 22.1 g Carbs: 69 g Protein: 17.3 g Fiber: 10.6 g

189. Asparagus Rice Pilaf

Preparation Time: 10 minutes | **Cooking Time:** 35 minutes | **Servings:** 4

Ingredients:

1 1/4 cups rice	1/2 pound asparagus, diced, boiled
2 ounces spaghetti, whole-grain, broken	1/4 cup minced white onion

1/2 teaspoon minced garlic

1/4 teaspoon ground black pepper

1/4 cup vegan butter

1/2 cup cashew halves

½ teaspoon salt

2 1/4 cups vegetable broth

Directions:

Take a saucepan, place it over medium-low heat, add butter and when it melts, stir in spaghetti and cook for 3 minutes until golden brown.

Add onion and garlic, cook for 2 minutes until tender, then stir in rice, cook for 5 minutes, pour in the broth, season with salt and black pepper, and bring it to a boil.

Switch heat to medium level, cook for 20 minutes, then add cashews and asparagus, and stir until combined.

Serve straight away.

Nutrition:

Calories: 249 Cal Fat: 10 g Carbs: 35.1 g Protein: 5.3 g Fiber: 1.8 g

190. Mexican Stuffed Peppers

Preparation Time: 10 minutes | **Cooking Time:** 40 minutes | **Servings:** 4

Ingredients:

2 cups cooked rice

15 ounces cooked black beans

1 tablespoon olive oil

14.5 ounce diced tomatoes

1 teaspoon garlic salt

1/2 teaspoon salt

1/2 cup chopped onion

4 large green bell peppers, destemmed, cored

1 tablespoon salt

1/2 teaspoon ground cumin

1 teaspoon red chili powder

2 cups shredded vegan Mexican cheese blend

Directions:

Boil the bell peppers in salty water for 5 minutes until softened and then set aside until required.

Heat oil over medium heat in a skillet pan, then add onion and cook for 10 minutes until softened.

Transfer the onion mixture in a bowl, add remaining ingredients, reserving ½ cup cheese blended, stir until mixed, and then fill this mixture into the boiled peppers.

Arrange the peppers in the square baking dish, sprinkle them with remaining cheese and bake for 30 minutes at 350 degrees F.

Serve straight away.

Nutrition:

Calories: 509 Cal Fat: 22.8 g Carbs: 55.5 g Protein: 24 g Fiber: 12 g

191. Quinoa and Black Bean Chili

Preparation Time: 10 minutes | **Cooking Time:** 32 minutes | **Servings:** 10

Ingredients:

1 cup quinoa, cooked

1 medium white onion, peeled, chopped

1 green bell pepper, deseeded, chopped

1 tablespoon minced chipotle peppers in adobo sauce

1 jalapeno pepper, deseeded, minced

2 teaspoons minced garlic

¾ teaspoon salt

1 tablespoon red chili powder

1 tablespoon olive oil

38 ounces cooked black beans

1 cup of frozen corn

1 zucchini, chopped

1 red bell pepper, deseeded, chopped

28 ounces crushed tomatoes

1/3 teaspoon ground black pepper

1 teaspoon dried oregano

1 tablespoon ground cumin

1/4 cup chopped cilantro

Directions:

Take a large pot, place it over medium heat, add oil, and when hot, add onion and cook for 5 minutes.

Then stir in garlic, cumin, and chili powder, cook for 1 minute, add remaining ingredients except for corn and quinoa, stir well and simmer for 20 minutes at medium-low heat until cooked.

Then stir in corn and quinoa, cook for 5 minutes until hot and then top with cilantro.

Serve straight away.

Nutrition:

Calories: 233 Cal Fat: 3.5 g Carbs: 42 g Protein: 11.5 g Fiber: 11.8 g

192. Mushroom Risotto

Preparation Time: 10 minutes | **Cooking Time:** 35 minutes | **Servings:** 4

Ingredients:

1 cup of rice	3 small white onions, peeled, chopped
1 teaspoon minced celery	1 ½ cups sliced mushrooms
½ teaspoon minced garlic	1 teaspoon minced parsley
½ teaspoon salt	¼ teaspoon ground black pepper
1 tablespoon olive oil	1 teaspoon vegan butter
¼ cup vegan cashew cream	1 cup grated vegan Parmesan cheese
1 cup of coconut milk	5 cups vegetable stock

Directions:

Take a large skillet pan, place it over medium-high heat, add oil, and when hot, add onion and garlic and cook for 5 minutes.

Transfer to a plate, add celery and parsley into the pan, stir in salt and black pepper, and cook for 3 minutes.

Then switch heat to medium-low level, stir in mushrooms, cook for 5 minutes, then pour in cream and milk, stir in rice until combined, and bring the mixture to simmer.

Pour in vegetable stock, one cup at a time until it has absorbed, and, when done, stir in cheese and butter.

Serve straight away.

Nutrition:

Calories: 439 Cal Fat: 19.5 g Carbs: 48.7 g Protein: 17 g Fiber: 2 g

193. Quinoa with Chickpeas and Tomatoes

Preparation Time: 10 minutes | **Cooking Time:** 0 minute | **Servings:** 6

Ingredients:

1 tomato, chopped	1 cup quinoa, cooked
½ teaspoon minced garlic	¼ teaspoon ground black pepper
½ teaspoon salt	1/2 teaspoon ground cumin
4 teaspoons olive oil	3 tablespoons lime juice
1/2 teaspoon chopped parsley	

Directions:

Take a large bowl, place all the ingredients in it, except for the parsley, and stir until mixed. Garnish with parsley and serve straight away.

Nutrition:

Calories: 185 Cal Fat: 5.4 g Carbs: 28.8 g Protein: 6 g Fiber: 4.5 g

194. Barley Bake

Preparation Time: 10 minutes | **Cooking Time:** 98 minutes | **Servings:** 6

Ingredients:

1 cup pearl barley	1 medium white onion, peeled, diced
2 green onions, sliced	1/2 cup sliced mushrooms
1/8 teaspoon ground black pepper	1/4 teaspoon salt
1/2 cup chopped parsley	1/2 cup pine nuts
1/4 cup vegan butter	29 ounces vegetable broth

Directions:

Place a skillet pan over medium-high heat, add butter and when it melts, stir in onion and barley, add nuts and cook for 5 minutes until light brown.

Add mushrooms, green onions, and parsley, sprinkle with salt and black pepper, cook for 1 minute and then transfer the mixture into a casserole dish.

Pour in broth, stir until mixed and bake for 90 minutes until barley is tender and has absorbed all the liquid.

Serve straight away.

Nutrition:

Calories: 280 Cal Fat: 14.2 g Carbs: 33.2 g Protein: 7.4 g Fiber: 7 g

195. Zucchini Risotto

Preparation Time: 10 minutes | **Cooking Time:** 30 minutes | **Servings:** 6

Ingredients:

2 cups Arborio rice	10 sun-dried tomatoes, chopped
1 medium white onion, peeled, chopped	1 tablespoon chopped basil leaves
1/2 medium zucchini, sliced	1 teaspoon dried thyme
1/3 teaspoon ground black pepper	1 tablespoon vegan butter
6 tablespoons grated vegan Parmesan cheese	7 cups vegetable broth, hot

Directions:

Take a large pot, place it over medium heat, add butter and when it melts, add onion and cook for 2 minutes.

Stir in rice, cook for another 2 minutes until toasted, and then stir in broth, 1 cup at a time until absorbed completely and creamy mixture comes together.

Then stir in remaining ingredients until combined, taste to adjust seasoning, and serve.

Nutrition:

Calories: 363 Cal Fat: 4.1 g Carbs: 71.2 g Protein: 9.1 g Fiber: 3.1 g

196. Lemony Quinoa

Preparation Time: 10 minutes | **Cooking Time:** 0 minute | **Servings:** 6

Ingredients:

1 cup quinoa, cooked	1/4 of medium red onion, peeled, chopped
1 bunch of parsley, chopped	2 stalks of celery, chopped
1/4 teaspoon of sea salt	1/4 teaspoon cayenne pepper
1/2 teaspoon ground cumin	1/4 cup lemon juice
1/4 cup pine nuts, toasted	

Directions:

Take a large bowl, place all the ingredients in it, and stir until combined.

Serve straight away.

Nutrition:

Calories: 147 Cal Fat: 4.8 g Carbs: 21.4 g Protein: 6 g Fiber: 3 g

197. Cuban Beans and Rice

Preparation Time: 10 minutes | **Cooking Time:** 55 minutes | **Servings:** 6

Ingredients:

1 cup uncooked white rice	1 green bell pepper, cored, chopped
15.25 ounces cooked kidney beans	1 cup chopped white onion
4 tablespoons tomato paste	1 teaspoon minced garlic
1 teaspoon salt	1 tablespoon olive oil
2 ½ cups vegetable broth	

Directions:

Take a saucepan, place it over medium heat, add oil, and when hot, add onion, garlic, and bell pepper and cook for 5 minutes until tender.

Then stir in salt and tomatoes, switch heat to the low level and cook for 2 minutes.

Then stir in rice and beans, pour in the broth, stir until mixed and cook for 45 minutes until rice has absorbed all the liquid.

Serve straight away.

Nutrition:

Calories: 258 Cal Fat: 3.2 g Carbs: 49.3 g Protein: 7.3 g Fiber: 5 g

198. Brown Rice, Broccoli, and Walnut

Preparation Time: 5 minutes | **Cooking Time:** 18 minutes | **Servings:** 4

Ingredients:

1 cup of brown rice	1 medium white onion, peeled, chopped
1 pound broccoli florets	½ cup chopped walnuts, toasted

½ teaspoon minced garlic	⅛ teaspoon ground black pepper
½ teaspoon salt	1 tablespoon vegan butter
1 cup vegetable broth	1 cup shredded vegan cheddar cheese

Directions:

Take a saucepan, place it over medium heat, add butter and when it melts, add onion and garlic and cook for 3 minutes.

Stir in rice, pour in the broth, bring the mixture to boil, then switch heat to medium-low level and simmer until rice has absorbed all the liquid. Meanwhile, take a casserole dish, place broccoli florets in it, sprinkle with salt and black pepper, cover with a plastic wrap, and microwave for 5 minutes until tender.

Place cooked rice in a dish, top with broccoli, sprinkle with nuts and cheese, and then serve.

Nutrition:

Calories: 368 Cal Fat: 23 g Carbs: 30.4 g Protein: 15.1 g Fiber: 5.7 g

199. Pecan Rice

Preparation Time: 5 minutes | **Cooking Time:** 10 minutes | **Servings:** 4

Ingredients:

1/4 cup chopped white onion	1/4 teaspoon ground ginger
1/2 cup chopped pecans	1/4 teaspoon salt
2 tablespoons minced parsley	1/4 teaspoon ground black pepper
1/4 teaspoon dried basil	2 tablespoons vegan margarine
1 cup brown rice, cooked	

Directions:

Take a skillet pan, place it over medium heat, add margarine and when it melts, add all the ingredients except for rice and stir until mixed. Cook for 5 minutes, then stir in rice until combined and continue cooking for 2 minutes. Serve straight away.

Nutrition:

Calories: 280 Cal Fat: 16.1 g Carbs: 31 g Protein: 4.3 g Fiber: 3.8 g

200. Broccoli and Rice Stir Fry

Preparation Time: 5 minutes | **Cooking Time:** 10 minutes | **Servings:** 8

Ingredients:

16 ounces frozen broccoli florets, thawed	3 green onions, diced
½ teaspoon salt	¼ teaspoon ground black pepper
2 tablespoons soy sauce	1 tablespoon olive oil
1 ½ cups white rice, cooked	

Directions:

Take a skillet pan, place it over medium heat, add broccoli, and cook for 5 minutes until tender-crisp.

Then add scallion and other ingredients, toss until well mixed, and cook for 2 minutes until hot.

Serve straight away.

Nutrition:

Calories: 187 Cal Fat: 3.4 g Carbs: 33 g Protein: 6.3 g Fiber: 2.3 g

201. Lentil, Rice and Vegetable Bake

Preparation Time: 10 minutes | **Cooking Time:** 40 minutes | **Servings:** 6

Ingredients:

1/2 cup white rice, cooked	1 cup red lentils, cooked
1/3 cup chopped carrots	1 medium tomato, chopped
1 small onion, peeled, chopped	1/3 cup chopped zucchini
1/3 cup chopped celery	1 ½ teaspoon minced garlic
½ teaspoon ground black pepper	1 teaspoon dried basil
1 teaspoon ground cumin	1 teaspoon dried oregano
½ teaspoon salt	1 teaspoon olive oil
8 ounces tomato sauce	

Directions:
Take a skillet pan, place it over medium heat, add oil, and when hot, add onion and garlic and cook for 5 minutes.

Then add remaining vegetables, season with salt, black pepper, and half of each cumin, oregano, and basil, and cook for 5 minutes until vegetables are tender.

Take a casserole dish, place lentils and rice in it, top with vegetables, spread with tomato sauce and sprinkle with remaining cumin, oregano, and basil, and bake for 30 minutes until bubbly. Serve straight away.

Nutrition:
Calories: 187 Cal Fat: 1.5 g Carbs: 35.1 g Protein: 9.7 g Fiber: 8.1 g
\

202. Tangy Tofu Meatloaf

Preparation Time: 10 minutes | **Cooking Time:** 40 minutes | **Servings:** 6

Ingredients:

2 ½ lb ground tofu	Salt and ground black pepper to taste
3 tbsp flaxseed meal	2 large eggs
2 tbsp olive oil	1 lemon,1 tbsp juiced
¼ cup freshly chopped parsley	¼ cup freshly chopped oregano
4 garlic cloves, minced	Lemon slices to garnish

Directions:
Preheat the oven to 400 F and grease a loaf pan with cooking spray. Set aside.

In a large bowl, combine the tofu, salt, black pepper, and flaxseed meal. Set aside.

In a small bowl, whisk the eggs with the olive oil, lemon juice, parsley, oregano, and garlic. Pour the mixture onto the mix and combine well.

Spoon the tofu mixture into the loaf pan and press to fit into the pan. Bake in the middle rack of the oven for 30 to 40 minutes.

Remove the pan, tilt to drain the meat's liquid, and allow cooling for 5 minutes.

Slice, garnish with some lemon slices, and serve with braised green beans.

Nutrition:
Calories:238, Total Fat:26.3g, Saturated Fat:14.9g, Total Carbs:1g, Dietary Fiber:0g, Sugar:0g, Protein:1g, Sodium:183mg

203. Vegan Bacon-Wrapped Tofu with Buttered Spinach

Preparation Time: 5 minutes | **Cooking Time:** 20 minutes | **Servings:** 4

Ingredients:
For the bacon-wrapped tofu:

4 tofu	8 slices vegan bacon
Salt and black pepper to taste	2 tbsp olive oil

For the buttered spinach:

2 tbsp butter	1 lb spinach
4 garlic cloves	Salt and ground black pepper to taste

Directions:
For the bacon-wrapped tofu:
Preheat the oven to 450 F.

Wrap each tofu with two vegan bacon slices, season with salt and black pepper, and place on the baking sheet. Drizzle with the olive oil and bake in the oven for 15 minutes or until the vegan bacon browns and the tofu cooks within.
For the buttered spinach:
Meanwhile, melt the butter in a large skillet, add and sauté the spinach and garlic until the leaves wilt, 5 minutes. Season with salt and black pepper. Remove the tofu from the oven and serve with the buttered spinach.

Nutrition:
Calories:260, Total Fat:24.7g, Saturated Fat:14.3g, Total Carbs:4g, Dietary Fiber:0g, Sugar:2g, Protein:6g, Sodium:215mg

204. Seitan Zoodle Bowl

Preparation Time: 15 minutes | **Cooking Time:** 13 minutes | **Servings:** 4

Ingredients:

5 garlic cloves, minced, divided	¼ tsp pureed onion
Salt and ground black pepper to taste	2 ½ lb Seitan, cut into strips
2 tbsp avocado oil	3 large eggs, lightly beaten

¼ cup vegetable broth 2 tbsp coconut aminos
1 tbsp white vinegar ½ cup freshly chopped scallions
1 tsp red chili flakes 4 medium zucchinis, spiralized
½ cup toasted pine nuts, for topping

Directions:

In a medium bowl, combine half of the pureed garlic, onion, salt, and black pepper. Add the seitan and mix well.

Heat the avocado oil in a large, deep skillet over medium heat and add the seitan. Cook for 8 minutes. Transfer to a plate.

Pour the eggs into the pan and scramble for 1 minute. Spoon the eggs to the side of the seitan and set aside.

Reduce the heat to low and in a medium bowl, mix the vegetable broth, coconut aminos, vinegar, scallions, remaining garlic, and red chili flakes. Mix well and simmer for 3 minutes. Stir in the seitan, zucchini, and eggs. Cook for 1 minute and turn the heat off. Adjust the taste with salt and black pepper.

Spoon the zucchini food into serving plates, top with the pine nuts and serve warm.

Nutrition:

Calories:687, Total Fat:54.5g, Saturated Fat:27.4g, Total Carbs:9g, Dietary Fiber:2g, Sugar:4g, Protein:38g, Sodium:883mg

205. Tofu Parsnip Bake

Preparation Time: 5 minutes | **Cooking Time:** 44 minutes | **Servings:** 4

Ingredients:

6 vegan bacon slices, chopped — 2 tbsp butter
½ lb parsnips, peeled and diced — 2 tbsp olive oil
1 lb ground tofu — Salt and ground black pepper to taste
2 tbsp butter — 1 cup full-fat heavy cream
2 oz dairy-free cream cheese (vegan), softened — 1 ¼ cups grated cheddar cheese
¼ cup chopped scallions

Directions:

Preheat the oven to 300 F and lightly grease a baking dish with cooking spray. Set aside.

Put the vegan bacon in a medium pot and fry on both sides until brown and crispy, 7 minutes. Spoon onto a plate and set aside.

Melt the butter in a large skillet and sauté the parsnips until softened and lightly browned. Transfer to the baking sheet and set aside.

Heat the olive oil in the same pan and cook the tofu (seasoned with salt and black pepper). Spoon onto a plate and set aside too.

Add the butter, full-fat heavy cream, cashew cream, two-thirds of the cheddar cheese, salt, and black pepper to the pot. Melt the ingredients over medium heat with frequent stirring, 7 minutes.

Spread the parsnips in the baking dish, top with the tofu, pour the full-fat heavy cream mixture over, and scatter the top with the vegan bacon and scallions.

Sprinkle the remaining cheese on top, and bake in the oven until the cheese melts and is golden, 30 minutes.

Remove the dish, spoon the food into serving plates, and serve immediately.

Nutrition:

Calories:534, Total Fat:56g, Saturated Fat:34.6g, Total Carbs:4g, Dietary Fiber:1g, Sugar:1g, Protein:7g, Sodium:430mg

206. Squash Tempeh Lasagna

Preparation Time: 15 minutes | **Cooking Time:** 40 minutes | **Servings:** 4

Ingredients:

2 tbsp butter
1 ½ lb ground tempeh — Salt and ground black pepper to taste
1 tsp garlic powder — 1 tsp onion powder
2 tbsp coconut flour — 1 ½ cup grated mozzarella cheese
1/3 cup parmesan cheese — 2 cups crumbled cottage cheese
1 large egg, beaten into a bowl — 2 cups unsweetened marinara sauce
1 tbsp dried Italian mixed herbs — ¼ tsp red chili flakes
4 large yellow squash, sliced — ¼ cup fresh basil leaves

Directions:

Preheat the oven to 375 F and grease a baking dish with cooking spray. Set aside.

Melt the butter in a large skillet over medium heat and cook the tempeh until brown, 10 minutes. Set aside to cool.

In a medium bowl, mix the garlic powder, onion powder, coconut flour, salt, black pepper, mozzarella cheese, half of the parmesan cheese, cottage cheese, and egg. Set aside.

In another bowl, combine the marinara sauce, mixed herbs, and red chili flakes. Set aside.

Make a single layer of the squash slices in the baking dish; spread a quarter of the egg mixture on top, a layer of the tempeh, then a quarter of the marinara sauce. Repeat the layering process in the same ingredient proportions and sprinkle the top with the remaining parmesan cheese.

Bake in the oven until golden brown on top, 30 minutes.

Remove the dish from the oven, allow cooling for 5 minutes, garnish with the basil leaves, slice, and serve.

Nutrition:

Calories:194, Total Fat:17.4g, Saturated Fat:2.1g, Total Carbs:7g, Dietary Fiber:3g, Sugar:2g, Protein:7g, Sodium:72mg

207. Bok Choy Tofu Skillet

Preparation Time: 10 minutes | **Cooking Time:** 18 minutes | **Servings:** 4

Ingredients:

2 lb tofu, cut into 1-inch cubes	Salt and ground black pepper to taste
4 vegan bacon slices, chopped	1 tbsp coconut oil
1 orange bell pepper, deseeded, cut into chunks	2 cups baby bok choy
2 tbsp freshly chopped oregano	2 garlic cloves, pressed

Directions:

Season the tofu with salt and black pepper, and set aside.

Heat a large skillet over medium heat and fry the vegan bacon until brown and crispy. Transfer to a plate.

Melt the coconut oil in the skillet and cook the tofu until golden-brown and cooked through, 10 minutes. Remove onto the vegan bacon plate and set aside.

Add the bell pepper and bok choy to the skillet and sauté until softened, 5 minutes. Stir in the vegan bacon, tofu, oregano, and garlic. Season with salt and black pepper and cook for 3 minutes or until the flavors incorporate. Turn the heat off.

Plate the dish and serve with cauliflower rice.

Nutrition:

Calories:273, Total Fat:18.7g, Saturated Fat:7.9g, Total Carbs:15g, Dietary Fiber:4g, Sugar:8g, Protein:15g, Sodium:341mg

208. Fennel and Chickpeas Provençal

Preparation Time: 10 minutes | **Cooking Time:** 50 minutes | **Servings:** 4

Ingredients:

15 ounces cooked chickpeas	3 fennel bulbs, sliced
1 medium onion, peeled, sliced	15 ounces diced tomatoes
10 black olives, pitted, cured	10 Kalamata olives, pitted
1 ½ teaspoon minced garlic	1 teaspoon salt
1/8 teaspoon ground black pepper	1 teaspoon Herbes de Provence
1/2 teaspoon red pepper flakes	2 tablespoons olive oil
1/2 cup water	2 tablespoons chopped parsley

Directions:

Take a saucepan, place it over medium-high heat, add oil, and when hot, add onion, fennel, and garlic and cook for 20 minutes until softened.

Then add remaining ingredients except for olives and chickpeas, bring the mixture to boil, switch heat to medium-low level and simmer for 15 minutes.

Then add remaining ingredients, cook for 10 minutes until hot, garnish stew with parsley and serve.

Nutrition:
Calories: 395 Cal Fat: 13 g Carbs: 56 g Protein: 16 g Fiber: 13 g

209. Tofu Fajita Bowl

Preparation Time: 5minutes | **Cooking Time:** 10minutes | **Servings:** 4

Ingredients:

2 tbsp olive oil	1½ lb tofu, cut into strips
Salt and ground black pepper to taste	2 tbsp Tex-Mex seasoning
1 small iceberg lettuce, chopped	2 large tomatoes, deseeded and chopped
2 avocados, halved, pitted, and chopped	1 green bell pepper, deseeded and thinly sliced
1 yellow onion, thinly sliced	4 tbsp fresh cilantro leaves
½ cup shredded dairy-free parmesan cheese blend	1 cup plain unsweetened yogurt

Directions:
Heat the olive oil in a medium skillet over medium heat, season the tofu with salt, black pepper, and Tex-Mex seasoning. Fry in the oil on both sides until golden and cooked, 5 to 10 minutes. Transfer to a plate.

Divide the lettuce into 4 serving bowls, share the tofu on top, and add the tomatoes, avocados, bell pepper, onion, cilantro, and cheese.

Top with dollops of plain yogurt and serve immediately with low carb tortillas.

Nutrition:
Calories:263, Total Fat:26.4g, Saturated Fat:8.8g, Total Carbs:4g, Dietary Fiber:1g, Sugar:3g, Protein:4g, Sodium:826mg

210. Indian Style Tempeh Bake

Preparation Time: 10minutes | **Cooking Time:** 26minutes | **Servings:** 4

Ingredients:

3 tbsp unsalted butter	6 tempeh, cut into 1-inch cubes
Salt and ground black pepper to taste	2 ½ tbsp garam masala
1 cup baby spinach, tightly pressed	1¼ cups coconut cream
1 tbsp fresh cilantro, finely chopped	

Directions:
Preheat the oven to 350 F and grease a baking dish with cooking spray. Set aside.

Heat the ghee in a medium skillet over medium heat, season the tempeh with salt and black pepper, and cook in the oil on both sides until golden on the outside, 6 minutes.

Mix in half of the garam masala and transfer the tempeh (with juices into the baking dish.

Add the spinach, and spread the coconut cream on top. Bake in the oven for 20 minutes or until the cream is bubbly.

Remove the dish, garnish with cilantro, and serve with cauliflower couscous.

Nutrition:
Calories:598, Total Fat:56g, Saturated Fat:18.8g, Total Carbs12:g, Dietary Fiber:3g, Sugar:5g, Protein:15g, Sodium:762mg

211. Tofu- Seitan Casserole

Preparation Time: 10minutes | **Cooking Time:** 20minutes | **Servings:** 4

Ingredients:

1 tofu, shredded	7 oz seitan, chopped
8 oz dairy-free cream cheese (vegan	1 tbsp Dijon mustard
1 tbsp plain vinegar	10 oz shredded cheddar cheese
Salt and ground black pepper to taste	

Directions:
Preheat the oven to 350 F and grease a baking dish with cooking spray. Set aside.

Spread the tofu and seitan in the bottom of the dish.

In a small bowl, mix the cashew cream, Dijon mustard, vinegar, and two-thirds of the cheddar cheese. Spread the mixture on top of the tofu and seitan, season with salt and black pepper, and cover with the remaining cheese.

Bake in the oven for 15 to 20 minutes or until the cheese melts and is golden brown.

Remove the dish and serve with steamed collards.

Nutrition:

Calories475:, Total Fat:41.2g, Saturated Fat:12.3g, Total Carbs:6g, Dietary Fiber:3g, Sugar:2g, Protein:24g, Sodium:755mg

212. Ginger Lime Tempeh

Preparation Time: 10 minutes | **Cooking Time:** 40 minutes | **Servings:** 4

Ingredients:

5 kaffir lime leaves	1 tbsp cumin powder
1 tbsp ginger powder	1 cup plain unsweetened yogurt
2 lb tempeh	Salt and ground black pepper to taste
1 tbsp olive oil	2 limes, juiced

Directions:

In a large bowl, combine the kaffir lime leaves, cumin, ginger, and plain yogurt. Add the tempeh, season with salt, and black pepper, and mix to coat well. Cover the bowl with a plastic wrap and marinate in the refrigerator for 2 to 3 hours.

Preheat the oven to 350 F and grease a baking sheet with cooking spray.

Take out the tempeh and arrange it on the baking sheet. Drizzle with olive oil, lime juice, cover with aluminum foil, and slow-cook in the oven for 1 to 1 ½ hours or until the tempeh cooks within.

Remove the aluminum foil, turn the broiler side of the oven on, and brown the top of the tempeh for 5 to 10 minutes.

Take out the tempeh and serve warm with red cabbage slaw.

Nutrition:

Calories:285, Total Fat:25.6g, Saturated Fat:13.6g, Total Carbs:7g, Dietary Fiber:2g, Sugar:2g, Protein:11g, Sodium:772mg

213. Tofu Mozzarella

Preparation Time: 10minutes | **Cooking Time:** 35minutes | **Servings:** 4

Ingredients:

1½ lb tofu halved lengthwise	Salt and ground black pepper to taste
2 eggs	2 tbsp Italian seasoning
1 pinch red chili flakes	½ cup sliced Pecorino Romano cheese
¼ cup fresh parsley, chopped	4 tbsp butter
2 garlic cloves, minced	2 cups crushed tomatoes
1 tbsp dried basil	Salt and ground black pepper to taste
½ lb sliced mozzarella cheese	

Directions:

Preheat the oven to 400 F and grease a baking dish with cooking spray. Set aside.

Season the tofu with salt and black pepper; set aside.

In a medium bowl, whisk the eggs with the Italian seasoning, and red chili flakes. On a plate, combine the Pecorino Romano cheese with parsley.

Melt the butter in a medium skillet over medium heat.

Quickly dip the tofu in the egg mixture and then dredge generously in the cheese mixture. Place in the butter and fry on both sides until the cheese melts and is golden brown, 8 to 10 minutes. Place on a plate and set aside.

Sauté the garlic in the same pan and mix in the tomatoes. Top with the basil, salt, and black pepper, and cook for 5 to 10 minutes. Pour the sauce into the baking dish.

Lay the tofu pieces in the sauce and top with the mozzarella cheese. Bake in the oven for 10 to 15 minutes or until the cheese melts completely.

Remove the dish and serve with a leafy green salad.

Nutrition:

Calories:140, Total Fat:13.2g, Saturated Fat:7.1g, Total Carbs:2g, Dietary Fiber:0g, Sugar:0g, Protein:3g, Sodium:78mg1

214. Seitan Meatza with Kale

Preparation Time: 10minutes | **Cooking Time:** 22minutes | **Servings:** 4

Ingredients:

1 lb ground seitan	Salt and black pepper to taste
2 cups powdered Parmesan cheese	¼ tsp onion powder

¼ tsp garlic powder

1 tsp white vinegar

¼ cup baby kale, chopped roughly

½ cup unsweetened tomato sauce

½ tsp liquid smoke

1 cup mozzarella cheese

Directions:

Preheat the oven to 400 F and line a medium pizza pan with parchment paper and grease with cooking spray. Set aside.

In a medium bowl, combine the seitan, salt, black pepper, and parmesan cheese. Spread the mixture on the pizza pan to fit the shape of the pan. Bake in the oven for 15 minutes or until the meat cooks.

Meanwhile in a medium bowl, mix the onion powder, garlic powder, tomato sauce, vinegar, and liquid smoke. Remove the meat crust from the oven and spread the tomato mixture on top. Add the kale and sprinkle with the mozzarella cheese.

Bake in the oven for 7 minutes or until the cheese melts.

Take out from the oven, slice, and serve warm.

Nutrition:

Calories:601, Total Fat:51.8g, Saturated Fat:16.4g, Total Carbs:18g, Dietary Fiber:5g, Sugar:3g, Protein:23g, Sodium:398mg

215. Broccoli Tempeh Alfredo

Preparation Time: 10minutes | **Cooking Time:** 15minutes | **Servings:** 4

Ingredients:

6 slices tempeh, chopped

4 tofu, cut into 1-inch cubes

4 garlic cloves, minced

1 ½ cups full-fat heavy cream

¼ cup shredded parmesan cheese

2 tbsp butter

Salt and ground black pepper to taste

1 cup baby kale, chopped

1 medium head broccoli, cut into florets

Directions:

Put the tempeh in a medium skillet over medium heat and fry until crispy and brown, 5 minutes. Spoon onto a plate and set aside.

Melt the butter in the same skillet, season the tofu with salt and black pepper, and cook on

both sides until golden-brown. Spoon onto the tempeh's plate and set aside.

Add the garlic to the skillet, sauté for 1 minute.

Mix in the full-fat heavy cream, tofu, and tempeh, and kale, allow simmering for 5 minutes or until the sauce thickens.

Meanwhile, pour the broccoli into a large safe-microwave bowl, sprinkle with some water, season with salt, and black pepper, and microwave for 2 minutes or until the broccoli softens.

Spoon the broccoli into the sauce, top with the parmesan cheese, stir and cook until the cheese melts. Turn the heat off.

Spoon the mixture into a serving platter and serve warm.

Nutrition:

Calories:193, Total Fat:20.1g, Saturated Fat:12.5g, Total Carbs:3g, Dietary Fiber:0g, Sugar:2g, Protein:1g, Sodium:100mg

216. Avocado Seitan

Preparation Time: 10 minutes | **Cooking Time:** 2 hours 15 minutes | **Servings:** 4

Ingredients:

1 white onion, finely chopped

3 tbsp coconut oil

3 tbsp chili pepper

Salt and ground black pepper to taste

1 large avocado, halved and pitted

¼ cup vegetable stock

3 tbsp tamari sauce

1 tbsp red wine vinegar

2 lb Seitan

½ lemon, juiced

Directions:

In a large pot, combine the onion, vegetable stock, coconut oil, tamari sauce, chili pepper, red wine vinegar, salt, black pepper. Add the seitan, close the lid, and cook over low heat for 2 hours.

Scoop the avocado pulp into a bowl, add the lemon juice, and using a fork, mash the avocado into a puree. Set aside.

When ready, turn the heat off and mix in the avocado. Adjust the taste with salt and black pepper. Spoon onto a serving platter and serve warm.

Nutrition:

Calories:412, Total Fat:43g, Saturated Fat:37g, Total Carbs:9g, Dietary Fiber:3g, Sugar:0g, Protein:5g, Sodium:12mg

217. Jamaican Jerk Tempeh

Preparation Time: 15 minutes | **Cooking Time:** 45 minutes | **Servings:** 4

Ingredients:

½ cup plain unsweetened yogurt

2 tbsp Jamaican jerk seasoning

2 lb tempeh

¼ cup almond meal

2 tbsp melted butter

Salt and black pepper to taste

3 tbsp tofu

Directions:

Preheat the oven to 350 F and grease a baking sheet with cooking spray.

In a large bowl, combine the plain yogurt, butter, Jamaican jerk seasoning, salt, and black pepper. Add the tempeh and toss to coat evenly. Allow marinating for 15 minutes.

In a food processor, blend the tofu with the almond meal until finely combined. Pour the mixture onto a wide plate.

Remove the tempeh from the marinade, shake off any excess liquid, and coat generously in the tofu mixture. Place on the baking sheet and grease lightly with cooking spray.

Bake in the oven for 40 to 45 minutes or until golden brown and crispy, turning once.

Remove the tempeh and serve warm with red cabbage slaw and parsnip fries.

Nutrition:

Calories:684, Total Fat:68g, Saturated Fat:12.1g, Total Carbs:13g, Dietary Fiber:4g, Sugar:1g, Protein:13g, Sodium:653mg

218. Zucchini Seitan Stacks

Preparation Time: 15 minutes | **Cooking Time:** 18 minutes | **Servings:** 4

Ingredients:

1 ½ lb seitan

Salt and black pepper to taste

4 tbsp olive oil

½ cup vegetable broth

3 tbsp almond flour

2 large zucchinis, cut into 2-inch slices

2 tsp Italian mixed herb blend

Directions:

Preheat the oven to 400 F.

Cut the seitan into strips and set aside.

In a zipper bag, add the almond flour, salt, and black pepper. Mix and add the seitan slices. Seal the bag and shake to coat the seitan with the seasoning.

Grease a baking sheet with cooking spray and arrange the zucchinis on the baking sheet. Season with salt and black pepper, and drizzle with 2 tablespoons of olive oil.

Using tongs, remove the seitan from the almond flour mixture, shake off the excess flour, and put two to three seitan strips on each zucchini.

Season with the herb blend and drizzle again with olive oil.

Cook in the oven for 8 minutes; remove the sheet and carefully pour in the vegetable broth. Bake further for 5 to 10 minutes or until the seitan cooks through.

Remove from the oven and serve warm with low carb bread.

Nutrition:

Calories:582, Total Fat:49.7g, Saturated Fat:18.4g, Total Carbs:8g, Dietary Fiber:3g, Sugar:2g, Protein:31g, Sodium:385mg

219. Curried Tofu Meatballs

Preparation Time: 5 minutes | **Cooking Time:** 25 minutes | **Servings:** 4

Ingredients:

3 lb ground tofu

2 green bell peppers, deseeded and chopped

2 tbsp melted butter

2 tbsp hot sauce

1 tbsp red curry powder

1 medium yellow onion, finely chopped

3 garlic cloves, minced

1 tsp dried parsley

Salt and ground black pepper to taste

3 tbsp olive oil

Directions:

Preheat the oven to 400 F and grease a baking sheet with cooking spray.

In a bowl, combine the tofu, onion, bell peppers, garlic, butter, parsley, hot sauce, salt, black pepper, and curry powder. With your hands, form a 1-inch tofu ball from the mixture and place it on the greased baking sheet.

Drizzle the olive oil over the meat and bake in the oven until the tofu balls are brown on the outside and cook within, 20 to 25 minutes.

Remove the dish from the oven and plate the tofu ball.

Garnish with some scallions and serve warm on a bed of spinach salad with herbed vegan paneer cheese dressing.

Nutrition:
Calories:506, Total Fat:45.6g, Saturated Fat:18.9g, Total Carbs:11g, Dietary Fiber:1g, Sugar:1g, Protein:19g, Sodium:794mg

220. Spicy Mushroom Collard Wraps

Preparation Time: 10 minutes | **Cooking Time:** 16 minutes | **Servings:** 4

Ingredients:

2 tbsp avocado oil	1 large yellow onion, chopped
2 garlic cloves, minced	Salt and ground black pepper to taste
1 small jalapeño pepper, deseeded and finely chopped	1 ½ lb mushrooms, cut into 1-inch cubes
1 cup cauliflower rice	2 tsp hot sauce
8 collard leaves	¼ cup plain unsweetened yogurt for topping

Directions:
Heat 2 tablespoons of avocado oil in a large deep skillet; add and sauté the onion until softened, 3 minutes.

Pour in the garlic, salt, black pepper, and jalapeño pepper; cook until fragrant, 1 minute.

Mix in the mushrooms and cook both sides, 10 minutes.

Add the cauliflower rice and hot sauce. Sauté until the cauliflower slightly softens, 2 to 3 minutes. Adjust the taste with salt and black pepper.

Lay the collards on a clean flat surface and spoon the curried mixture onto the middle part of the leaves, about 3 tablespoons per leaf. Spoon the plain yogurt on top, wrap the leaves, and serve immediately.

Nutrition:
Calories:380, Total Fat:34.8g, Saturated Fat:19.9g, Total Carbs:10g, Dietary Fiber:5g, Sugar:5g, Protein:10g, Sodium:395mg

221. Pesto Tofu Zoodles

Preparation Time: 5minutes | **Cooking Time:** 12minutes | **Servings:** 4

Ingredients:

2 tbsp olive oil	1 medium white onion, chopped
1 garlic clove, minced	2 (14 oz blocks firm tofu, pressed and cubed
1 medium red bell pepper, deseeded and sliced	6 medium zucchinis, spiralized
Salt and black pepper to taste	¼ cup basil pesto, olive oil-based
2/3 cup grated parmesan cheese	½ cup shredded mozzarella cheese
Toasted pine nuts to garnish	

Directions:
Heat the olive oil in a medium pot over medium heat; sauté the onion and garlic until softened and fragrant, 3 minutes.

Add the tofu and cook until golden on all sides then pour in the bell pepper and cook until softened, 4 minutes.

Mix in the zucchinis, pour the pesto on top, and season with salt and black pepper. Cook for 3 to 4 minutes or until the zucchinis soften a little bit. Turn the heat off and carefully stir in the parmesan cheese.

Dish into four plates, share the mozzarella cheese on top, garnish with the pine nuts, and serve warm.

Nutrition:
Calories:79, Total Fat:6.2g, Saturated Fat:3.7g, Total Carbs:5g, Dietary Fiber:2g, Sugar:3g, Protein:2g, Sodium:54mg

222. Cheesy Mushroom Pie

Preparation Time: 12minutes | **Cooking Time:** 43minutes | **Servings:** 4

Ingredients:
For the pie crust:

¼ cup almond flour + extra for dusting	3 tbsp coconut flour
½ tsp salt	¼ cup butter, cold and crumbled

3 tbsp erythritol

1 ½ tsp vanilla extract

4 whole eggs

For the filling:

2 tbsp butter

1 medium yellow onion

2 garlic cloves, minced

2 cups mixed mushrooms, chopped

1 green bell pepper, deseeded and diced

1 cup green beans, cut into 3 pieces each

Salt and black pepper to taste

¼ cup coconut cream

1/3 cup vegan sour cream

½ cup almond milk

2 eggs, lightly beaten

¼ tsp nutmeg powder

1 tbsp chopped parsley

1 cup grated parmesan cheese

Directions:

For the pastry crust:

Preheat the oven to 350 F and grease a pie pan with cooking spray

In a large bowl, mix the almond flour, coconut flour, and salt.

Add the butter and mix with an electric hand mixer until crumbly. Add the erythritol and vanilla extract until mixed in. Then, pour in the eggs one after another while mixing until formed into a ball.

Flatten the dough on a clean flat surface, cover in plastic wrap, and refrigerate for 1 hour.

After, lightly dust a clean flat surface with almond flour, unwrap the dough, and roll out the dough into a large rectangle, ½ - inch thickness and fit into a pie pan.

Pour some baking beans onto the pastry and bake in the oven until golden. Remove after, pour the beans, and allow cooling.

For the filling:

Meanwhile, melt the butter in a skillet and sauté the onion and garlic until softened and fragrant, 3 minutes. Add the mushrooms, bell pepper, green beans, salt, and black pepper; cook for 5 minutes.

In a medium bowl, beat the coconut cream, vegan sour cream, milk, and eggs. Season with black pepper, salt, and nutmeg. Stir in the parsley and cheese.

Spread the mushroom mixture in the baked pastry and spread the cheese filling on top. Place the pie in the oven and bake for 30 to 35 minutes or until a toothpick inserted into the pie comes out clean and golden on top.

Remove, let cool for 10 minutes, slice, and serve with roasted tomato salad.

Nutrition:

Calories:120, Total Fat:9.2g, Saturated Fat:2.3g, Total Carbs:7g, Dietary Fiber:3g, Sugar:3g, Protein:5g, Sodium:17mg

223. Tofu Scallopini with Lemon

Preparation Time: 5minutes | **Cooking Time:** 21minutes | **Servings:** 4

Ingredients:

1 ½ lb thin cut tofu chops, boneless

Salt and ground black pepper to taste

1 tbsp avocado oil

3 tbsp butter

2 tbsp capers

1 cup vegetable broth

½ lemon, juiced + 1 lemon, sliced

2 tbsp freshly chopped parsley

Directions:

Heat the avocado oil in a large skillet over medium heat. Season the tofu chops with salt and black pepper; cook in the oil on both sides until brown and cooked through 12 to 15 minutes. Transfer to a plate, cover with another plate and keep warm.

Add the butter to the pan to melt and cook the capers until hot and sizzling stirring frequently to avoid burning for 3 minutes.

Pour in the vegetable broth and lemon juice, use a spatula to scrape any bits stuck to the bottom of the pan, and allow boiling until the sauce reduces by half.

Add the tofu back to the sauce, arrange the lemon slices on top, and sprinkle with half of the parsley. Allow simmering for 3 minutes.

Plate the food, garnish with the remaining parsley, and serve warm with creamy mashed cauliflower.

Nutrition:

Calories:214, Total Fat:15.6g, Saturated Fat:2.5g, Total Carbs:12g, Dietary Fiber:2g, Sugar:6g, Protein:9g, Sodium:280mg

224. Tofu Chops with Green Beans and Avocado Sauté

Preparation Time: 10minutes | **Cooking Time:** 22 minutes | **Servings:** 4

Ingredients:

For the tofu chops:

2 tbsp avocado oil	4 slices firm tofu
Salt and ground black pepper to taste	

For the green beans and avocado sauté:

2 tbsp avocado oil	1 ½ cups green beans
2 large avocados, halved, pitted, and chopped	Salt and ground black pepper to taste
6 green onions, chopped	1 tbsp freshly chopped parsley

Directions:

For the tofu chops:

Heat the avocado oil in a medium skillet, season the tofu with salt and black pepper, and fry in the oil on both sides until brown, and cooked through for 12 to 15 minutes. Transfer to a plate and set aside in a warmer for serving.

For the green beans and avocado sauté:

Heat the avocado oil in a medium skillet, add and sauté the green beans until sweating and slightly softened for 10 minutes. Mix in the avocados (don't worry if they mash up a bit), season with salt and black pepper, and half of the green onions. Warm the avocados for 2 minutes. Turn the heat off.

Dish the sauté into serving plates, garnish with the remaining green onions and parsley, and serve with the tofu chops.

Nutrition:

Calories:503, Total Fat:41.9g, Saturated Fat:14.5g, Total Carbs:18g, Dietary Fiber:2g, Sugar:4g, Protein:19g, Sodium:314mg

225. Mushroom in Tortillas

Preparation Time: 15minutes | **Cooking Time:** 6hours, 64minutes | **Servings:** 4

Ingredients:

For the mushrooms:	2 tbsp olive oil
½ cup sliced yellow onion	2 lb mushroom
4 tbsp ras el hanout seasoning	Salt to taste
3 ½ cups vegetable broth	For the keto tortillas:
5 tbsp psyllium husk powder	1¼ cups almond flour
1 tsp salt	2 eggs, cracked into a bowl
1 cup of water	2 tbsp butter, for frying

Directions:

For the mushroom:

In a large pot, heat the olive oil and sauté the onion for 3 minutes or until softened. Season the mushrooms with ras el hanout, salt, and place in the onion. Sear on each side for 3 minutes and pour the vegetable broth on top. Cover the lid, reduce the heat to low, and cook for 4 to 5 hours or until the mushroom softens. After, open the lid and shred the mushroom with two forks. Cook further over low heat for 1 hour to allow the spices to penetrate the meat strands. Turn the heat off and using a slotted spoon, transfer the meat onto a plate. Set aside in a warmer for serving.

For the keto tortillas:

In a medium bowl, combine the psyllium husk powder, almond flour, and salt. Mix in the eggs until a thick dough forms and then the water. Separate the dough into 8 or 10 pieces.

Lay a parchment paper on a flat surface, grease with a little cooking spray, and put a dough piece on top. Cover with another parchment paper and, using a rolling pin, flatten the dough into a circle. Repeat the same process for the remaining dough balls.

Melt a quarter of the butter in a large skillet over medium heat and fry the flattened dough one after another on both sides until light brown and cooked through, 40 minutes in total.

Transfer the keto tortillas to serving plates, spoon the shredded meat onto the keto tortillas and top with some leafy greens. Serve immediately.

Nutrition:

Calories:345, Total Fat:26.1g, Saturated Fat:15.4g, Total Carbs:11g, Dietary Fiber:5g, Sugar:5g, Protein:20g, Sodium:402mg

226. Hazelnuts and Cheese Stuffed Zucchinis

Preparation Time: 15minutes | **Cooking Time:** 20minutes | **Servings:** 4

Ingredients:

2 tbsp olive oil	1 cup cauliflower rice
¼ cup vegetable broth	1 ¼ cup diced tomatoes
1 medium red onion, chopped	¼ cup pine nuts
¼ cup hazelnuts	4 tbsp chopped cilantro
1 tbsp balsamic vinegar	1 tbsp smoked paprika
4 medium zucchinis, halved	1 cup grated parmesan cheese

Directions:

Preheat the oven to 350 F.

Pour the cauliflower rice and vegetable broth into a medium pot and cook over medium heat for 5 minutes or until softened. Turn the heat off, fluff the cauliflower rice, and allow cooling.

Scoop the flesh out of the zucchini halves using a spoon and chop the pulp. Brush the inner parts of the vegetable with olive oil.

In a bowl, mix the cauliflower rice, tomatoes, red onion, pine nuts, hazelnuts, cilantro, balsamic vinegar, paprika, zucchini pulp, salt, and black pepper.

Spoon the mixture into the zucchini halves, drizzle with more olive oil, and sprinkle the cheese on top.

Place the stuffed vegetables on a baking sheet and bake in the oven for 15 to 20 minutes or until the cheese has melted and golden.

Remove, allow cooling, and serve.

Nutrition:

Calories:197, Total Fat:15.6g, Saturated Fat:9.3g, Total Carbs:5g, Dietary Fiber:0g, Sugar:1g, Protein:9g, Sodium:1179mg

227. Tempeh Stuffed Mushrooms

Preparation Time: 5minutes | **Cooking Time:** 20minutes | **Servings:** 4

Ingredients:

2 tbsp butter	½ lb ground tempeh
Salt and ground black pepper to taste	1 tsp paprika
3 tbsp fresh chives, finely chopped	7 oz cashew cream
12 medium portabella mushrooms, stalks removed	¼ cup shredded Soy cheese

Directions:

Preheat the oven to 400 F and grease a baking sheet with cooking spray. Set aside.

Melt the butter in a medium skillet over medium heat; add the tempeh, season with salt, black pepper, and paprika. Cook until brown, 10 minutes while frequently stirring to break any lumps that form. Turn the heat off and mix in two-thirds of the chives and all the cashew cream until evenly combined.

Place the mushrooms on the baking sheet and spoon the mixture into the mushrooms. Top with the Soy cheese and bake in the oven until the mushrooms turn golden and the cheese melted, 10 minutes.

Remove the stuffed mushrooms onto serving plates, garnish with the remaining chives, and serve immediately.

Nutrition:

Calories:159, Total Fat:14.6g, Saturated Fat:7.9g, Total Carbs:3g, Dietary Fiber:0g, Sugar:0g, Protein:5g, Sodium:94mg

228. Mushroom and Vegan Bacon Lettuce Wraps

Preparation Time: 10minutes | **Cooking Time:** 15minutes | **Servings:** 4

Ingredients:

8 vegan bacon slices, chopped	2 tbsp olive oil
½ cup sliced cremini mushrooms	Salt and ground black pepper to taste
1½ lb crumbled tempeh	1 iceberg lettuce, leaves separated and washed
1 cup shredded cheddar cheese	

Directions:

In a large skillet, add the bacon and cook over medium heat until brown and crispy. Transfer onto a paper-towel-lined plate and set aside.

Add 1 tablespoon of olive oil to the skillet to heat and sauté the mushrooms. Season with salt and black pepper; allow cooking for 5 minutes or until softened.

Add the remaining oil to the skillet to heat and cook the tempeh (season with salt and black pepper until brown, 10 minutes, while breaking the lumps that form. Turn the heat off.

Divide the tempeh into the lettuce leaves, sprinkle with the cheddar cheese, top with the vegan bacon and mushrooms. Wrap the leaves and serve immediately with mayonnaise.

Nutrition:
Calories:447, Total Fat:43.6g, Saturated Fat:26.4g, Total Carbs:13g, Dietary Fiber:1g, Sugar:0g, Protein:10g, Sodium:1403mg

229. Mushroom in Thai Curry Sauce

Preparation Time: 15minutes | **Cooking Time:** 25minutes, 30seconds | **Servings:** 4

Ingredients:

6 tbsp butter	1 medium canon cabbage, shredded
Salt and ground black pepper to taste	1 lb mushrooms
1 celery, chopped	1 tbsp red curry powder
1 ¼ cups coconut cream	

Directions:
Melt 2 tablespoons of butter in a medium skillet, add and sauté the cabbage until soft and slightly golden, and season with salt and black pepper, 5 minutes. Spoon the cabbage onto a plate and set aside.

Melt 2 tablespoons of butter in the skillet, season the mushroom with salt and black pepper, and fry in the fat until brown on the outside and cooked within, 10 minutes. Remove onto a plate and set aside.

Add the remaining butter to the skillet and once melted, sauté the celery until softened. Mix in the curry powder, heat for 30 seconds, and stir in the coconut cream. Allow simmering for 5 to 10 minutes. Season with salt and black pepper.

Put the meat in the sauce and spoon some sauce over the mushroom. Turn the heat off.

Serve the mushroom and curry sauce with the buttered cabbage.

Nutrition:
Calories:310, Total Fat:24.5g, Saturated Fat:11.8g, Total Carbs:10g, Dietary Fiber:2g, Sugar:5g, Protein:16g, Sodium:136mg

230. Baked Camembert Cheese with Seitan and Pecans

Preparation Time: 8minutes | **Cooking Time:** 22minutes | **Servings:** 4

Ingredients:

9 oz whole Camembert cheese	3 tbsp olive oil
½ lb seitan chops, cut into small cubes	Salt and ground black pepper to taste
2 oz pecans	1 garlic clove, minced
1 tbsp freshly chopped parsley	

Directions:
Preheat the oven to 400 F.

While the cheese is in its box, using a knife, score around the top and side of about a ¼ -inch into the cheese and take off the top layer of the skin. Place the cheese on a baking tray and melt in the oven for 8 to 10 minutes.

Remove the cheese from the oven after.

For the topping:

Meanwhile, heat the olive oil in a medium skillet over medium heat, season the seitan with salt and black pepper, and fry in the oil until brown on all sides with a little crust, 10 to 12 minutes. Transfer to a medium mixing bowl and add the pecans, garlic, and parsley.

Spoon the mixture onto the cheese and bake in the oven for 10 minutes or until the cheese softens and nuts toasts.

Serve warm with low carb bread or steamed asparagus.

Nutrition:
Calories:266, Total Fat:24.9g, Saturated Fat:4.7g, Total Carbs:6g, Dietary Fiber:1g, Sugar:2g, Protein:7g, Sodium:232mg

231. Cheesy Tempeh Burrito Bowl

Preparation Time: 10minutes | **Cooking Time:** 15minutes | **Servings:** 4

Ingredients:

1 tbsp butter	1 lb ground tempeh
½ cup vegetable broth	4 tbsp taco seasoning
Salt and ground black pepper to taste	½ cup sharp cheddar cheese, shredded
½ cup sour cream	¼ cup sliced black olives
1 avocado, cubed	¼ cup tomatoes, diced
1 green onion, sliced	1 tbsp fresh cilantro, chopped

Directions:

Melt the butter in a large skillet over medium heat. Add and cook the tempeh until brown while breaking any lumps that form, 10 minutes.

Mix in the vegetable broth, taco seasoning, salt, and black pepper; cook until most of the liquid has evaporated, 5 minutes.

Mix in half of the cheddar cheese and allow melting. Turn the heat off.

Spoon the dish into a large serving bowl and top with olives, avocado, tomatoes, green onion, and cilantro.

Serve warm with low carb tortillas.

Nutrition:

Calories:530, Total Fat:57.5g, Saturated Fat:8.9g, Total Carbs:3g, Dietary Fiber:1g, Sugar:1g, Protein:3g, Sodium:8mg

232. Tofu Casserole with Cottage Cheese

Preparation Time: 5 minutes | **Cooking Time:** 5 minutes | **Servings:** 4

Ingredients:

2 tbsp avocado oil	1½ lb crumbled tofu
Salt and black pepper to taste	¼ cup sliced Kalamata olives
½ cup cottage cheese, crumbled	2 garlic cloves, minced
½ cup unsweetened marinara sauce	1 ¼ cups heavy cream

Directions:

Preheat the oven to 400 F and lightly grease a casserole dish with cooking spray. Set aside.

Heat the avocado oil in a deep, medium skillet over medium heat, add the tofu, season with salt and black pepper, and cook until brown, 10 minutes. Stir frequently.

Transfer and spread the tofu in the bottom of the casserole dish. Scatter the olives, cottage cheese, and garlic on top.

In a medium bowl, mix the marinara sauce and heavy cream, and pour the mixture all over the other Ingredients.

Bake in the oven until the top is bubbly and lightly brown, 20 to 30 minutes.

Remove after and dish into serving plates.

Serve warm with a leafy green salad.

Nutrition:

Calories:511, Total Fat:46.4g, Saturated Fat:7.5g, Total Carbs:13g, Dietary Fiber:4g, Sugar:5g, Protein:16g, Sodium:153mg

233. Egg Roll and Tofu Bowl

Preparation Time: 15minutes | **Cooking Time:** 15minutes | **Servings:** 4

Ingredients:

2 tbsp sesame oil	2 large eggs
2 tbsp minced garlic	½ tsp ginger puree
1 medium white onion, diced	1 lb ground tofu
Salt and ground black pepper to taste	1 habanero pepper, chopped
1 small green cabbage, shredded	5 scallions, chopped
3 tbsp coconut aminos	1 tbsp white vinegar
2 tbsp sesame seeds	

Directions:

Heat 1 tablespoon of sesame oil in a medium skillet over medium heat and scramble the eggs until set, 1 minute. Transfer to a plate and set aside.

Heat the remaining sesame oil in the same skillet and sauté the garlic, ginger, and onion in the same skillet until softened and fragrant, 4 minutes.

Add the ground tofu, season with salt, black pepper, and habanero pepper. Cook until the tofu turns brown, 10 minutes.

Mix in the cabbage, scallions, coconut aminos, and vinegar and cook until the cabbage is tender. Stir in the eggs and adjust the taste with salt and black pepper.

Dish the food, garnish with the sesame seeds and serve with low carb tortillas.

Nutrition:
Calories:319, Total Fat:23.1g, Saturated Fat:13.4g, Total Carbs:7g, Dietary Fiber:2g, Sugar:4g, Protein:21g, Sodium:1060mg

234. Pizza Alla Puttanesca

Preparation Time: 15 minutes | **Cooking Time:** 30-120 minutes | **Servings:** 6

Ingredients:
Dough:

1½ cups unbleached all-purpose flour	½ cup warm water, or as needed
1 tablespoon olive oil	1½ teaspoons instant yeast
½ teaspoon salt	½ teaspoon Italian seasoning

Sauce:

½ cup crushed tomatoes	½ cup shredded vegan mozzarella cheese
¼ cup pitted green olives, sliced	¼ cup pitted kalamata olives, sliced
1 tablespoon chopped fresh flat-leaf parsley	1 tablespoon capers, rinsed and drained
¼ teaspoon garlic powder	¼ teaspoon sugar
¼ teaspoon dried basil	¼ teaspoon dried oregano
¼ teaspoon hot red pepper flakes	Salt and freshly ground black pepper

Directions:
Get a bowl to mix your dough. Whisk together the flour, yeast, salt, and seasoning.

Add the oil slowly whilst stirring, then add water little by little until the dough ball is formed.

Knead the dough on a floured surface for 2 minutes.

Shape it and put it in a warm bowl to rise for an hour.

Whilst the dough rises, mix the sauce. Combine tomatoes, olives, capers, parsley, basil, oregano, garlic powder, sugar, red pepper, salt, and pepper.

Oil a tray that will fit in your instant pot and stretch the dough to fit it.

Spread the sauce over the dough.

Insert the tray into your instant pot and cook for 10 minutes on steam.

Release the pressure quickly and sprinkle the mozzarella on top at the end.

Nutrition:
Calories:680, Total Fat:71.8g, Saturated Fat:20.9g, Total Carbs:10g, Dietary Fiber:7g, Sugar:2g, Protein:3g, Sodium:525mg

235. Seitan Fajitas

Preparation Time: 40 minutes | **Cooking Time:** 30-120 minutes | **Servings:** 6

Ingredients:

1lb seitan, cut into strips	2 tablespoons tomato paste
1½ cups tomato salsa	1 tablespoon chili powder
1 tablespoon soy sauce	2 large bell peppers (any color), seeded and cut into ¼-inch-thick strips
1 large yellow onion, thinly sliced	1 garlic clove, minced
Salt and freshly ground black pepper	2 tablespoons freshly squeezed lime juice
1 ripe Hass avocado, peeled, pitted, and diced, for garnish	1 large ripe tomato, diced, for garnish

Directions:
Mix the tomato paste, salsa, chili powder, and soy sauce until combined well.

Put the bell peppers, onion, and garlic in your instant pot.

Put your seitan strips on top. Try and avoid touching them.

Pour the tomato mix over everything.

Seal and cook on Poultry for 30 minutes.

Depressurize naturally, stir in the lime to taste.

Serve and top with avocado and tomato.

Nutrition:
Calories: 140 Cal Fat: 0.9 g Carbs: 27.1 g Protein: 6.3 g Fiber: 6.2 g

236. Zesty Stuffed Bell Peppers

Preparation Time: 30 minutes | **Cooking Time:** 30-120 minutes | **Servings:** 4

Ingredients:

4 large bell peppers (any color or a combination	1 (14-ounce can tomato sauce
2 cups cooked brown or white rice	1½ cups cooked pinto beans or black beans or 1 (15-ounce) can beans, rinsed and drained
1 cup fresh or thawed frozen corn kernels	1 cup diced fresh tomatoes or 1 (14-ounce can diced tomatoes, drained
2 teaspoons olive oil (optional	4 garlic cloves, minced
4 scallions, chopped	1 tablespoon chili powder
2 teaspoons minced chipotle chiles in adobo	1½ teaspoon ground cumin
1¼ teaspoon dried oregano	½ teaspoon sugar
Salt and freshly ground black pepper	

Directions:

Warm the oil in your instant pot, leaving the lid open.

When the oil is hot, add the garlic and scallions and soften for 3 minutes.

Add the chili powder and a teaspoon of both the cumin and the oregano.

Put the garlic mixture in a bowl to one side. Add the rice, beans, corn, tomatoes, and chiles with a little salt and pepper. Mix well.

Top and hollow your bell peppers.

Fill the peppers evenly with the mix and set them in the steamer basket of your instant pot.

Mix the tomato sauce, remaining cumin, remaining oregano, sugar, and salt in the base of your instant pot.

Lower the steamer basket, seal, and cook on Steam for 24 minutes.

Depressurize fast and serve immediately.

Nutrition:
Calories: 140 Cal Fat: 0.9 g Carbs: 27.1 g Protein: 6.3 g Fiber: 6.2 g

237. Moroccan Stuffed Peppers

Preparation Time: 30 minutes | **Cooking Time:** 30-120 minutes | **Servings:** 4

Ingredients:

4 large bell peppers (assorted colors look great	2 cups boiling water or vegetable broth
2 cups couscous	1 cup cooked chickpeas or 1 (15-ounce can chickpeas
1 medium-size yellow onion, minced	2 carrots, peeled and minced
1 large zucchini, minced	3 garlic cloves, minced
3 tablespoons tomato paste	2 teaspoons olive oil
2 teaspoons harissa or hot chili paste	2 teaspoons ground coriander
1 teaspoon paprika	1 teaspoon ground cinnamon
½ tablespoon ground cumin	1 teaspoon salt
¼ teaspoon freshly ground black pepper	1 tablespoon minced fresh flat-leaf parsley leaves, for garnish

Directions:

Top and hollow the peppers. Remove the stems, then chop the tops and keep the diced pepper.

Warm the oil in your instant pot.

When hot, add the onion and soften for 4 minutes.

Add the carrots, pepper tops, zucchini, garlic, and cook for 2 more minutes.

Add the harissa, tomato paste, coriander, cinnamon, cumin, paprika, salt, and pepper.

Add the couscous and water, stir well.

Add the chickpeas and stir again.

Pack the stuffing into the peppers and put them in the steamer basket of your instant pot.

Put a cup of water in your instant pot. Lower the steamer basket.

Seal and cook on Steam for 24 minutes.

Depressurize naturally and serve immediately, topped with parsley.

Nutrition:
Calories:680, Total Fat:71.8g, Saturated Fat:20.9g, Total Carbs:10g, Dietary Fiber:7g, Sugar:2g, Protein:3g, Sodium:525mg

238. Tempeh Chops with Caramelized Onions and Brie Cheese

Preparation Time: 10minutes | **Cooking Time:** 35minutes | **Servings:** 4

Ingredients:

3 tbsp olive oil	2 large red onions, sliced
2 tbsp balsamic vinegar	1 tsp sugar-free maple syrup
Salt and ground black pepper to taste	4 mushroom chops
4 slices brie cheese	2 tbsp freshly chopped mint leaves

Directions:
Heat 1 tablespoon of olive oil in a medium skillet over medium heat until starting to smoke. Reduce the heat to low and sauté the onions until golden brown. Pour in the vinegar, maple syrup, and salt. Cook with frequent stirring to prevent burning until the onions caramelize, 20 minutes. Transfer to a plate and set aside.

Heat the remaining olive oil in the same skillet, season the mushroom with salt and black pepper, and cook in the oil until cooked and brown on the outside, 10 to 12 minutes.

Put a brie slice on each meat and top with the caramelized onions. Allow the cheese to melt for 2 to 3 minutes.

Carefully spoon the meat with topping onto serving plates and garnish with the mint leaves. Serve immediately with buttered radishes.

Nutrition:
Calories:680, Total Fat:71.8g, Saturated Fat:20.9g, Total Carbs:10g, Dietary Fiber:7g, Sugar:2g, Protein:3g, Sodium:525mg

239. Brown Rice Stir Fry with Vegetables

Preparation Time: 10-75 minutes | **Cooking Time:** 25 minutes | **Servings:** 4

Ingredients:

1 handful fresh parsley, chopped	1/2 zucchini, chopped
2 tablespoons olive oil	2 tablespoons soy sauce
1/2 bell pepper, chopped	1/2 cup brown rice, uncooked
4 garlic cloves, minced	1 cup red cabbage, chopped
1/8 teaspoon cayenne powder	1/2 broccoli head, chopped
Sesame seeds, for garnish	

Directions:
Cook the brown rice as per the package instructions.

Bring water to a boil in a frying pan and then add veggies and make sure they are fully covered with water. Cook for 1-2 minutes on high heat, and then drain the water and set aside.

Add oil to the wok pan and heat over high heat and then add garlic along with parsley and cayenne powder. Cook for a minute stirring frequently and then add the drained veggies, tamari, and the cooked rice.

Cook for 1-2 minutes and then garnish with sesame seeds if desired. Serve and enjoy!

Nutrition:
Calories: 140 Cal Fat: 0.9 g Carbs: 27.1 g Protein: 6.3 g Fiber: 6.2 g

240. Grilled Veggie Skewers

Preparation Time: 10-75 minutes | **Cooking Time:** 15 minutes | **Servings:** 4-6

Ingredients:

1 red onion, peeled, chopped	2 tablespoons avocado oil
2 portobello mushrooms, chopped	1 sweet potato, chopped
2 bell peppers, chopped	6 baby red potatoes, quartered
Salt and black pepper, to taste	4 ears corn

Directions:
Preheat the oven to 375F and add the sweet potato to a cooking pot along with the quartered potatoes and water. Bring to a boil and cook until lightly tender for about 10 minutes. When done, drain the water and let cool a bit.

Thread the vegetables onto skewers, and then brush them evenly with oil. When done, season the vegetables generously with salt and pepper on each side.

Cook the vegetables for about 10-15 minutes until tender and cooked through. Flip halfway. Place the corn directly on the vegetables to cook together.

When done, serve and enjoy with the desired sauce.

Nutrition:
Calories:680, Total Fat:71.8g, Saturated Fat:20.9g, Total Carbs:10g, Dietary Fiber:7g, Sugar:2g, Protein:3g, Sodium:525mg

241. Eggplant Teriyaki Bowls

Preparation Time: 10-75 minutes | **Cooking Time:** 45 minutes | **Servings:** 4

Ingredients:

1 carrot, shredded	1 chunky eggplant
¼ cup edamame beans, frozen	1 lime, ½ sliced, ½ juiced
2 spring onions, chopped	1 ½ tablespoon vegetable oil
1 handful radishes, sliced	1 tablespoon caster sugar
1 garlic clove, crushed	½ cup jasmine rice
2 tablespoons sesame seeds, toasted	1 small ginger, grated
2 tablespoons soy sauce	

Directions:
Add 2 cups of water to a cooking pan, add rice and salt to taste. Bring to a boil, cook for a minute, and then close the lid. Reduce the heat to low and cook for 10 minutes until cooked through. Turn off the heat and steam for an additional 10 minutes.

Add a tablespoon of oil to a bowl and toss the eggplant in it. Preheat the wok pan, add the eggplant, and cook for 5 minutes, stirring often, until slightly softened and charred. Add the

carrots to the wok along with garlic, ginger, and spring onions, and then fry for 2-3 minutes.

In a small bowl, whisk the sugar along with soy sauce and a cup of water, and then add it into the wok. Simmer until the eggplant is very soft, for about 10-15 minutes.

Add water to the pan and bring to a boil and then add the frozen edamame beans, remove the beans, drain and rinse them well under running water. Add the radishes to a bowl, drain the beans again, and then add them to the radishes. Squeeze lime juice on top and toss well until combined.

Serve the rice in the bowls and then scoop the eggplant and sauce on top along with the beans and radishes. Sprinkle with sesame seeds and garnish with the lime slices. Enjoy

Nutrition:
Calories: 140 Cal Fat: 0.9 g Carbs: 27.1 g Protein: 6.3 g Fiber: 6.2 g

242. Quinoa and Black Bean Chilli

Preparation Time: 10-75 minutes | **Cooking Time:** 45 minutes | **Servings:** 8

Ingredients:

3 cups vegetable stock	1 onion, chopped
1 cup quinoa, rinsed, drained	1 red chili, chopped
2 teaspoons ground cumin	1 lb. tomatoes, chopped
olive oil spray	1 teaspoon smoked paprika
1 small avocado, sliced	½ teaspoon chili powder
2 garlic cloves, crushed	1 lb. black beans, rinsed, drained
Coriander leaves, to serve	

Directions:
Generously grease the cooking pan with oil and place over medium heat and then add the onion, red chili, and garlic. Fry the ingredients until soft, and then add spices and stir.

Add the vegetable stock into the pan along with quinoa, black beans, and tomatoes, and then adjust the seasonings if needed.

Close the lid and simmer until quinoa is tender, for about 30 minutes.

When done, garnish with coriander leaves and top with the avocado slices. Serve and enjoy!

Nutrition:
Calories: 140 Cal Fat: 0.9 g Carbs: 27.1 g Protein: 6.3 g Fiber: 6.2 g

243. Broccoli Mac and Cheese

Preparation Time: 10-75 minutes | **Cooking Time:** 20 minutes | **Servings:** 4

Ingredients:

8 oz. whole-grain macaroni elbows, cooked	1 head of broccoli, florets
1 ½ tablespoon avocado oil	1 onion, chopped
1 cup potato, peeled and grated	3 cloves garlic, minced
½ teaspoon garlic powder	½ teaspoon onion powder
½ teaspoon dry mustard powder	1 small pinch of red pepper flakes
⅔ cup raw cashews	1 cup water, or more if needed
¼ cup nutritional yeast	3 teaspoons apple cider vinegar
salt	

Directions:
Place a large pot over medium heat. Add salt and water and bring to a boil.

Add broccoli and cook for 5 minutes. Once done, drain excess liquid and set aside in a large mixing bowl.

Place a large skillet over medium heat. Add oil.

Add onion, salt and cook for about 5 minutes.

Add potatoes, garlic, garlic powder, onion powder, mustard powder, salt, red pepper flakes and cook for 60 seconds.

Add cashews, water, bring the mixture to a simmer, reduce the heat, and let it cook until potatoes are tender. Remove from the heat.

Pour the mixture into a food processor, add nutritional yeast, vinegar, and pulse until the mixture is smooth, adding water if necessary.

Serve cooked pasta in bowls, topped with the blended mixture.

Nutrition:
Calories:680, Total Fat:71.8g, Saturated Fat:20.9g, Total Carbs:10g, Dietary Fiber:7g, Sugar:2g, Protein:3g, Sodium:525mg

244. Butternut Squash Linguine with Fried Sage

Preparation Time: 10-75 minutes | **Cooking Time:** 25 minutes | **Servings:** 4

Ingredients:

3 cups butternut squash, peeled, seeded, and chopped	2 cups vegetable broth
12 oz. whole-grain fettuccine, cooked, 1 cup cooking liquid saved	1 onion, chopped
2 garlic cloves, pressed	2 tablespoons olive oil
1 tablespoon fresh sage, chopped	⅛ teaspoon red pepper flakes
salt and pepper	

Directions:
Place a large pan over medium heat. Add oil.

Add sage and cook it until crispy. Season with salt and set aside.

Return the same pan to medium heat, add butternut, onion, garlic, red pepper flakes, salt, and pepper. Cook for about 10 minutes.

Add broth and bring to a boil, then reduce the heat and let it cook for 20 minutes.

Place a pot of salty water over medium heat.

Cool the squash mixture and blend the mixture until smooth with a mixer.

Add pasta, ¼ cup reserved pasta liquid to the pan, return pan to medium heat and cook for 3 minutes.

Nutrition:
Calories: 140 Cal Fat: 0.9 g Carbs: 27.1 g Protein: 6.3 g Fiber: 6.2 g

245. Paella

Preparation Time: 10-75 minutes | **Cooking Time:** 1 hour | **Servings:** 6

Ingredients:

15 oz. diced tomatoes, drained	2 cups short-grain brown rice

1 ½ cups cooked chickpeas

3 cups vegetable broth

⅓ cup dry white wine

1 14 oz. artichokes, drained and chopped

½ cup Kalamata olives pitted and halved

¼ cup parsley, chopped

½ cup peas

3 tablespoons extra-virgin olive oil, divided

1 onion, chopped

6 garlic cloves, pressed or minced

2 teaspoons smoked paprika

½ teaspoon saffron threads, crumbled

2 bell peppers, stemmed, seeded, and sliced

2 tablespoons lemon juice

salt and pepper

Directions:

Preheat the oven to 350F.

Place a large skillet over medium heat and add 2 tablespoons of oil.

Add onion, salt and cook for 5 minutes.

Add garlic, paprika and cook for ½ a minute.

Add tomatoes and stir well. Cook until the mixture starts to thicken.

Add rice and cook for 1 minute while stirring.

Add chickpeas, broth, wine, saffron, and salt to taste. Increase the heat and bring the mixture to a boil. Remove from the heat.

Cover and immediately transfer to an oven on the lower rack. Bake for 1 hour.

Prepare a baking sheet by lining it with parchment paper. Combine artichokes, peppers, olives, 1 tablespoon olive oil, salt, and pepper. Mix well and roast vegetables on the upper rack in the oven for 45 minutes.

Add parsley and lemon juice to the baking pan and mix well.

Sprinkle the roasted vegetables and peas on the baked rice.

Nutrition:

Calories: 140 Cal Fat: 0.9 g Carbs: 27.1 g Protein: 6.3 g Fiber: 6.2 g

246. Spicy Thai Peanut Sauce Over Roasted Sweet Potatoes and Rice

Preparation Time: 10-75 minutes | **Cooking Time:** 1 hour 30 minutes | **Servings:** 4

Ingredients:

For the spicy Thai peanut sauce:

½ cup creamy peanut butter

¼ cup reduced-sodium tamari

3 tablespoons apple cider vinegar

2 tablespoons honey or maple syrup

1 teaspoon grated fresh ginger

2 cloves garlic, pressed

¼ teaspoon red pepper flakes

2 tablespoons water

For the roasted vegetables:

2 sweet potatoes, peeled and sliced

1 bell pepper, cored, deseeded, and sliced

about 2 tablespoons coconut oil (or olive oil)

¼ teaspoon cumin powder

salt

For the rice and garnishes:

1 ¼ cup jasmine brown rice

2 green onions, sliced

a handful of cilantro, torn

a handful of peanuts, crushed

Directions:

Place a pot of water on medium heat and bring it to a boil.

Preheat the oven to 425F.

On a rimmed baking sheet, mix sweet potato, 1 tablespoon coconut oil, cumin, and salt. Roast in the middle rack for about 35 minutes.

On another baking sheet, mix bell pepper with 1 teaspoon coconut oil, salt and mix well, Roast on the top rack for about 20 minutes until tender.

When water is boiling in the pot add rice and mix well. Cook for about 30 minutes and drain excess liquid. Once done, cover and let it sit for 10 minutes, fluff it after.

Mix sauce ingredients in a small bowl and set aside.

Divide rice, roasted vegetables in bowls and top with sauce, green onions, cilantro, and peanuts before serving.

Nutrition:
Calories:680, Total Fat:71.8g, Saturated Fat:20.9g, Total Carbs:10g, Dietary Fiber:7g, Sugar:2g, Protein:3g, Sodium:525mg

247. Butternut Squash Chipotle Chili With Avocado

Preparation Time: 10-75 minutes | **Cooking Time:** 20 minutes | **Servings:** 4

Ingredients:

3 cups black beans, cooked	14 oz. can diced tomatoes, including the liquid
2 cups vegetable broth	1 onion, chopped
2 bell peppers, chopped	1 small butternut squash, cubed
4 garlic cloves, minced	2 tablespoons olive oil
1 tablespoon chili powder	½ tablespoon chopped chipotle pepper in adobo
1 teaspoon ground cumin	¼ teaspoon ground cinnamon
1 bay leaf	2 avocados, diced
3 corn tortillas for crispy tortilla strips	salt

Directions:
Place a stockpot over medium heat. Add oil.
Add and cook onion, bell peppers, and butternut squash for about 5 minutes.
Reduce the heat, add garlic, chili powder, ½ tablespoon chopped chipotle peppers, cumin, and cinnamon. Cook for ½ a minute.
Add bay leaves, black beans, tomatoes, and their juices and broth. Mix well. Cook for about 1 hour.
Remove bay leaf when done cooking.
Slice corn tortillas into thin little strips.
Place a pan over medium heat and add olive oil.
Add tortilla strips and season with salt. Cook until crispy for about 7 minutes. Remove from the heat and place in a bowl covered with a paper towel to drain excess oil.
Serve chili in bowls, topped with crispy tortilla chips and avocado.

Nutrition:
Calories: 140 Cal Fat: 0.9 g Carbs: 27.1 g Protein: 6.3 g Fiber: 6.2 g

248. Chickpea Biryani

Preparation Time: 10-75 minutes | **Cooking Time:** 40 minutes | **Servings:** 6

Ingredients:

4 cups veggie stock	2 cups basmati rice, rinsed
1 can chickpeas, drained, rinsed	½ cup raisins
1 large onion, thinly sliced	2 cups thinly sliced veggies (bell pepper, zucchini, and carrots)
3 garlic cloves, chopped	1 tablespoon ginger, chopped
1 tablespoon cumin	1 tablespoon coriander
1 teaspoon chili powder	1 teaspoon cinnamon
½ teaspoon cardamom	½ teaspoon turmeric
2 tablespoons olive oil salt	1 bay leaf

Directions:
Place a large skillet over medium-high heat. Add oil.
Sauté onions for about 5 minutes.
Reduce the heat to medium, add vegetables, garlic, and ginger. Cook for 5 minutes. Scoop 1 cup of this mixture and set aside.
Add spices, bay leaf, and rice. Stir for about 1 minute.
Add stock and salt to taste.
Add chickpeas, raisins, and 1 cup of vegetables. Bring the mixture to a simmer over high heat.
Lower the heat, cover tightly, and let it simmer for ½ an hour. Remove from the heat when rice is done.

Nutrition:
Calories: 140 Cal Fat: 0.9 g Carbs: 27.1 g Protein: 6.3 g Fiber: 6.2 g

249. Chinese Eggplant

Preparation Time: 10-75 minutes | **Cooking Time:** 45 minutes | **Servings:** 4

Ingredients:

1 ½ lbs. eggplants, chopped	2 cups of water

2 tablespoons cornstarch

4 tablespoons peanut oil

4 cloves garlic, chopped

2 teaspoons ginger, minced

10 dried red chilies

salt

For the Szechuan sauce:

1 teaspoon Szechuan peppercorns

¼ cup of soy sauce

1 tablespoon garlic chili paste

1 tablespoon sesame oil

1 tablespoon rice vinegar

1 tablespoon Chinese cooking wine

3 tablespoons coconut sugar

½ teaspoon five-spice

Directions:

Place chopped eggplants in a shallow bowl. Add water and 2 teaspoons of salt. Stir cover and let it sit for about 15 minutes.

Meanwhile, place a small pan over medium heat. Toast the Szechuan peppercorns for about 2 minutes and crush them.

Add crushed peppercorns to a medium bowl, add soy, chili paste, sesame oil, rice vinegar, Chinese cooking vinegar, coconut sugar, and five spices.

Drain excess liquid from the eggplants and toss in the corn starch.

Place a large skillet over medium heat, add eggplants and cook them until golden. Set aside. Add 1 tablespoon of oil to the skillet placed over medium heat. Cook garlic and ginger for 2 minutes. Add dried chilies and cook for 1 minute. Add the Szechuan sauce and bring the mixture to a simmer in 20 seconds.

Add back eggplants and cook for about 60 seconds.

Nutrition:

Calories:680, Total Fat:71.8g, Saturated Fat:20.9g, Total Carbs:10g, Dietary Fiber:7g, Sugar:2g, Protein:3g, Sodium:525mg

250. Black Pepper Tofu with Bok Choy

Preparation Time: 10-75 minutes | **Cooking Time:** 30 minutes | **Servings:** 2

Ingredients:

12 oz. firm tofu, cubed

1/3 cup cornstarch for dredging

2 tablespoons coconut oil

1 teaspoon freshly cracked peppercorns

1 shallot, sliced

4 cloves garlic, chopped

6 oz. baby bok choy, sliced into 4 slices

For the black pepper sauce:

2 tablespoons soy sauce

2 tablespoons Chinese cooking wine

2 tablespoons water

1 teaspoon brown sugar

½ teaspoon freshly cracked peppercorns

1 teaspoon chili paste

Directions:

In a small bowl, combine wok sauce ingredients and mix well until sugar dissolves. Set aside.

Place cornstarch in a shallow bowl and dredge tofu in the cornstarch. Set aside.

Place a large skillet over medium heat. Heat 1 tablespoon coconut oil.

Add peppercorns and toast for about 1 minute.

Add tofu and cook on all sides for about 6 minutes. Set tofu aside.

Add the remaining coconut oil. Add shallots, garlic, and bok choy. Cook for 8 minutes.

Add back the tofu and cook for less than a minute.

Nutrition:

Calories: 140 Cal Fat: 0.9 g Carbs: 27.1 g Protein: 6.3 g Fiber: 6.2 g

251. Spaghetti Alla Puttanesca

Preparation Time: 10-75 minutes | **Cooking Time:** 30 minutes | **Servings:** 4

Ingredients:

For the Puttanesca sauce:

28 oz. can chunky tomato sauce

⅓ cup chopped Kalamata olives

⅓ cup capers

1 tablespoon Kalamata olive brine

1 tablespoon caper brine

3 cloves garlic, minced

¼ teaspoon red pepper flakes

1 tablespoon olive oil

½ cup parsley leaves, chopped and divided

salt and pepper

For the pasta:

8 oz. whole-grain spaghetti

6 oz. zucchini noodles

Directions:

Place a medium skillet over medium heat.

Add tomato sauce, olives, capers, olive brine, caper brine, garlic, and red pepper flakes. Bring the mixture to a boil, reduce the heat, and let it simmer for 20 minutes. Remove from the heat and set aside.

Place a pot over medium heat. Add water, salt, spaghetti, and cook as directed on the package. When done, drain excess water.

Pour the sauce over pasta and mix well.

Add zucchini noodles before serving.

Nutrition:

Calories: 140 Cal Fat: 0.9 g Carbs: 27.1 g Protein: 6.3 g Fiber: 6.2 g

252. Thai Red Curry

Preparation Time: 10-75 minutes | **Cooking Time:** 40 minutes | **Servings:** 4

Ingredients:

1 ¼ cups brown jasmine rice, rinsed	1 tablespoon coconut oil
1 cup onion, chopped	1 tablespoon fresh ginger, ginger
2 cloves garlic, minced	1 red bell pepper, sliced
1 yellow bell pepper, sliced	3 carrots, peeled and sliced
2 tablespoons Thai red curry paste	1 14 oz. can coconut milk
½ cup of water	1 ½ cups packed kale, chopped
1 ½ teaspoon coconut sugar	1 tablespoon tamari
2 teaspoons fresh lime juice	

Directions:

Place a large pot over medium heat and add water. Bring it to a boil.

Add rice, salt and cook for 30 minutes. Remove from the heat, cover, and let it sit for 10 minutes.

Place a large pan over medium heat. Add oil.

Cook onion and salt for about 5 minutes.

Add garlic, ginger and cook for about ½ a minute.

Add bell peppers, carrots and cook for about 5 minutes.

Add curry paste and cook for an additional 2 minutes.

Add coconut milk, water, kale, sugar, tamari, and lime juice. Remove from the heat.

Nutrition:

Calories:680, Total Fat:71.8g, Saturated Fat:20.9g, Total Carbs:10g, Dietary Fiber:7g, Sugar:2g, Protein:3g, Sodium:525mg

253. Salisbury Steak and Mushroom Gravy

Preparation Time: 30 minutes | **Cooking Time:** 30-120 minutes | **Servings:** 4

Ingredients:

4 palm-sized pieces of beef seitan	1 1/2 tablespoons vegan chicken-flavored bouillon
8 ounces mushrooms, chopped	1/2 teaspoon garlic powder
1/2 teaspoon basil	1 bay leaf
1/8 teaspoon celery salt	1/8 teaspoon seasoned salt
1/4 teaspoon pepper	1 cup of water
1 cup non-dairy milk	2 tablespoons olive oil
1/2 cup plus 3 tablespoons flour	

Directions:

Make a coating for the seitan by mixing the garlic powder, celery salt, ½ cup flour, basil, seasoned salt, and pepper in a bowl. Make sure the seitan is wet before coating it with the flour mixture.

Heat the oil in the instant pot on the sauté setting. Brown the seitan steaks on each side, then set aside.

Add the water, mushrooms, bay leaf, and bouillon to the instant pot, then place the seitan on top. Seal the lid and cook on high for 4 minutes, before letting the pressure release naturally.

Remove the lid and discard the bay leaf. Return to the sauté setting.

Remove the steaks, then stir in the non-dairy milk. Add the flour to thicken the gravy, then add the steaks. Simmer for 10 minutes. Add additional flour if needed.

Serve with a side of mashed potatoes smothered in your mushroom gravy.

Nutrition:
Calories: 140 Cal Fat: 0.9 g Carbs: 27.1 g Protein: 6.3 g Fiber: 6.2 g

254. Stuffed Sweet Onions

Preparation Time: 45 minutes | **Cooking Time:** 30-120 minutes | **Servings:** 5

Ingredients:

10 medium-sized sweet onions	1 lb portobello mushrooms, chopped
1 medium-sized eggplant, finely chopped	3 tbsp olive oil
1 tbsp dried mint	1 tsp cayenne pepper
½ tsp cumin powder	1 tsp salt
½ cup tomato paste	¼ cup fresh parsley, finely chopped

Directions:
Cut a ¼-inch slice from the top of each onion and trim a small amount from the bottom end. This will make the onions stand upright. Place onions in a microwave-safe dish and add about 1 cup of water. Cover with a tight lid and microwave on High for 2-3 minutes. Remove onions from a dish and cool slightly. Now carefully remove the inner layers of onions with a sharp knife, leaving about a ¼-inch onion shell. In a large bowl, combine chopped mushrooms, eggplant, olive oil, mint, cayenne pepper, cumin powder, salt, and tomato paste. Use 1 tablespoon of the mixture to fill the onions.

Grease the bottom of the stainless steel insert with some oil and gently place onions. Add 2 cups of water or vegetable stock and seal the lid. Press the 'Manual' button and set the timer for 15 minutes.

When done, release the pressure naturally and open the lid. Sprinkle with parsley before serving.

Nutrition:
Calories: 140 Cal Fat: 0.9 g Carbs: 27.1 g Protein: 6.3 g Fiber: 6.2 g

255. Lemony Roasted Vegetable Risotto

Preparation Time: 30 minutes | **Cooking Time:** 15-120 minutes | **Servings:** 4

Ingredients:

3 1/2 Cups Butternut Squash, peeled, cubed	1/1/2 Cups Zucchini, diced
1 large Carrot, peeled, chopped	2 Tablespoons Olive Oil
Sea Salt + Pepper to taste	1 Onion, diced
2 Garlic Cloves, minced	6 cups Vegetable Broth
1 Tablespoon Vegan Butter	2 cups Arborio Rice
1/2 Cup Baby Spinach	1 Teaspoon Lemon Zest
2 Tablespoons lemon juice, more to taste	

Directions:
Preheat the oven to 400 degrees F. Line a baking tray with parchment paper. Add butternut squash, zucchini, and carrot to the tray. Coat with 1 teaspoon of olive oil, salt, and pepper, toss well.

Roast in the oven for 15-20 minutes or until squash is soft when poked with a fork. When done, remove from the oven and set aside.

Press saute mode on the instant pot. Add remaining olive oil, and when hot, cook onions and garlic for 2-3 minutes or until onions become semi-transparent.

Add rice and stir for 1-2 minutes to coat.

Add broth, and vegan butter. Stir to combine.

Turn the instant pot off. Cover and seal. Press the manual button and adjust the time to 7 minutes.

When done cooking, release the pressure and stir well.

Return to saute mode, add spinach and roasted vegetables.

Stir until the spinach has wilted. Taste and add salt and pepper as needed.

Top with lemon juice and zest.

Best when served fresh and warm.

Enjoy!

Nutrition:
Calories: 140 Cal Fat: 0.9 g Carbs: 27.1 g Protein: 6.3 g Fiber: 6.2 g

256. Thai Coconut Peanut Tofu

Preparation Time: 26 minutes | **Cooking Time:** 15-120 minutes | **Servings:** 4

Ingredients:

1 cup Creamy Natural Peanut Butter	1 Can (about 1 1/2 cups) light Coconut Milk
1/2 Cup Vegetable Broth	2 Teaspoons Curry Powder
2 Tablespoons Coconut Sugar	2 Teaspoons Ground Cumin Powder
1/4 Teaspoon Sea Salt, add more to taste	1-2 Tablespoons Coconut Oil (or Olive or Sesame Oil
1 Bunch Green Onions, sliced (reserve half for garnish	2 Tablespoons minced Fresh Ginger
1 cup Carrots, shredded	1/4 Cup Roasted Cashews, salted or unsalted
1 Pinch Cayenne Pepper	2 Tablespoons Tamari (or Soy Sauce
3 Teaspoons Rice Vinegar	1 Package (200 GramsExtra-Firm Tofu, cubed
1 Lemon, juiced	

Directions:
In a bowl, mix peanut butter, coconut milk, broth, curry powder, coconut sugar, cumin, and sea salt. Make sure ingredients are mixed completely. Set aside.

Press saute mode on the instant pot. When it is hot, add the coconut oil, half of the green onions, ginger, and garlic.

Add a pinch of salt and saute for 2-3 minutes, stirring frequently.

Add the carrots, cashews, cayenne, and saute for 2 minutes more.

Add the peanut butter mixture into the pot and stir well.

Then add tamari or soy sauce and rice vinegar. Stir to combine.

Lastly, add tofu to the pot and mix.

Cover and turn off saute mode. Press the manual button, change the pressure to high and let cook for 2 minutes.

Quick-release when 2 minutes are done.

Return to saute mode and let simmer to let tofu infuse with flavor. Add more broth if too thick.

Add lemon juice and serve over rice, quinoa, or steamed vegetables.

Garnish with the rest of the green onions and enjoy!

Nutrition:
Calories: 140 Cal Fat: 0.9 g Carbs: 27.1 g Protein: 6.3 g Fiber: 6.2 g

257. Vegan Butter Curry Tofu

Preparation Time: 77 minutes | **Cooking Time:** 15-120 minutes | **Servings:** 4-5

Ingredients:

1 1/2 Cups Coconut Yogurt	4 Cloves Garlic, minced
1 Teaspoon Fresh Ginger, grated	Sea Salt
1 Package Extra-Firm Tofu, cubed	1/2 Cup Vegan Butter
1 Teaspoon Cumin Seeds	1 Onion, diced
2 Teaspoons Garam Masala	2 Teaspoons Curry Powder
1 Teaspoon Paprika	1 Teaspoon Cinnamon
2 Teaspoons Cayenne (optional	1 6 Ounce Can Tomato Paste
1 14 Ounce Can Coconut Milk	1 cup Vegetable Broth
Cilantro, for garnish	Cooked Jasmine or Basmati Rice
Naan (optional	

Directions:
In a bowl, make a marinade by mixing coconut yogurt, garlic, ginger, and sea salt. Add tofu and toss to coat. Refrigerate for 1 hour.

After the marinade is ready, spread out the tofu in a single layer on a baking sheet. Broil until tofu starts to turn brown on all sides, about 20 minutes, turning tofu every 5 minutes. Set aside when done.

Turn on the instant pot to saute mode and melt butter.

Add cumin seeds and cook for 1 minute.

Add onions and cook until soft (2-3 minutes
Add garam masala, curry powder, paprika, cinnamon, and cayenne (optional). Stir.
Stir in tomato paste, coconut milk, and broth.
Set instant pot to manual mode and cook for 12 minutes.
When finished, let the pressure naturally release for 5 minutes, then quick release.
Stir in tofu.
Top tofu and sauce over rice and garnish with cilantro and serve with naan (optional
Enjoy!

Nutrition:
Calories: 140 Cal Fat: 0.9 g Carbs: 27.1 g Protein: 6.3 g Fiber: 6.2 g

258. Thai Coconut Rice

Preparation Time: 30 minutes | **Cooking Time:** 15-120 minutes | **Servings:** 4

Ingredients:

1 Cup White Sticky Rice or Jasmine Rice, rinsed	1 1/2 Cups Water
1 14 Ounce Can Coconut Milk	1/2 Teaspoon Sea Salt
1/2 Teaspoon Organic Cane Sugar	Sesame Seeds (optional

Directions:
Add 2 cups of water to the inner pot and insert trivet.
In an oven-safe bowl add rice and 1 1/2 cups of water.
Place the bowl on a trivet, close the lid, and seal. Pressure cook on high for 15 minutes.
On a stovetop, simmer coconut milk, sugar, and salt.
When rice is done cooking, allow pressure to release naturally then quick release.
Open and remove the bowl.
Pour half of the coconut sauce into the rice and stir well.
Top with sesame seeds optional and more coconut sauce.
Enjoy!

Nutrition:
Calories: 140 Cal Fat: 0.9 g Carbs: 27.1 g Protein: 6.3 g Fiber: 6.2 g

259. Cauliflower Alfredo

Preparation Time: 25 minutes | **Cooking Time:** 15-120 minutes | **Servings:** 6

Ingredients:

2 Tablespoons Vegan Butter	1/2 Onion, chopped
4 Cloves Garlic, minced	1 Cup Vegetable
1 head cauliflower, stem and leaves removed, chopped	2 Teaspoons Garlic Powder
Sea Salt	1/4 Cup Plain Unsweetened Almond Milk
1 Package Pasta (fettuccini, linguini, or spaghetti	Sun-Dried Tomatoes (optional
Fresh Parsley (Optional	

Directions:
On saute mode on the instant pot, melt vegan butter. Saute onion and minced garlic for 2-3 minutes.
Add broth and cauliflower.
Cover the pot and seal it.
Set to manual for 6 minutes.
On a stovetop, cook pasta according to package directions. Set aside.
When the instant pot is done cooking, allow to naturally release pressure for 10 minutes, then quick release.
Use an immersion blender to blend ingredients or puree with a standard blender.
Add garlic powder and sea salt. Blend. Taste and add more garlic and salt to taste.
One tablespoon at a time, add almond milk to desired consistency.
Serve with pasta and top with sun-dried tomatoes and fresh parsley (optional
Enjoy!

Nutrition:
Calories: 140 Cal Fat: 0.9 g Carbs: 27.1 g Protein: 6.3 g Fiber: 6.2 g

260. Shredded Squash

Preparation Time: 12 minutes | **Cooking Time:** 15-120 minutes | **Servings:** 3

Ingredients:
1 Cup Water
1 Squash, washed, halved, and seeds removed

Directions:

Place the metal tripod (trivet into the instant pot and 1 cup of water.

Put one squash on top of the other with cut sides facing up.

Close the lid and seal.

Cook in manual mode, high pressure, for 5 minutes.

Let the pressure release for 5 minutes. Quick-release and open.

Shred the squash with a fork to see if it is done. If it does not shred easily, cook on high pressure for an additional 1-2 minutes.

Serve with favorite store-bought pasta sauce or drizzle with olive oil and fresh garlic

Enjoy!

Nutrition:
Calories: 140 Cal Fat: 0.9 g Carbs: 27.1 g Protein: 6.3 g Fiber: 6.2 g

261. Butternut Squash Risotto

Preparation Time: 20 minutes | **Cooking Time:** 15-120 minutes | **Servings:** 8

Ingredients:

3 Tablespoons Extra Virgin Olive Oil

1 1/2 Pound Butternut Squash, peeled, halved, seeds removed and cubed

2 Teaspoons Ground Sage

Sea Salt and Black Pepper

1 Onion, diced

5 1/2 Cups Vegetable Broth

4 Tablespoons Vegan Butter

2 1/2 cups Arborio Rice

1 cup Dry White Wine (optional

1 Tablespoon Nutritional Yeast (optional

Directions:
On the saute feature, heat olive oil and add squash, sage, salt, and pepper. Cook for 9 minutes.
Add onion and cook for 1 minute.
Add vegan butter, wine(optional), and broth. Stir to combine.
Add rice and stir.
Close the lid and seal.
On manual mode, set time to 5 minutes.
When done, quick release.
Stir in the nutritional yeast and allow to sit for 5 minutes to thicken.
Serve warm. Enjoy!

Nutrition:
Calories: 140 Cal Fat: 0.9 g Carbs: 27.1 g Protein: 6.3 g Fiber: 6.2 g

262. Thai Green Curry with Spring Vegetables

Preparation Time: 10-75 minutes | **Cooking Time:** 45 minutes | **Servings:** 4

Ingredients:

1 cup brown basmati rice, rinsed

2 teaspoons coconut oil

1 onion, diced

1 tablespoon fresh ginger, chopped

2 cloves garlic, chopped

2 cups asparagus, sliced

1 cup carrots, peeled and sliced

2 tablespoons Thai green curry paste

14 oz. full-fat coconut milk (I used full-fat coconut milk for a richer curry)

½ cup of water

1 ½ teaspoon coconut sugar

2 cups packed baby spinach, chopped

1 ½ teaspoon fresh lime juice
salt

1 ½ teaspoons tamari

Directions:
Place a pot over medium heat. Add water and bring it to a boil.
Add rice, salt to taste and cook for 30 minutes.
When done, cover the rice and set aside for more than 10 minutes.
Place a large skillet over medium heat. Add oil.
Cook onion, garlic, ginger, and a pinch of salt.

Add asparagus, carrots and cook for 3 minutes. Add curry paste and cook for an additional 2 minutes.

Add coconut milk, ½ cup water, sugar, and bring this mixture to a simmer. Reduce the heat and let it cook for 10 minutes until vegetables are tender.

Add spinach and let it cook for ½ a minute. Remove from the heat and season with rice vinegar and tamari.

Nutrition:
Calories: 140 Cal Fat: 0.9 g Carbs: 27.1 g Protein: 6.3 g Fiber: 6.2 g

263. Tamarind Potato Curry

Preparation Time: 10-75 minutes | **Cooking Time:** 1 hour | **Servings:** 4

Ingredients:

26.5 oz. potatoes, peeled and cubed	1 onion
1 garlic clove	1-inch ginger, chopped
1 green chili, chopped	oil for frying
1 teaspoon cumin seeds	½ teaspoon fennel seeds
1 teaspoon ground coriander	1 teaspoon chili powder
14 oz. plum tomatoes	2 teaspoon brown sugar
2 tablespoons tamarind paste	1 handful coriander leaves
rice or naan bread, to serve	

Directions:
Place a pot of water over medium heat. Add salt and potatoes. Bring to a boil.

Place onion, garlic, ginger, chili, and 2 tablespoons water in a food processor. Pulse until smooth.

Place a pan over medium heat. Add oil.

Toast cumin and fennel seeds until they pop.

Add spices, puree, and cook for 5 minutes.

Add tomatoes, sugar, tamarind, and let it simmer for 10 minutes.

Add potatoes and some water. Cover and let it cook until tender.

Serve with rice or naan bread.

Nutrition:
Calories: 140 Cal Fat: 0.9 g Carbs: 27.1 g Protein: 6.3 g Fiber: 6.2 g

264. West African Stew with Sweet Potato and Greens

Preparation Time: 10-75 minutes | **Cooking Time:** 1 hour | **Servings:** 4

Ingredients:

1/5 cup crunchy peanut butter	1/3 cup coconut cream
3 cups vegetable stock	21 oz. sweet potatoes, cubed
2 cups okra, halved	1 cup loosely packed kale, chopped
2 onions, 1 roughly chopped and 1 diced	1-inch ginger, chopped
3 garlic cloves	1 scotch bonnet chili
4 tablespoons tomato purée	sunflower oil
2 teaspoons coriander seeds, toasted and crushed	2 teaspoons ground cumin
salt	

Directions:
Combine roughly chopped onion, ginger, garlic, scotch bonnet, tomato puree, and peanut butter in a blender. Blend for 1 minute until paste forms.

Place a cast-iron pan over medium heat. Add 2 tablespoons of sunflower oil.

Add diced onions and cook for 5 minutes. Season with salt.

Add spices, peanut sauce, and cook for 5 minutes.

Add coconut cream, stock, and bring it to a simmer for about 10 minutes.

Add cubed sweet potatoes, cover, and cook for about 15 minutes.

Add okra, kale and cook for 10 additional minutes.

Remove from heat before serving.

Nutrition:
Calories:680, Total Fat:71.8g, Saturated Fat:20.9g, Total Carbs:10g, Dietary Fiber:7g, Sugar:2g, Protein:3g, Sodium:525mg

265. Jackfruit Tamales

Preparation Time: 1 Hour, 45 minutes | **Cooking Time:** 15-120 minutes | **Servings:** 10

Ingredients:

10-15 Corn Husks	1 Tablespoon Olive Oil
1 Onion, chopped	1 Tablespoon Garlic, minced
2 Teaspoons Cumin	1/2 Teaspoon Chili Powder
4 Cups Vegetable Broth, plus 1/2 Cup for jackfruit filling	1 20 Ounce Can Green Jackfruit, drained
4 Cups Masa Harina Flour	2 Teaspoons Baking Powder
1 Teaspoon Sea Salt, plus more to taste for jackfruit filling	1 cup Coconut Oil, melted

Directions:

Soak the corn husks in hot water in the sink for 1 hour.

On the stovetop, heat 1 tablespoon olive oil, add onions, garlic, cumin, and chili powder. Cook until onions are soft.

Add 1/2 cup of broth. Stir until combined.

Add jackfruit and simmer for a few minutes stirring occasionally.

Shred jackfruit and cook for 5 minutes or until liquid has cooked down.

In a bowl, whisk masa harina, baking powder, and sea salt. Then add coconut oil.

Add the broth 1/4 cup at a time until the dough is soft and spongy, but not sticky.

One at a time, remove the corn husk from the sink and lay on a flat surface, and spread out a scoop of masa into the middle of the husk about 1/4 inch thick.

Place a spoonful of jackfruit mixture onto the masa and take the two sides of the husk and let the masa surround the filling, then roll. Fold over one end and secure with a strip of the corn husk.

Pour 2 cups of water into the instant pot and insert the steam rack.

Vertically line the tamales around the instant pot with the open side up.

When the pot is filled, place a corn husk on top. Close the lid and seal.

Cook on manual setting for 40 minutes on low pressure.

They are done when the tamale easily separates from the corn husk. Cook for 10 more minutes if needed.

Remove the steamer and allow to cool a little uncovered for up to 10 minutes.

Enjoy!

Nutrition:

Calories: 140 Cal Fat: 0.9 g Carbs: 27.1 g Protein: 6.3 g Fiber: 6.2 g

266. Red Beans and Rice

Preparation Time: 55 minutes | **Cooking Time:** 15-120 minutes | **Servings:** 6

Ingredients:

1 Pound Seitan (optional	1/4 cup Olive oil
1 Large Onion, diced	1 Celery Rib, chopped
1 Large Bell Pepper, diced	2 Tablespoons Garlic, minced
Sea Salt and Pepper	2 Teaspoons Paprika
2 Teaspoons Store-Bought Cajun Seasoning	1 Sprig Fresh Thyme
2 Bay Leaves	1 Pound Dry Red Kidney Beans, thoroughly rinsed
7 Cups Vegetable Broth or Water	3 Cups Cooked Brown Rice

Directions:

On saute setting, add olive oil. When hot, add onion, celery, bell pepper, and garlic. Cook for 2-3 minutes or until soft.

Add salt and pepper, paprika, cajun seasoning, thyme, and bay leaves. Stir well for 1 minute.

Add beans and broth or water. Stir.

Cover, seal and set to manual on high pressure for 28 minutes.

During this time, cook rice on the stovetop.

When time is up, quickly release and remove the lid.

If using seitan, add at this time, cover, and seal again. Cook for another 15 minutes on manual setting at high pressure. Allow pressure to release on its own when done cooking.

Serve hot over rice. Enjoy!

Nutrition:

Calories: 140 Cal Fat: 0.9 g Carbs: 27.1 g Protein: 6.3 g Fiber: 6.2 g

267. Teriyaki Seitan Cauliflower Rice Bowl

Preparation Time: 15 minutes | **Cooking Time:** 15-120 minutes | **Servings:** 4

Ingredients:

1 Tablespoon Sesame Oil	1 Clove Garlic, minced
1/2 Inch Ginger Root, peeled, minced	1 Pound Seitan or 1 Package Extra Firm Tofu
1/2 Cup Vegetable Broth	4 Cups Cauliflower Florets
1/4 Cup Store-Bought Teriyaki Sauce	2 Cups Edamame, shelled and cooked (frozen and thawed is okay
1 Avocado, sliced	4 Green Onions, chopped
Sesame Seeds(optional	Extra Teriyaki Sauce(optional

Directions:

On the Saute setting, add sesame oil. When the oil is hot, cook garlic and ginger until brown for about 30 seconds to 1 minute.

Add the seitan or tofu and cook for 1-2 minutes then add broth.

Place the steaming basket over the seitan and add the cauliflower florets to the basket. Close the lid and seal.

Cook on high pressure for 1 minute, then quick release when done.

Remove the steaming basket. Also, remove the remaining contents of seitan or tofu and liquid from the instant pot to a separate container or bowl.

Add the cauliflower back to the bottom of the instant pot and use a mash potato masher to break down the cauliflower into rice.

To the seitan or tofu, add teriyaki sauce and stir until combined well.

Top cauliflower with seitan or tofu, edamame, avocado, green onions, sesame seeds(optional), and extra teriyaki sauce(optional). Serve immediately and enjoy!

Nutrition:

Calories: 140 Cal Fat: 0.9 g Carbs: 27.1 g Protein: 6.3 g Fiber: 6.2 g

268. Pasta With Mushroom Tomato Sauce

Preparation Time: 15 minutes | **Cooking Time:** 15-120 minutes | **Servings:** 5

Ingredients:

5-6 Cups Mushrooms, chopped	1/4 cup Onion, diced
2 Cloves Garlic, minced	1 Teaspoon Dried Basil
1 Teaspoon Dried Parsley	1 Teaspoon Dried Oregano
3/4 Teaspoon Sea Salt	1 Jar 25.5 Ounces Pasta Sauce
2 Cups Water	1 Package or 8 Ounces Whole Wheat or Gluten-Free Pasta

Directions:

On saute mode add mushrooms, onions, garlic, dried basil, parsley, oregano, and sea salt. Mushrooms will release liquid as they cook down. Cook for 3-4 minutes.

Add sauce, water, and pasta. All ingredients should be covered in liquid. Add more water if needed to cover all ingredients.

Place lid on instant pot and cook on manual mode on high pressure for 9 minutes.

Quick-release when time is done.

Serve hot. Enjoy!

Nutrition:

Calories: 140 Cal Fat: 0.9 g Carbs: 27.1 g Protein: 6.3 g Fiber: 6.2 g

269. Fragrant Vegetable Rice

Preparation Time: 29 minutes | **Cooking Time:** 15-120 minutes | **Servings:** 4

Ingredients:

3 Tablespoons Sesame Oil	2 Teaspoons Fresh Ginger, grated or minced
1 Tablespoon Sesame Seeds	1 Clove Garlic, minced
1 Yellow Onion, chopped	1/2 Pound Fresh Asparagus, trimmed and cut into 1-inch pieces
1 Bell Pepper, chopped	2 Cups Mushrooms, sliced

3 Tablespoons Tamari or Soy Sauce	1 Tablespoon Vegan Butter
1 1/2 Cups Water	3/4 Cups Jasmine or Basmati Rice

Directions:

Add two tablespoons of sesame oil to the instant pot. On the saute setting, cook ginger, sesame seeds, and garlic for 1 minute.

Add onions and cook for 1 minute.

Add bell pepper, asparagus, and mushrooms. Cook for 2 minutes.

Add tamari or soy sauce and vegan butter. Stir to combine.

Mix in rice and water and stir well.

Cover the instant pot and seal. Pressure cook for 4 minutes.

When done, allow it to naturally release for 10 minutes.

Serve hot. Enjoy!

Nutrition:

Calories: 140 Cal Fat: 0.9 g Carbs: 27.1 g Protein: 6.3 g Fiber: 6.2 g

270. Mexican Quinoa Bowl

Preparation Time: 25 minutes | **Cooking Time:** 15-120 minutes | **Servings:** 2

Ingredients:

1 cup Quinoa	1 Cup Salsa, any store brand
1 Cup Water	1 15 Ounce Can Black Beans, thoroughly drained and rinsed
2 Cups Corn Kernels, thawed if using frozen	Sea Salt and Pepper
1 lime, zested and juiced	1/2 cup Cilantro, chopped
1 Romaine Lettuce Heart, chopped	1/2 Pint Grape Tomatoes, sliced lengthwise
1/2 cup Red Onion, diced	1 Avocado, sliced

Directions:

Add quinoa, salsa, water, beans, corn, sea salt, and pepper to the instant pot. Close lid and seal. Press the Rice button or cook on a manual setting for 12 minutes on low pressure. When done cooking, allow pressure to release on its own.

Remove lid and fluff quinoa with a fork.

Add lime zest and juice, cilantro, and more salt and pepper if needed. Toss well.

Serve warm and top with lettuce, tomatoes, red onion, and avocado.

Enjoy!

Nutrition:

Calories: 140 Cal Fat: 0.9 g Carbs: 27.1 g Protein: 6.3 g Fiber: 6.2 g

271. Vegan Mac And Cheese

Preparation Time: 13 minutes | **Cooking Time:** 15-120 minutes | **Servings:** 4-6

Ingredients:

1 Pound Dry Macaroni or any dry short pasta	4 Cups Water
1 1/2 Cups Unsweetened Plain Almond Milk	2 Tablespoons All-Purpose Flour or Tapioca Starch
2-3 Cups Shredded Vegan Cheese	Sea Salt
2 Tablespoons Vegan Butter	2 Tablespoons Mustard Powder or Nutritional Yeast

Directions:

Add macaroni or other dry pasta, water, and salt to the instant pot.

Close lid and seal.

On the manual setting, set to 4 minutes.

While the instant pot is cooking, whisk almond milk and flour or tapioca starch until combined. Set aside.

When done, quick release valve and open when steam is gone.

Turn instant pot on saute mode.

Stir in almond milk and flour mixture, vegan butter, cheese, mustard powder, or nutritional yeast. Stir well.

When the cheese is melted, turn off the instant pot, taste and add more salt if needed, serve and enjoy!

Nutrition:

Calories: 140 Cal Fat: 0.9 g Carbs: 27.1 g Protein: 6.3 g Fiber: 6.2 g

272. Refried Beans

Preparation Time: 55 minutes | **Cooking Time:** 15-120 minutes | **Servings:** 8

Ingredients:

1 Tablespoon Olive Oil	1 cup Onions, diced
3 Cloves Garlic, minced	1 Jalapeno, seeds removed and minced
Sea Salt	Pinch Cayenne Pepper(optional
1 pound dry Black or Pinto Beans, thoroughly rinsed	6 Cups Vegetable Broth or Water
1 Teaspoon Cumin	1 Tablespoon Chili Powder
1 Teaspoon Oregano	Fresh Cilantro, Chopped

Directions:

On the saute setting, heat oil and add onions, garlic, jalapenos, and sea salt, and cayenne pepper(optional). Cook for 3-4 minutes until soft and browned.

Add beans, vegetable broth or water, cumin, chili powder, and oregano to the instant pot. Cover with lid and secure.

On the bean/chili mode, cook for 45 minutes or manual mode, high pressure for 35 minutes.

When done, allow the pressure to release naturally or use the quick release.

Reserve 2 1/2 cups of liquid and drain the rest.

Use a potato masher and mash to desired consistency. If using a blender, add beans and blend with reserved liquid.

Stir in cilantro. Serve warm. Enjoy!

Nutrition:
Calories: 140 Cal Fat: 0.9 g Carbs: 27.1 g Protein: 6.3 g Fiber: 6.2 g

273. Cajun Vegan Shrimps

Preparation Time: 10 minutes | **Cooking Time:** 30-120 minutes | **Servings:** 6

Ingredients:

½ cup of coconut oil	½ cup chopped onion
½ cup chopped carrots	10oz. vegan shrimps
1 green bell pepper, seeded, chopped	¼ cup all-purpose flour
1 cup of water	4 tablespoons lemon juice
Salt and pepper, to taste	3 cloves garlic
2 teaspoons Cajun seasoning	¼ cup chopped cilantro
4 cups cooked brown rice, to serve with	

Directions:

Heat coconut oil in an Instant pot on Sauté.

Add vegetables and cook for 5 minutes.

Sprinkle veggies with flour and cook for 1 minute.

Add water and stir until smooth.

Add remaining ingredients, except the rice, and season to taste.

Cover and select Manual.

High-pressure 4 minutes.

Use a quick pressure release method.

Serve over rice.

Nutrition:
Calories: 140 Cal Fat: 0.9 g Carbs: 27.1 g Protein: 6.3 g Fiber: 6.2 g

274. Seitan Delicacy

Preparation Time: 15 minutes | **Cooking Time:** 30-120 minutes | **Servings:** 6

Ingredients:

2 tablespoons vegetable oil	1 tablespoon tomato puree
2 cups vegetable stock	2 cups red wine
1lb. cooked and sliced seitan	1 cup carrots, sliced
½ cup onion, sliced	2 tablespoons all-purpose flour
Salt and pepper, to taste	2 cups sliced brown mushrooms
1 bay leaf	2 cloves garlic, minced
1 ½ cup peeled pearl onions	1 tablespoon coconut oil
1 teaspoon dried thyme	

Directions:

Heat oil into Instant Pot on Sauté.

Add onions and carrots. Cook for 5 minutes.

Add garlic and spices. Cook for 1 minute.

Sprinkle it with flour and cook for 1 minute.

Pour in the stock and simmer for 2 minutes.

Toss in remaining ingredients.
Lock the lid into place and select Manual.
High-pressure 8 minutes.
Use a natural pressure release method.
Serve warm.

Nutrition:
Calories: 140 Cal Fat: 0.9 g Carbs: 27.1 g Protein: 6.3 g Fiber: 6.2 g

275. Eggplant Caponata

Preparation Time: 42 minutes | **Cooking Time:** 30-120 minutes | **Servings:** 8

Ingredients:

4-5 eggplants, sliced	2 medium-sized onions, peeled and chopped
10 large, fresh tomatoes, roughly chopped	7.5 oz green olives
7.5 oz capers	1 medium-sized chili pepper
2 stalks of celery	½ cup of oil
3 tablespoons of red wine vinegar	Salt to taste
1 tsp of sugar	½ tbsp of basil, dry

Directions:
Chop the eggplants into bite-sized pieces and season with some salt. Allow it to stand for about 30 minutes and rinse well.
Plug your instant pot and add the eggplants in the stainless steel insert. Add all the remaining ingredients and securely close the lid. Adjust the steam release handle and press the "Manual" button. Set the timer for 12 minutes and cook on high pressure.
When done, press the "Cancel" button and release the pressure naturally.
Open the pot and serve warm.

Nutrition:
Calories: 140 Cal Fat: 0.9 g Carbs: 27.1 g Protein: 6.3 g Fiber: 6.2 g

276. Potato Mushrooms Pot

Preparation Time: 15 minutes | **Cooking Time:** 30-120 minutes | **Servings:** 6

Ingredients:

2 tablespoons vegetable oil	½ lb. potatoes, peeled, cubed
1lb. sliced shiitake mushrooms	1lb. sliced cremini mushrooms
4 cups vegetable stock	4 cloves garlic, minced
Salt and pepper, to taste	1 lb. sliced oyster mushrooms
½ cup red wine	1 tablespoon coconut aminos
¼ cup chopped onion	1 teaspoon thyme

Directions:
Heat vegetable oil into Instant pot on Sauté.
Add onions and cook for 4 minutes.
Add garlic and cook for 1 minute.
Stir in mushrooms and cook for 1 minute.
Add remaining ingredients.
Lock the lid into place and select Manual.
High-pressure 9 minutes.
Use a quick pressure release method.
Serve warm.

Nutrition:
Calories: 140 Cal Fat: 0.9 g Carbs: 27.1 g Protein: 6.3 g Fiber: 6.2 g

277. Black Bean, Chorizo & Enchilada Lasagna

Preparation Time: 15 minutes | **Cooking Time:** 30-120 minutes | **Servings:** 6

Ingredients:

12 ounces soy chorizo	1 medium-size sweet potato, thinly sliced
1 can of black beans	2 cups enchilada sauce
1 package of corn tortillas	1/4 teaspoon cumin
1/4 teaspoon chili powder	

Directions:
Season the chorizo with cumin and chili powder. Oil the instant pot and pour a quarter of the sauce into the bottom. Add a single layer of tortilla, then add a third of the chorizo, sweet potatoes, and black beans. Repeat the layers,

finishing with one more layer of tortillas and sauce.

Seal the lid and cook on high for 4 minutes. Serve with vegan sour cream for garnish.

Nutrition:
Calories: 140 Cal Fat: 0.9 g Carbs: 27.1 g Protein: 6.3 g Fiber: 6.2 g

278. Yellow Split Pea with Lemon

Preparation Time: 40 minutes | **Cooking Time:** 30-120 minutes | **Servings:** 5

Ingredients:

2 cups split yellow peas	1 cup onions, finely chopped
1 large carrot, sliced	2 large potatoes, chopped
3 tbsp olive oil	¼ cup freshly squeezed lemon juice
3 garlic cloves, crushed	1 tsp cayenne pepper
½ tsp salt	4 cups vegetable stock

Directions:
Plug your instant pot and press the "Sautee" button. Heat the olive oil in the stainless steel insert and add onions. Stir-fry for one minute. Add the remaining vegetables and continue to cook for 5-6 minutes. Stir in the cayenne pepper and season with salt.

Finally, pour in the vegetable stock and close the lid. Set the steam release handle and set the "Manual" mode for 25 minutes.

When done, press the "Cancel" button and perform a quick release. Open the lid and stir in the lemon juice.

Serve immediately.

Nutrition:
Calories: 140 Cal Fat: 0.9 g Carbs: 27.1 g Protein: 6.3 g Fiber: 6.2 g

279. Spicy White Peas

Preparation Time: 30 minutes | **Cooking Time:** 30-120 minutes | **Servings:** 4

Ingredients:

1 lb of white peas	4 slices of vegan bacon
1 large onion, finely chopped	1 small chili pepper, finely chopped
2 tbsp of all-purpose flour	2 tbsp of coconut oil
1 tbsp of cayenne pepper	3 bay leaves, dried
1 tsp of salt	½ tsp of freshly ground black pepper

Directions:
Plug your instant pot and press the "Saute" button. Melt the coconut oil in the stainless steel insert. Add chopped onion and stir-fry until translucent.

Add bacon, peas, finely chopped chili pepper, bay leaves, salt, and pepper. Gently stir in two tablespoons of flour and add 3 cups of water.

Close the lid and set the steam release handle. Press the "Manual" button and set the timer for 15 minutes. Cook on high pressure.

When done, press the "Cancel" button and release the steam naturally. Turn off the instant pot.

Let it chill for 10 minutes before serving. Enjoy!

Nutrition:
Calories: 140 Cal Fat: 0.9 g Carbs: 27.1 g Protein: 6.3 g Fiber: 6.2 g

280. Stuffed Potatoes

Preparation Time: 60 minutes | **Cooking Time:** 30-120 minutes | **Servings:** 3

Ingredients:

6 small potatoes, whole	¼ cup olive oil
3 garlic cloves, crushed	¼ cup crumbled tofu
1 tsp fresh rosemary, finely chopped	½ tsp dried thyme
2 oz button mushrooms, sliced	1 tsp salt

Directions:
Rinse well the potatoes and drain in a large colander. Rub with salt and place in your instant pot.

Add enough water to cover and seal the lid. Press the "Manual" button and set the timer for 30 minutes.

When you hear the cooker's end signal, perform a quick release and open. Gently remove the potatoes and chill for a while keeping them whole.

Meanwhile, in a medium-sized bowl, combine olive oil with crushed garlic, tofu, rosemary, thyme, and mushrooms. Press the "Sautee" button and add the mixture. Gently simmer until mushrooms soften and cheese melts. Remove from the cooker.

Now, cut the top of each potato and spoon out the middle. Fill with the tofu mixture and serve immediately.

Enjoy!

Nutrition:
Calories:680, Total Fat:71.8g, Saturated Fat:20.9g, Total Carbs:10g, Dietary Fiber:7g, Sugar:2g, Protein:3g, Sodium:525mg

281. Seitan with Tomatillo Sauce

Preparation Time: 15 minutes | **Cooking Time:** 30-120 minutes | **Servings:** 10

Ingredients:

4 cups cubed chicken-flavored seitan	1 2/3 pounds tomatillos, husked and chopped
1 can green chilis	3 cloves garlic, minced
1/4 cup apple cider vinegar	1 teaspoon salt
2 teaspoons chili powder	1/2 teaspoon cumin
1/4 teaspoon coriander	1 teaspoon olive oil
1/4 cup water	Juice of 1 lime

Directions:
Add everything except the seitan to a food processor and blend to make the sauce.

Add the sauce and the seitan to the instant pot. Seal the lid and cook on high for 4 minutes, then let the pressure release naturally.

Serve in warm tortillas or over a bed of rice.

Nutrition:
Calories: 140 Cal Fat: 0.9 g Carbs: 27.1 g Protein: 6.3 g Fiber: 6.2 g

282. Garlic Shiitake

Preparation Time: 45 minutes | **Cooking Time:** 30-120 minutes | **Servings:** 4

Ingredients:

1 lb shiitake mushrooms	2 large potatoes, finely chopped
4 garlic cloves, crushed	2 tbsp oil
1 tsp garlic powder	1 tbsp cumin seeds
½ tsp chili powder	1 large zucchini, chopped
1 cup onions	2 cups vegetable stock
1 cup tomato sauce	

Directions:
With the cooker's lid off, heat the olive oil on the "Sautee" mode. Add cumin seeds and stir-fry for one minute. Now, add onions, chili powder, crushed garlic, and garlic powder. Cook for 3 minutes, stirring constantly.

Add mushrooms and continue to cook on "Sautee" mode for 3 minutes.

Finally, add the remaining ingredients and seal the lid. Press the "Manual" button and set the timer for 20 minutes.

When done, press the "Cancel" button and release the steam pressure naturally.

Open the lid and serve immediately.

Enjoy!

Nutrition:
Calories: 140 Cal Fat: 0.9 g Carbs: 27.1 g Protein: 6.3 g Fiber: 6.2 g

283. Stuffed Bell Peppers

Preparation Time: 35 minutes | **Cooking Time:** 30-120 minutes | **Servings:** 4

Ingredients:

5 bell peppers, seeds removed	1 medium-sized onion, peeled and finely chopped
7oz button mushrooms, sliced	4 garlic cloves, peeled and crushed
4 tbsp of extra-virgin olive oil	1 tsp of salt
¼ tsp of freshly ground black pepper	¼ cup of rice
½ tbsp. of Cayenne pepper	2 cups vegetable stock

Directions:

With the cooker's lid off, heat two tablespoons of olive oil on the "Sautee" mode. Add onions and garlic and stir-fry until translucent. Press the "Cancel" button and set it aside.

Rinse well each bell pepper and pat dry with some kitchen paper. Remove the stem along with seeds.

In a small bowl, combine rice with the mixture from your pot. Add mushrooms and stir all well. Season with salt, pepper, and cayenne pepper. Stuff each bell pepper with this mixture. Gently place them in your instant pot, filled side up, and pour in the broth.

Seal the lid and set the steam release handle. Press the "Manual" mode and set the timer for 15 minutes.

When done, press the "Cancel" button and release the pressure naturally.

Enjoy!

Nutrition:

Calories:680, Total Fat:71.8g, Saturated Fat:20.9g, Total Carbs:10g, Dietary Fiber:7g, Sugar:2g, Protein:3g, Sodium:525mg

284. Chickpeas with Onions

Preparation Time: 35 minutes | **Cooking Time:** 30-120 minutes | **Servings:** 5

Ingredients:

1 lb chickpeas, soaked	3 large purple onions, peeled and sliced
2 large tomatoes, roughly chopped	3 oz parsley, chopped
2 cups vegetable broth	1 tbsp cayenne pepper
3 tbsp almond butter	2 tbsp olive oil
1 tsp salt	½ tsp freshly ground black pepper

Directions:

Plug your instant pot and heat the oil in the stainless steel insert. Press the "Sautee" button and add onions. Stir-fry for five minutes. Now, add soaked chickpeas, chopped tomatoes, chopped parsley, and vegetable broth. Stir in the cayenne pepper, salt, and freshly ground black pepper.

Close the lid and set the steam release handle. Press the "Stew" button and cook for 30 minutes.

When done, press the "Cancel" button and turn off the pot. Perform a quick release and open the pot.

Serve chickpeas warm.

Nutrition:

Calories: 140 Cal Fat: 0.9 g Carbs: 27.1 g Protein: 6.3 g Fiber: 6.2 g

285. Portobello Mushrooms with Green Peas

Preparation Time: 65 minutes | **Cooking Time:** 30-120 minutes | **Servings:** 4

Ingredients:

8 oz Portobello mushrooms, sliced	1 cup green peas
1 cup pearl onions, minced	2 large carrots
½ cup celery stalks, chopped	2 garlic cloves, crushed
2 large potatoes, chopped	1 tbsp apple cider vinegar
1 tsp rosemary	1 tbsp cayenne pepper
1 tsp salt	½ tsp pepper, freshly ground
2 tbsp almond butter	3 cups vegetable stock

Directions:

Set your instant pot to "Saute" mode. Add onions, carrots, celery stalks, and garlic. Sprinkle some salt, pepper, rosemary, and cayenne pepper. Stir-fry for a few minutes.

Now, add the remaining ingredients and seal the lid. Set the steam release handle and press the "Manual" mode. Set the timer for 30 minutes.

When done, press the "Cancel" button and release the pressure naturally.

Open the lid and serve immediately.

Nutrition:

Calories:680, Total Fat:71.8g, Saturated Fat:20.9g, Total Carbs:10g, Dietary Fiber:7g, Sugar:2g, Protein:3g, Sodium:525mg

286. One-Pot Quinoa

Preparation Time: 20 minutes | **Cooking Time:** 30-120 minutes | **Servings:** 2

Ingredients:

4 cups of water	2 cups quinoa

3 garlic cloves, minced 2 tbsp rice vinegar
2 tbsp soy sauce 1tsp grated ginger
2 tbsp sugar 8 oz bag of frozen vegetables (Asian-style

Directions:
Combine all the ingredients (except for frozen vegetables in Instant Pot. Cover the pot with a lid. Set steam release handle to 'sealing' and set Instant Pot to manual to 1 minute over high pressure.
Once done, allow it to naturally release pressure for 10 minutes. Change steam release handle to 'venting' to release any remaining steam. Open the lid. Then add thawed frozen veggies and mix well.

Nutrition:
Calories: 140 Cal Fat: 0.9 g Carbs: 27.1 g Protein: 6.3 g Fiber: 6.2 g

287. Instant Pot Hot Dogs

Preparation Time: 35 minutes | **Cooking Time:** 30-120 minutes | **Servings:** 4

Ingredients:
For Marinade: ¼ cup of soy sauce
¼ cup of water 1 tbsp rice vinegar
½ tsp liquid smoke ½ tsp garlic powder
½ tsp onion powder For Topping:
Ketchup, mustard, etc For Hot Dog:
4 large carrots 4 oil-free vegan hot dog buns

Directions:
Place trivet in the inner pot. Pour in 1½ cups water. Place 4 carrots on a trivet and cover the pot with a lid. Switch the manual button for 3 minutes over high pressure. Set steam release handle to 'sealing'.
When the timer beeps, change the steam release handle to 'venting' to release the steam immediately.
Mix the marinade ingredients in a container. Add carrots along with the marinade. Let it marinate for 24 hours.
Take them from marinade and transfer them to Instant Pot. Pour in marinade and switch on the sauté button. Switch adjust button to get 'high' temperature setting. Sauté it for 10 minutes.

Serve carrot dogs over desired oil-free hot dog buns topped with favorite sauces.

Nutrition:
Calories:680, Total Fat:71.8g, Saturated Fat:20.9g, Total Carbs:10g, Dietary Fiber:7g, Sugar:2g, Protein:3g, Sodium:525mg

288. Curried Potato and Cauliflower (Indian Aloo Gobi

Preparation Time: 40 minutes | **Cooking Time:** 30-120 minutes | **Servings:** 2

Ingredients:
1 head cauliflower 1½ lbs potatoes, peeled and then chopped
2 cups of water 1 red onion, chopped finely
1 tsp salt 3 garlic cloves, minced
1 tsp ground coriander 1 tsp garam masala
1 tsp chili powder 1/2 tsp turmeric
1 tsp grated ginger

Directions:
Steam the cauliflower head in Instant Pot for 2 minutes on a trivet with 1½ cups water. Immediately release pressure and take the trivet out from the Instant Pot. Allow it to cool. Empty the pot of water.
Sauté onions, ginger, and garlic for 5 minutes along with ½ cup water (using the sauté function). Once the timer beeps, switch on the 'Keep Warm/Cancel' button. Add 1½ cups water to the inner pot. Add potatoes and all spices. Mix everything around using a spoon.
Cover the pot with a lid and switch on the manual button for 8 minutes over high pressure. Set steam release handle to 'sealing'. Once finished cooking, allow pressure to release naturally for about 5-10 minutes. In the meanwhile, chop cauliflower into bite-size bits. Using the steam release handle to release the remaining steam after 5-10 minutes. Add cauliflower pieces and stir around using a spoon.

Nutrition:
Calories: 140 Cal Fat: 0.9 g Carbs: 27.1 g Protein: 6.3 g Fiber: 6.2 g

289. Corn Chorizo Pie

Preparation Time: 6 minutes | **Cooking Time:** 30-120 minutes | **Servings:** 6

Ingredients:

12 soft corn tortillas	1 crumbled vegan chorizo
1 onion, minced	1 teaspoon olive oil
2 canned chipotle chilies in adobo, minced	1½ cups corn kernels
1½ cups shredded vegan cheddar cheese	2 tablespoons chili powder
1 tablespoon tomato paste	1 tablespoon grated unsweetened dark chocolate
1 (15-ounce can vegan refried beans, stirred	1 teaspoon ground cumin
¼ teaspoon black pepper	1 teaspoon smoked paprika
1 teaspoon dark brown sugar	1 teaspoon dried oregano
8 ounces steamed diced tempeh, chopped seitan	½ teaspoon salt
1 (14.5-ounce) can crushed tomatoes	4 garlic cloves, minced
1½ cups cooked pinto beans	

Directions:

Add the onion, garlic, and oil to the instant pot.
Cook for 30 seconds and then add the tomato paste, cumin, chipotle chiles, chocolate, oregano, chili powder, paprika, brown sugar, and seasoning.
Add some water and cover with a lid.
Cook for 2 minutes and then add the tomatoes.
Cover and cook for 1 minute.
Add the tempeh, beans, corn, and mix well.
Cover and cook for another 5 minutes.
Serve hot.

Nutrition:
Calories: 140 Cal Fat: 0.9 g Carbs: 27.1 g Protein: 6.3 g Fiber: 6.2 g

290. Cheesy Tomato Gratin

Preparation Time: 10 minutes | **Cooking Time:** 30-120 minutes | **Servings:** 6

Ingredients:

1 (14.5-ounce) can petite diced tomatoes	1 cup shredded vegan mozzarella cheese
3 large potatoes, peeled and sliced	½ teaspoon smoked paprika
¼ cup vegetable broth	1 onion, minced
2 tablespoons chili powder	½ teaspoon ground cumin
¼ teaspoon cayenne pepper	3 garlic cloves, minced
1 teaspoon dried oregano	3 tablespoons tomato paste
Salt and black pepper	

Directions:

Add the onion, garlic to your instant pot.
Cover and cook for 30 seconds.
Add the broth, oregano, cumin, tomato paste, cayenne, paprika, and chili powder.
Add the tomatoes, and mix well.
Cook for 2 minutes.
Add the potato slices and cook for 4 minutes.
Add the cheese and cook for another minute.
Serve warm.

Nutrition:
Calories: 140 Cal Fat: 0.9 g Carbs: 27.1 g Protein: 6.3 g Fiber: 6.2 g

291. Sweet Potatoes and Onions with Jerk Sauce

Preparation Time: 6 minutes | **Cooking Time:** 30-120 minutes | **Servings:** 6

Ingredients:

2 sweet potatoes, peeled and diced	1 pound tempeh, diced
½ sweet onion, diced	¼ teaspoon cayenne pepper
1 garlic clove, crushed	¼ teaspoon paprika
2 scallions, coarsely chopped	2 teaspoons soy sauce
1 tablespoon ginger	2 tablespoons lime
1 teaspoon dried thyme	1 teaspoon dark brown sugar
1 hot green chile, seeded and chopped	½ teaspoon ground allspice

¼ teaspoon ground cinnamon	½ teaspoon salt
1 tablespoon rice vinegar	¼ teaspoon black pepper
⅓ cup water	½ large or 1 small Vidalia or other sweet onion, cut into ½-inch dice

Directions:

In a blender add the chile, scallions, ginger, garlic, and onion.

Blend for 30 seconds and add the soy sauce, cinnamon, cayenne, seasoning, vinegar, marmalade, allspice, sugar, and thyme.

Add some water and blend again.

Add the tempeh, onion, and potatoes to the instant pot.

Add the jerk sauce you made.

Mix well and cook for 5 minutes.

Serve warm.

Nutrition:

Calories: 140 Cal Fat: 0.9 g Carbs: 27.1 g Protein: 6.3 g Fiber: 6.2 g

292. Mushroom Marsala Rotini

Preparation Time: 25 minutes | **Cooking Time:** 15-120 minutes | **Servings:** 4

Ingredients:

3 Tablespoons Olive Oil	1 Small Onion, diced
4 Cloves Garlic, chopped	1/2 Pound Fresh Mushrooms, sliced
Sea Salt and Pepper	2 Tablespoons All-Purpose Flour
1/2 cup Marsala Wine	1 1/4 Teaspoon Better Than Bouillon No Beef Base Vegetarian
1 1/2 Cups Water	2 Tablespoons Vegan Butter

Directions:

On saute mode, add olive oil, when hot add onions, garlic, mushrooms, and season with sea salt. Cook for 3-4 minutes stirring frequently until fragrant.

Stir in flour and cook for 1 minute.

Add wine and deglaze the pot.

Add No Beef Base, water, and vegan butter. Stir to combine.

Turn the pot on to manual mode, seal, and set it to 5 minutes.

Quick-release and uncover.

Turn on saute mode and stir until the sauce becomes the desired consistency.

Enjoy!

Nutrition:

Calories: 140 Cal Fat: 0.9 g Carbs: 27.1 g Protein: 6.3 g Fiber: 6.2 g

293. Seitan with Apple Brandy Gravy

Preparation Time: 50 minutes | **Cooking Time:** 30-120 minutes | **Servings:** 4

Ingredients:

4 chicken-flavored seitan breasts	2 apples, peeled and sliced
1/4 cup brandy	1 3/4 cups apple cider
2 tablespoons olive oil	1 small onion, chopped
1 1/2 tablespoons vegan chicken-flavored bouillon	2 cloves garlic, minced
1 teaspoon dried thyme	1/8 teaspoon cinnamon
1/8 teaspoon nutmeg	Salt and pepper, to taste
3 tablespoons flour	

Directions:

Heat the olive oil on the sauté setting and cook the onion for 5 minutes. Add the garlic and cook for an additional minute.

Add the rest of the ingredients, except for the flour. Seal the lid and cook on high for 4 minutes. Let the pressure release naturally, then remove the lid and switch to the sauté setting.

Remove the seitan and cover it with foil to keep warm. Whisk in 2 to 3 tablespoons of flour to thicken the sauce and simmer for 30 minutes.

Add the seitan to reheat in the sauce for a few minutes right before you are ready to serve. Serve with a baked potato.

Nutrition:

Calories: 140 Cal Fat: 0.9 g Carbs: 27.1 g Protein: 6.3 g Fiber: 6.2 g

294. Kalamata Olive Seitan

Preparation Time: 15 minutes | **Cooking Time:** 30-120 minutes | **Servings:** 4

Ingredients:

6 chicken-flavored seitan breasts

1 stalk celery, minced

1 cup red wine

1/2 cup water

1/4 teaspoon ground thyme

1/2 teaspoon fresh ground pepper

1 cup pitted and sliced Kalamata olives

10 ounces grape tomatoes, halved

1 tablespoon tomato paste

1/2 teaspoon fennel seeds, crushed

2 cloves garlic, minced

Directions:

Spray the instant pot with nonstick spray. Combine all the ingredients.

Seal the lid and cook on high for 4 minutes, then allow pressure to release naturally. Serve with a leafy green salad.

Nutrition:

Calories: 140 Cal Fat: 0.9 g Carbs: 27.1 g Protein: 6.3 g Fiber: 6.2 g

295. Italian Mushroom Tofu Strata

Preparation Time: 12 minutes | **Cooking Time:** 30-120 minutes | **Servings:** 4

Ingredients:

8 ounces Italian bread, toasted, diced

½ cup chopped roasted red bell pepper

2 cups crumbled firm tofu

8 ounces cremini mushrooms, chopped

¼ teaspoon ground turmeric

½ teaspoon dried basil

2 teaspoons olive oil (optional

1 onion, minced

½ cup chopped fresh basil

2 tablespoons nutritional yeast

½ teaspoon onion powder

Salt and black pepper

3 plum tomatoes, chopped

1 cup vegetable broth

3 garlic cloves, minced

2 medium-size zucchini, thinly sliced

Directions:

Add the yeast, tofu, onion, basil, seasoning, turmeric, and broth in a blender.

Blend until smooth.

Combine the bell pepper, tomatoes, and basil in a bowl.

In another bowl combine the zucchini, garlic, mushroom, and bread.

Add half the tomato mixture into your instant pot.

Then add the zucchini mixture. Add the remaining tomato mixture on top of the zucchini mixture.

Finally, add the tofu mixture on top

Cook with the lid on for about 8 minutes.

Serve hot.

Nutrition:

Calories:680, Total Fat:71.8g, Saturated Fat:20.9g, Total Carbs:10g, Dietary Fiber:7g, Sugar:2g, Protein:3g, Sodium:525mg

Chapter 3: Side Dishes

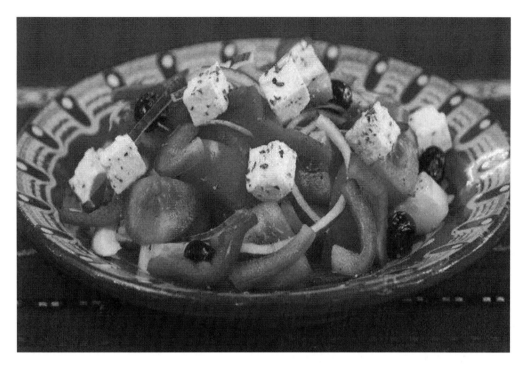

296. Coconut Mushroom Dumplings

Preparation Time: 10minutes | **Cooking Time:** 12minutes | **Servings:** 4

Ingredients:

1 lb ground mushroom	2 scallions, chopped
1 small cucumber, deseeded and grated	4 garlic cloves, minced
1 tsp freshly pureed ginger	1 tsp red chili flakes
2 tbsp tamari sauce	2 tbsp sesame oil
3 tbsp coconut oil, for frying	

Directions:

In a medium bowl, combine the mushroom, scallions, cucumber, garlic, ginger, red chili flakes, tamari sauce, and sesame oil. Using your hands, form 1-inch oval shapes out of the mixture and place them on a plate.

Heat the coconut oil in a medium skillet over medium heat; fry the dumplings for 12 minutes until brown on both sides and cooked

Transfer to a paper towel-lined plate to drain grease and serve with creamy spinach puree.

Nutrition:

Calories:439, Total Fat:31.9g, Saturated Fat:12.2g, Total Carbs:9g, Dietary Fiber:4g, Sugar:1g, Protein:36g, Sodium:574mg

297. Balsamic Beans Salad

Preparation Time: 10 minutes | **Cooking Time:** 00 minutes | **Servings:** 4

Ingredients:

1 cup of frozen green beans	1/4 cup chopped almonds
1/2 cup chopped green onions	3/4 cup mayonnaise
2 tablespoons balsamic vinegar	Black pepper to taste

Directions:

Place beans in a colander, and run warm water over them until they are thawed. Place in a large bowl.

Toast almonds in a skillet over medium heat. Then combine with beans.

Stir in onions, and mayonnaise. Mix in balsamic vinegar, and season with pepper. Cover, and refrigerator.

Nutrition:
Calories145, Total Fat 10.9g, Saturated Fat 2.6g, Cholesterol 14mg, Sodium 263mg, Total Carbohydrate 9.4g, Dietary Fiber 1.5g, Total Sugars 3.1g, Protein 3.3g, Calcium 67mg, Iron 1mg, Potassium 94mg, Phosphorus 44mg

298. Kale and Cauliflower Salad

Preparation Time: 10 minutes | **Cooking Time:** 00 minutes | **Servings:** 4

Ingredients:
- ½ cup lemon juice
- 1 teaspoon honey
- ¼ teaspoon ground black pepper
- ½ cup roasted cauliflower
- 1 tablespoon olive oil
- 1/8 teaspoon salt
- 1 bunch kale, cut into bite-size pieces
- ½ cup dried cranberries

Directions:
Whisk lemon juice, olive oil, honey, salt, and black pepper in a large bowl. Add kale, cauliflower, and cranberries; toss to combine.

Nutrition:
Calories 76, Total Fat 5g, Saturated Fat 1.2g, Cholesterol 2mg, Sodium 131mg, Total Carbohydrate 5.9g, Dietary Fiber 1.3g, Total Sugars 2.8g, Protein 1.8g, Calcium 59mg, Iron 1mg, Potassium 146mg, Phosphorus 88mg

299. Kale and Cucumber Salad

Preparation Time: 05 minutes | **Cooking Time:** 10 minutes | **Servings:** 4

Ingredients:
- 2 tablespoons olive oil
- 2 tablespoons water
- 1 tablespoon soy sauce
- 8 cups thinly sliced kale, packed
- 3 tablespoons lemon juice
- 1 tablespoon minced garlic
- 2 teaspoons honey
- 1 cucumber, peeled and sliced

Directions:
Combine olive oil, lemon juice, water, garlic, soy sauce, and honey in a small bowl. Stir until smooth.

Place kale and cucumbers in a large bowl. Pour dressing over kale; toss until combined.
Marinate for a minimum of 20 minutes, tossing occasionally.
Serve.

Nutrition:
Calories 80, Total Fat 2.9g, Saturated Fat 0.4g, Cholesterol 0mg, Sodium 115mg, Total Carbohydrate 13g, Dietary Fiber 1.1g, Total Sugars 5.6g, Protein 2g, Calcium 78mg, Iron 1mg, Potassium 231mg, Phosphorus156mg

300. Black Bean Meatball Salad

Preparation Time: 10 minutes | **Cooking Time:** 25 minutes | **Servings:** 4

Ingredients:
For the Meatballs:
- 1/2 cup quinoa, cooked
- 3 cloves of garlic, peeled
- 1 teaspoon ground dried coriander
- 1 teaspoon smoked paprika
- 1 cup cooked black beans
- 1 small red onion, peeled
- 1 teaspoon ground dried cumin

For the Salad:
- 1 large sweet potato, peeled, diced
- 1 teaspoon minced garlic
- 1/3 cup almonds
- ½ teaspoon salt
- 1 lemon, juiced
- 1 cup coriander leaves
- 1/3 teaspoon ground black pepper
- 1 1/2 tablespoons olive oil

Directions:
Prepare the meatballs and for this, place beans and puree in a blender, pulse until pureed, and place this mixture in a medium bowl.
Add onion and garlic, process until chopped, add to the bean mixture, add all the spices, stir until combined, and shape the mixture into uniform balls.
Bake the balls on a greased baking sheet for 25 minutes at 350 degrees F until browned.
Meanwhile, spread sweet potatoes on a baking sheet lined with baking paper, drizzle with ½ tablespoon oil, toss until coated, and bake for 20 minutes with the meatballs.

Prepare the dressing, and for this, place the remaining ingredients for the salad in a food processor and pulse until smooth.

Place roasted sweet potatoes in a bowl, drizzle with the dressing, toss until coated, and then top with meatballs.

Serve straight away.

Nutrition:
Calories: 140 Cal Fat: 8 g Carbs: 8 g Protein: 10 g Fiber: 4 g

301. Kale Slaw

Preparation Time: 10-75 minutes | **Cooking Time:** 15 minutes | **Servings:** 4

Ingredients:

1 small bunch kale, chopped	½ small head cabbage, shredded
¼ onion, thinly sliced	¼ cup tender herbs (cilantro, basil, parsley, chives)
¼ cup olive oil	4 tablespoons lemon juice
2 garlic cloves, minced	salt, pepper, and chili flakes

Directions:
Combine kale, cabbage, herbs, and onions in a large bowl.

Add olive oil, lemon juice, minced garlic, salt, pepper and mix well.

Add chili flakes, toss well before serving.

Nutrition:
Calories: 140 Cal Fat: 0.9 g Carbs: 27.1 g Protein: 6.3 g Fiber: 6.2 g

302. Sweet Potatoes

Preparation Time: 29 minutes | **Cooking Time:** 15-120 minutes | **Servings:** 4

Ingredients:
4 Sweet Potatoes, scrubbed and rinsed
1 1/2 Cups Water
Optional Toppings:
Scrambled Tofu, Avocado, Tomatoes
Vegan Butter, Coconut Sugar, Cinnamon
Arugula, Olive Oil, Lemon, Sea Salt

Directions:
Add water to the instant pot.

Place the steaming tray inside and put potatoes on top.

Cover with lid and seal.

Pressure cook for 18 minutes in manual mode.

When done cooking, allow pressure to release on its own (about 15 minutes).

Remove the lid.

Serve immediately with desired toppings. Enjoy!

Nutrition:
Calories: 140 Cal Fat: 0.9 g Carbs: 27.1 g Protein: 6.3 g Fiber: 6.2 g

303. Baked Sweet Potatoes With Corn Salad

Preparation Time: 15-30 minutes | **Cooking Time:** 35 minutes | **Servings:** 4

Ingredients:
For the baked sweet potatoes:

3 tbsp olive oil	4 medium sweet potatoes, peeled and cut into ½-inch cubes
2 limes, juiced	Salt and black pepper to taste
¼ tsp cayenne pepper	2 scallions, thinly sliced

For the corn salad:

1 (15 oz) can sweet corn kernels, drained	½ tbsp, plant butter, melted
1 large green chili, deseeded and minced	1 tsp cumin powder

Directions:
For the baked sweet potatoes:
Preheat the oven to 400 F and lightly grease a baking sheet with cooking spray.

In a medium bowl, add the sweet potatoes, lime juice, salt, black pepper, and cayenne pepper. Toss well and spread the mixture on the baking sheet. Bake in the oven until the potatoes soften, 20 to 25 minutes.

Remove from the oven, transfer to a serving plate, and garnish with the scallions.

For the corn salad:
In a medium bowl, mix the corn kernels, butter, green chili, and cumin powder. Serve the sweet potatoes with the corn salad.

Nutrition:
Calories 372 Fats 20. 7g Carbs 41. 7g Protein 8. 9g

304. Cashew Siam Salad

Preparation Time: 10 minutes | **Cooking Time:** 3 minutes | **Servings:** 4

Ingredients:
Salad:
4 cups baby spinach, rinsed, drained
½ cup pickled red cabbage
Dressing:
1-inch piece ginger, finely chopped
1 tsp. chili garlic paste
1 tbsp. soy sauce
½ tbsp. rice vinegar
1 tbsp. sesame oil
3 tbsp. avocado oil
Toppings:
½ cup raw cashews, unsalted
¼ cup fresh cilantro, chopped

Directions:
Put the spinach and red cabbage in a large bowl. Toss to combine and set the salad aside.

Toast the cashews in a frying pan over medium-high heat, stirring occasionally until the cashews are golden brown. This should take about 3 minutes. Turn off the heat and set the frying pan aside.

Mix all the dressing ingredients in a medium-sized bowl and use a spoon to mix them into a smooth dressing.

Pour the dressing over the spinach salad and top with the toasted cashews.

Toss the salad to combine all ingredients and transfer the large bowl to the fridge. Allow the salad to chill for up to one hour – doing so will guarantee a better flavor. Alternatively, the salad can be served right away, topped with the optional cilantro. Enjoy!

Nutrition:
Calories 236 Carbohydrates 6. 1 g Fats 21. 6 g Protein 4. 2 g

305. Chickpea Curry

Preparation Time: 10 minutes | **Cooking Time:** 30 minutes | **Servings:** 2

Ingredients:
½ cup dried chickpeas rinsed
2 cups of water
1 tablespoon vegetable oil
½ teaspoon cumin seeds
1 small onion finely diced
½ teaspoon ginger powder
½ teaspoon garlic powder
½ tablespoon coriander powder
1 teaspoon salt
¼ teaspoon turmeric powder
1 tomato cored and finely diced,
½ cup parsley fresh, chopped
1/4 teaspoon garam masala

Directions:
In a bowl, combine the chickpeas and 2 cups of warm water and let soak for at least 4 hours or up to overnight. Drain the chickpeas and set them aside.

Select the High Sauté setting on the Instant Pot and heat the vegetable oil. Add the cumin seeds directly to the hot oil at the bottom edges of the Instant Pot and cook until they start to sizzle, about 1 minute. Add the chopped onions and cook, stirring occasionally, until translucent, about 5 minutes. Add the ginger powder and garlic powder and sauté until aromatic, about 1 minute. Add the coriander powder, salt, turmeric powder, and chickpeas; pour in the 2 cups water, and stir well.

Secure the lid and set the Pressure Release to Sealing. Press the Cancel button to reset the cooking program, then select the Pressure Cook or Manual setting and set the cooking time for 35 minutes at High Pressure.

Let the pressure release naturally; this will take 10 to 20 minutes. Open the pot and stir in the tomatoes and garam masala. Select the High Sauté setting and cook until the tomatoes soften about 5 minutes. Press the Cancel button to turn off the Instant Pot. Ladle into bowls, sprinkle with the parsley, and serve.

Nutrition:
Calories 202, Total Fat 9. 2g, Saturated Fat 1. 4g, Cholesterol 0mg, Sodium 1186mg, Total Carbohydrate 27. 9g, Dietary Fiber 7. 8g, Total Sugars 7. 3g, Protein 8. 2g

306. Easy Lentil and Vegetable Curry

Preparation Time: 10 minutes | **Cooking Time:** 45 minutes | **Servings:** 2

Ingredients:

3 ½ cups water	½ tablespoon butter
¼ teaspoon cumin seeds	½ teaspoon coriander seeds
¼ teaspoon turmeric powder	¼ teaspoon paprika
½ teaspoon garam masala	½ teaspoon garlic powder
¼ teaspoon ginger powder	¼ cup onion, finely chopped
2 cups chopped veggies of your choice (red pepper, carrot, cabbage, broccoli, etc.	¼ cup dried red lentils
1 1/2 cups vegetable stock	½ full-fat milk
¼ cup green peas	1 teaspoon lime juice
¼ teaspoon of sea salt	¼ teaspoon ground pepper

Directions:

Select the High Sauté setting on the Instant Pot and heat the butter. Add the cumin seeds directly to the melted butter at the bottom edges of the Instant Pot and cook until they start to sizzle, about 1 minute. Add the onion and cook, stirring occasionally, until translucent, about 5 minutes. Add the ginger powder and garlic powder and sauté until aromatic, about 1 minute. Add the coriander seeds, salt, paprika, turmeric powder, and chopped vegetables and red lentils; pour in the 1 1/2 cups water, and stir well.

Secure the lid and set the Pressure Release to Sealing. Press the Cancel button to reset the cooking program, then select the Pressure Cook or Manual setting and set the cooking time for 35 minutes at High Pressure.

Let the pressure release naturally; this will take 10 to 20 minutes. Open the Instant Pot and stir in the green peas and garam masala milk. Select the High Sauté setting and cook for 2 minutes. Press the Cancel button to turn off the Instant Pot. Ladle into bowls, sprinkle with the cilantro and lime juice, serve.

Nutrition:

Calories 200, Total Fat 4. 2g, Saturated Fat 2. 4g, Cholesterol 8mg, Sodium 331mg, Total Carbohydrate 31. 3g, Dietary Fiber 11. 9g, Total Sugars 5. 8g, Protein 9. 8g

307. Herbed Lentil Chili

Preparation Time: 10 minutes | **Cooking Time:** 20 minutes | **Servings:** 2

Ingredients:

1 tablespoon coconut oil	1 small onion chopped
½ teaspoon garlic powder	1 zucchini chopped
1 leek chopped	½ tablespoon paprika
¼ teaspoon cumin powder	¼ teaspoon coriander powder
½ teaspoon dried basil	¼ teaspoon dry mustard
1 cup crushed tomatoes	½ cup dry lentils
1 1/2 cups low sodium vegetable broth	Salt to taste
¼ teaspoon pepper	

Directions:

Select the "Sauté" setting on Instant Pot. Add coconut oil and let heat up. Add onions, garlic powder, zucchinis, and leeks. Sauté until onions are softened and lightly browned, about 4 minutes. Add paprika, cumin powder, coriander powder, basil, mustard and stir well for a minute or two. Add tomatoes, lentils, broth, salt to taste, and pepper.

Select "Cancel", then close the lid. Turn steam release handle to "Sealing" position. Select "Bean/Chili" and set the time for 14 minutes. Press "Cancel" and let Instant Pot naturally release pressure until float valve drops down and lid unlocks; alternatively, press "Cancel" and let Instant Pot naturally release for 10 minutes; then turn steam release valve to "Venting" until float valve drops down and lid unlocks.

Nutrition:

Calories 296, Calories from Fat 27, Fat 3g, Sodium 596mg, Potassium 935mg, Carbohydrates 49g, Fiber 22g, Sugar 6g, Protein 18g

308. Garbanzo Beans with Kale

Preparation Time: 05 minutes | **Cooking Time:** 30 minutes | **Servings:** 2

Ingredients:

½ cup dried garbanzo beans rinsed	2 cups of water
½ cup tomato paste	¼ teaspoon garlic powder
¼ teaspoon ginger powder	½ tablespoon curry powder
¼ teaspoon cinnamon powder	¼ teaspoon salt
¼ teaspoon ground black pepper	2 cups fresh kale

Directions:

Add garbanzo beans and water to the Instant Pot. Lock lid.

Press the beans button and cook for the default time of 30 minutes. When the timer beeps, let the pressure release naturally for 10 minutes. Quick-release any additional pressure until the float valve drops and then unlock the lid. Drain any extra liquid.

Stir in remaining ingredients. Switch to Low Pressure and simmer for 4 minutes to heat through and wilt kale.

Transfer mixture to a serving dish and serve warm.

Nutrition:

Calories 129, Total Fat 1. 8g, Saturated Fat 0. 1g, Cholesterol 0mg, Sodium 395mg, Total Carbohydrate 26. 6g, Dietary Fiber 6. 1g, Total Sugars 8. 1g, Protein 7. 1g

309. Three-Lentil Curry

Preparation Time: 10 minutes | **Cooking Time:** 25 minutes | **Servings:** 2

Ingredients:

½ tablespoon coconut oil	1 teaspoon garlic powder
1 teaspoon ginger powder	½ tablespoon garam masala
1 teaspoon cumin powder	¼ teaspoon turmeric powder
¼ teaspoon table salt	¼ teaspoon paprika
1 cinnamon stick 4-inch stick	2 green cardamom pods
1 bay leaf	½ cup red tomatoes chopped
¼ cup red lentils	¼ cup brown lentils
¼ cup green lentils	¼ cup
4 cups of water	1/2 cup coconut cream

Directions:

Press Sauté, set the time for 5 minutes.

Add coconut oil to the Instant Pot. Add the garlic powder, ginger powder, garam masala, cumin powder, turmeric powder, salt, paprika, cinnamon stick, cardamom pods, and bay leaves. Stir until fragrant, about 1 minute. Add the tomatoes and cook, stirring often, until it just begins to break down, 1 to 2 minutes.

Turn off the Sauté function. Stir in the red lentils, brown lentils, and green lentils until coated in the spices. Stir in the water and lock the lid onto the Instant Pot.

Press Pressure Cook on Max Pressure for 16 minutes with the Keep Warm setting off.

Use the Quick-release method to bring the Instant Pot pressure back to normal. Unlatch the lid and open the Instant Pot. Remove and discard the cinnamon stick, cardamom pods, and bay leaves. Stir in the cream until uniform, then set the lid askew over the Instant Pot for 5 minutes to blend the flavors. Stir again before serving.

Nutrition:

Calories 340, Total Fat 21. 1g, Saturated Fat 16. 3g, Cholesterol 0mg, Sodium 390mg, Total Carbohydrate 30. 8g, Dietary Fiber 10. 8g, Total Sugars 5. 7g, Protein 10. 4g

310. Baked Beans with Mustard

Preparation Time: 05 minutes | **Cooking Time:** 15 minutes | **Servings:** 2

Ingredients:

½ cup kidney beans rinsed and drained	½ cup pinto beans rinsed and drained
½ cup chickpea beans rinsed and drained	1 cup of water
1/2 cup tomato paste	1 teaspoon honey
½ tablespoon ground mustard	1 teaspoon paprika

Directions:

Add the kidney beans, pinto beans, chickpeas beans, water, tomato paste, honey, ground mustard, and paprika. Lock the lid into place and turn the valve to "Sealing. " Select Manual or Pressure Cook and adjust the pressure to High. Set the time for 8 minutes. When cooking ends, let the pressure release naturally for 15 minutes, then turn the valve to "Venting" to quickly release the remaining pressure. Unlock and remove the lid and stir well before serving.

Nutrition:

Calories 268, Total Fat 2. 7g, Saturated Fat 0. 3g, Cholesterol 0mg, Sodium 555mg, Total Carbohydrate 50. 6g, Dietary Fiber 13g, Total Sugars 11. 8g, Protein 14g

311. Rosemary Lentils, Beans Curry

Preparation Time: 10 minutes | **Cooking Time:** 30 minutes | **Servings:** 2

Ingredients:

1 cup of water	½ cup of brown rice
½ cup brown lentils	½ cup navy beans pre-soaked or quick-soaked
½ tablespoon rosemary	1 teaspoon garlic powder
½ cup chopped onions	½ cup low sodium vegetable broth

Directions:

In your Instant Pot, sauté the onions in the vegetable broth and garlic powder. First, heat the broth on medium and statue the onion for about 4 minutes until translucent then add the garlic powder for another 30 seconds.
Add the rest of the ingredients to Instant Pot, and stir it well.
Close the lid, and seal the vent Instant Pot. Set the cooker for 23 minutes, and cook at High pressure on the Manual setting.
Release the pressure naturally.
Serve and season as desired.

Nutrition:

Calories 269, Total Fat 1. 6g, Saturated Fat 0. 3g, Cholesterol 0mg, Sodium 255mg, Total Carbohydrate 55. 2g, Dietary Fiber 7. 4g, Total Sugars 1. 6g, Protein 9. 9g

312. Fava Beans

Preparation Time: 15 minutes | **Cooking Time:** 30 minutes | **Servings:** 2

Ingredients:

1 teaspoon olive oil	1 small onion, chopped
1 tomato, chopped	1 tablespoon tomato paste
1 cup of water	½ cup fava beans, drained
½ tablespoon ground cumin	1/2 teaspoons salt
1 1/2 teaspoons ground black pepper	½ teaspoon ground red pepper
1 tablespoon finely chopped parsley	

Directions:

In your Instant Pot, sauté olive oil and add onions. Cook and stir for 2 minutes. Add chopped tomatoes and tomato paste; cook until tomatoes are mushy, about 4 minutes.
Pour fava beans into Instant Pot. Add 1 cup water, cumin, salt, black pepper, and ground red pepper; stir well. Close the lid, and seal the vent Instant Pot. Set the cooker for 23 minutes, and cook at High pressure on the Manual setting.
Release the pressure naturally.
Stir in parsley.

Nutrition:

Calories 186, Total Fat 3. 5g, Saturated Fat 0. 5g, Cholesterol 0mg, Sodium 602mg, Total Carbohydrate 29. 9g, Dietary Fiber 11. 6g, Total Sugars 5. 5g, Protein 11. 4g

313. Spinach Split Pigeon Pea

Preparation Time: 15 minutes | **Cooking Time:** 15 minutes | **Servings:** 2

Ingredients:

½ cup split pigeon pea	1 cup spinach chopped
½ tablespoon vegetable oil	¼ teaspoon cumin seeds
1 green chili pepper sliced (optional	¼ teaspoon ginger powder
½ teaspoon garlic powder	1 tomato large, chopped

2 cups of water   ¼ teaspoon garam masala

¼ teaspoon salt   1/8 teaspoon turmeric powder

1/4 teaspoon red chili powder

Directions:
Start the Instant Pot in Sauté mode and heat vegetable oil in it. Add cumin seeds, green chili, ginger powder, and garlic powder.
Sauté for 30 seconds until garlic turns golden brown, then add chopped tomatoes and spices.
Add the split pigeon pea and water. Stir well. Press Cancel and close the Instant Pot lid with the vent in the Sealing position.
Press Manual or Pressure Cook mode for 3 minutes. When the Instant Pot beeps, do a Quick Pressure Release.
Open the lid and add chopped spinach and garam masala. Press Sauté mode. simmer for 2 minutes until the dal starts boiling and spinach is mixed with the lentils.
Spinach split pigeon pea is ready to be served.

Nutrition:
Calories 240, Total Fat 4. 8g, Saturated Fat 1g, Cholesterol 0mg, Sodium 325mg, Total Carbohydrate 38. 8g, Dietary Fiber 4. 5g, Total Sugars 5. 8g, Protein 13. 4g

314. **Mexican Beans**

Preparation Time: 15 minutes | **Cooking Time:** 35 minutes | **Servings:** 2

Ingredients:
½ cup dried pinto beans   2 cups of water

1 small onion, chopped   1 medium ripe tomato, chopped

1 fresh bell pepper, chopped   1 tablespoon fresh cilantro, chopped

Directions:
Select the High Sauté setting on the Instant Pot and add pinto beans, water, onion, ripe tomato, and bell pepper. Secure the lid and set the Pressure Release to Sealing. Press the Cancel button to reset the cooking program, then select the Pressure Cook or Manual setting and set the cooking time for 35 minutes at High Pressure.

Let the pressure release naturally; this will take 10 to 20 minutes.
Garnish with fresh cilantro.

Nutrition:
Calories 212, Total Fat 0. 9g, Saturated Fat 0. 1g, Cholesterol 0mg, Sodium 19mg, Total Carbohydrate 40. 4g, Dietary Fiber 9. 8g, Total Sugars 7. 1g, Protein 11. 9g

315. **Beans and Greens**

Preparation Time: 10 minutes | **Cooking Time:** 35 minutes | **Servings:** 2

Ingredients:
2 cups vegetable broth   ½ cup chopped spinach

1 cup red kidney beans   ½ cup black beans

¼ cup pinto beans,   ¼ cup chickpeas

1 tablespoon butter   ¼ tablespoon garlic powder

Salt to taste black pepper to taste

Directions:
Place broth and spinach into Instant Pot, and cook for 5 minutes, or until spinach is wilted. Mix in red kidney beans, black beans, chickpea and pinto beans and liquid, and butter. Season with garlic powder, salt, and black pepper. Secure the lid and set the Pressure Release to Sealing. Press the Cancel button to reset the cooking program, then select the Pressure Cook or Manual setting and set the cooking time for 30 minutes at high pressure.
Let the pressure release naturally; this will take 10 to 20 minutes.

Nutrition:
Calories 372, Total Fat 5. 3g, Saturated Fat 2. 3g, Cholesterol 8mg, Sodium 416mg, Total Carbohydrate 59. 4g, Dietary Fiber 14. 9g, Total Sugars 3. 6g, Protein

316. Soybean, Lentil, and Zucchini Curry

Preparation Time: 10 minutes | **Cooking Time:** 15 minutes | **Servings:** 2

Ingredients:

¼ tablespoon vegetable oil	1 cup finely chopped onions
¼ tablespoon curry paste	2 cups vegetable broth
½ cup finely chopped zucchini	½ tablespoon ginger powder
1/8 teaspoon ground red pepper	1 teaspoon garlic powder
½ cup dried small red lentils	½ cup yellow soybeans, rinsed and drained
1 tablespoon minced fresh parsley	¼ teaspoon salt
¼ teaspoon freshly ground black pepper Fresh coriander	2 tablespoons plain fat-free yogurt

Directions:

Press Sauté to preheat the Instant Pot. When the word "Hot" appears on the display, add the vegetable oil and sauté the onions for about 5 minutes, until the onions are translucent. Stir curry paste; cook for 1 minute. Add 1/2 cup broth, zucchini, ginger powder, red pepper, and garlic powder; cook 5 minutes or until zucchini is tender, stirring occasionally.

Add the remaining broth, lentils, and soybeans. Lock the lid in place. Press Manual and adjust to 4 minutes of cooking time.

When the beep sounds, quickly release the pressure by pressing Cancel and twist the steam handle to the Venting position.

Stir in cilantro, salt, and black pepper. Garnish with coriander leaves and yogurt, if desired.

Nutrition:

Calories 373, Total Fat 10g, Saturated Fat 1. 6g, Cholesterol 1mg, Sodium 1089mg, Total Carbohydrate 47g, Dietary Fiber 9. 5g, Total Sugars 6g, Protein 26. 5g

317. Spicy Navy Bean and Chard

Preparation Time: 05 minutes | **Cooking Time:** 20 minutes | **Servings:** 2

Ingredients:

½ tablespoon vegetable oil	¼ cup onions chopped
1 teaspoon garlic powder	2 cups vegetable broth
1 cup dried navy beans	½ cup chard stems removed, leaves sliced
1/8 teaspoon paprika	1/8 teaspoon sea salt

Directions:

Press Sauté to preheat the Instant pot. When the word "Hot" appears on the display, add the vegetable oil and sauté the onions and garlic powder for about 5 minutes, until the onions are translucent.

Add the navy beans and continue to stir. Stir in the first 2 cups of vegetable broth.

Lock the lid in place. Press Manual and adjust to 10 minutes of cooking time.

When the beep sounds, quickly release the pressure by pressing Cancel and twisting the steam handle to the Venting position.

Press Sauté and stir chopped green chard.

Cook, stirring constantly until the chard has wilted about 2 minutes.

Taste and add salt if you think it's needed, and pinch more paprika, if you like more spice.

Nutrition:

Calories 191, Total Fat 5. 8g, Saturated Fat 1. 1g, Cholesterol 0mg, Sodium 1190mg, Total Carbohydrate 23. 7g, Dietary Fiber 7. 6g, Total Sugars 2. 8g, Protein 12. 4g

318. Carrot and Soy Bean Stir Fry

Preparation Time: 15 minutes | **Cooking Time:** 20 minutes | **Servings:** 2

Ingredients:

¼ cup cauliflower florets	¼ cup broccoli florets
1/2 cup dried soybeans	1 large carrot, chopped
½ cup vegetable broth	1 tablespoon butter
1 onion, chopped	½ cup pumpkin, sliced

2 large mushrooms,
sliced
Salt and pepper to
taste

1 tablespoon garlic
powder

Directions:

Select the Sauté setting on the Instant Pot, add the butter, and heat for 1 minute. Add the onions, carrots, garlic powder, salt, pumpkin, broccoli, cauliflower, and mushrooms. Sauté for about 10 minutes, until the vegetables give up some of their liquid and begin to brown just a bit. Add vegetable broth and soybeans.

Lock the lid into place. Select Pressure Cook or Manual, and adjust the pressure to High and the time to 12 minutes. After cooking, let the pressure release naturally for 10 minutes, then quickly release any remaining pressure.

Unlock the lid.

Taste the soybeans and adjust the seasoning.

Serve and enjoy.

Nutrition:

Calories 291, Total Fat 5. 2g, Saturated Fat 3. 1g, Cholesterol 0mg, Sodium 1089mg, Total Carbohydrate 13. 7g, Dietary Fiber 4. 6g, Total Sugars 1g, Protein 22. 4g

319. Tomato Chickpeas Curry

Preparation Time: 15 minutes | **Cooking Time:** 20 minutes | **Servings:** 2

Ingredients:

1 tablespoon avocado
oil
1 1/2 teaspoons garlic
powder

1½ cups chickpeas
drained and rinsed
Freshly ground black
pepper

5 tomatoes, cored and
diced
½ tablespoon coarsely
chopped fresh
rosemary
½ teaspoon kosher
salt
3 cups of water

Directions:

Select the Sauté setting on the Instant Pot, add the avocado oil. Add the tomatoes and sauté for about 3 minutes until they start to break down and tomatoes become saucy. Add the garlic powder, rosemary and sauté for 1 minute more. Add water and chickpeas, salt, and pepper.

Lock the lid into place. Select Pressure Cook or Manual, and adjust the pressure to High and the

time to 12 minutes. After cooking, let the pressure release naturally for 10 minutes, then quickly release any remaining pressure.

Unlock the lid.

Serve and enjoy.

Nutrition:

Calories 434, Total Fat 7. 6g, Saturated Fat 0. 9g, Cholesterol 0mg, Sodium 621mg, Total Carbohydrate 74. 1g, Dietary Fiber 21. 6g, Total Sugars 19. 2g, Protein 22. 4g

320. Lemony Lentil and Greens

Preparation Time: 10 minutes | **Cooking Time:** 25 minutes | **Servings:** 2

Ingredients:

½ cup brown lentils,
rinsed
1 onion, diced
2 cups vegetable broth
1/4 teaspoon paprika

½ tablespoon butter

½ cup kale, chopped
Juice of 1 lemon

Directions:

Select the Sauté setting on the Instant Pot, add the butter, onions, sprinkle with a pinch of sea salt, and cook for 1 minute.

Next, add the chopped kale and paprika then stir together. Cook for another 2 minutes until the kale is slightly soft. Add the brown lentils to the Instant Pot along with the vegetable broth.

Lock the lid into place. Select Pressure Cook or Manual, and adjust the pressure to High and the time to 20 minutes. After cooking, let the pressure release naturally for 10 minutes, then quickly release any remaining pressure. Unlock the lid.

Squeeze the juice of a lemon into the pot and stir together.

Nutrition:

Calories 264, Total Fat 4. 9g, Saturated Fat 2. 3g, Cholesterol 8mg, Sodium 798mg, Total Carbohydrate 36. 8g, Dietary Fiber 16. 2g, Total Sugars 4g, Protein 18. 4g

321. Moroccan Red Lentil Curry

Preparation Time: 10 minutes | **Cooking Time:** 30 minutes | **Servings:** 2

Ingredients:

½ cup dry red lentils
1 small onion, diced
1 potato, peeled and chopped
1 tablespoon coconut oil
½ teaspoon turmeric powder
¼ teaspoon nutmeg
Juice of ½ lemon
Fresh cilantro for topping

½ leek, diced
½ zucchini, peeled and chopped
½ teaspoon garlic powder
½ teaspoon cumin
¼ teaspoon coriander powder
2 cups vegetable broth
Salt to taste (if needed

Directions:

Select Sauté and adjust to Normal or Medium heat. Add the coconut oil to the Instant Pot and heat until shimmering. Add onions and the leeks. Cook for 2 minutes.

Next add the zucchini, garlic powder, and potatoes along with the spices. Stir together and cook for 1 minute then pour in vegetable broth. Add red lentils. Lock the lid into place. Select Pressure Cook or Manual, and adjust the pressure to High and the time to 20 minutes. After cooking, let the pressure release naturally for 10 minutes, then quickly release any remaining pressure.

Unlock the lid. Squeeze in the lemon juice and stir together. Garnish with fresh cilantro.

Nutrition:

Calories 383, Total Fat 9. 3g, Saturated Fat 6. 5g, Cholesterol 0mg, Sodium 784mg, Total Carbohydrate 56. 6g, Dietary Fiber 19. 3g, Total Sugars 6. 5g, Protein 20. 9g

322. White Bean Spinach & Tomato Curry

Preparation Time: 15 minutes | **Cooking Time:** 25 minutes | **Servings:** 2

Ingredients:

1 teaspoon vegetable oil

1 small onion, diced

1 zucchini, peeled and diced
½ teaspoon dried basil
¼ teaspoon pepper
½ cup spinach chopped
½ cup tomatoes

½ teaspoon garlic, powder
¼ teaspoon salt
1/2 teaspoon crushed red pepper
1 cup white beans, drained and rinsed
1 1/2 cups vegetable broth

Directions:

Select the Sauté setting on the Instant Pot, add the vegetable oil, and heat for 1 minute. Add the onion and sauté for 2 minutes, then add the zucchini, garlic powder, tomatoes, and seasonings (salt, pepper, and basil) and continue to sauté for another 2 minutes.

Add the spinach to the Instant Pot and cook until it starts to wilt. Pour vegetable broth and white beans.

Select Pressure Cook or Manual, and adjust the pressure to High and the time to 20 minutes. After cooking, let the pressure release naturally for 10 minutes, then quickly release any remaining pressure.

Unlock the lid and Serve.

Nutrition:

Calories 418, Total Fat 4. 2g, Saturated Fat 0. 9g, Cholesterol 0mg, Sodium 708mg, Total Carbohydrate 70. 6g, Dietary Fiber 18. 1g, Total Sugars 6. 9g, Protein 28. 3g

323. Spinach, Red Lentil and Bean Curry

Preparation Time: 25 minutes | **Cooking Time:** 10 minutes | **Servings:** 2

Ingredients:

½ cup red lentils
1/4 container plain yogurt
¼ teaspoon turmeric powder
¼ tablespoons coconut oil
1 teaspoon garlic powder
1 cup fresh spinach, coarsely chopped

1/8 cup tomato puree
½ teaspoon garam masala
¼ teaspoon ground cumin
1 onion, chopped
½ teaspoon ginger powder
2 tomatoes, chopped

1 1/2 cups vegetable broth
½ teaspoon fresh cilantro, chopped
1 cup mixed beans

Directions:

In a bowl, stir together the tomato puree and yogurt. Season with garam masala, turmeric powder, ground cumin, and. Stir until creamy.

Select the Sauté setting on the Instant Pot, add the coconut oil, Stir in chopped onions, garlic powder, and ginger powder; cook until onions begin to brown. Stir in spinach; cook until dark green and wilted. Gradually stir in yogurt mixture. Then mix in the tomato puree and cilantro.

Stir lentils and mixed beans into the mixture pour vegetable broth mix well. Select Pressure Cook or Manual, and adjust the pressure to High and the time to 20 minutes. After cooking, let the pressure release naturally for 10 minutes, then quickly release any remaining pressure. Unlock the lid.

Serve and enjoy.

Nutrition:

Calories346, Total Fat 3. 1g, Saturated Fat 1. 9g, Cholesterol 2mg, Sodium 519mg, Total Carbohydrate 62. 4g, Dietary Fiber 25. 2g, Total Sugars 9. 7g, Protein 21. 8g

324. Coconut-Apple-Ginger Beans

Preparation Time: 25 minutes | **Cooking Time:** 22min | **Servings:** 2

Ingredients:

1 tablespoon vegetable oil
¼ teaspoon paprika
¼ teaspoon cumin seed
¼ teaspoon turmeric powder
1 small onion, finely chopped
¼ teaspoon garlic powder
1/8 teaspoon ginger powder
1 large apple
1 cup pinto beans
1 cup of coconut milk
½ tablespoon fresh lime juice
Kosher salt
Freshly ground pepper

Directions:

Select the Sauté setting on the Instant Pot, add the vegetable oil. Cook paprika, cumin seed, and turmeric powder, stirring, until fragrant, about

30 seconds. Add chopped onions, garlic powder, and ginger powder and cook, stirring, until softened, about 1 minute.

Add apples and pinto beans and stir to coat. Stir in coconut milk and 2 cups of water. Select Pressure Cook or Manual, and adjust the pressure to High and the time to 20 minutes. After cooking, let the pressure release naturally for 10 minutes, then quickly release any remaining pressure.

Unlock the lid. Add lime juice and season with salt and pepper.

Nutrition:

Calories 339, Total Fat 11. 2g, Saturated Fat 4. 5g, Cholesterol 0mg, Sodium 11mg, Total Carbohydrate 51. 3g, Dietary Fiber 11. 5g, Total Sugars 14. 9g, Protein 11. 6g

325. Lentil Chili

Preparation Time: 05 minutes | **Cooking Time:** 23 minutes | **Servings:** 2

Ingredients:

1 tablespoon butter
1 onion, chopped
½ teaspoon garlic powder
½ cup dry lentils
½ cup dry buckwheat
2 cups vegetable broth
1 cup tomatoes, chopped
1 teaspoon chili powder
1 teaspoon cumin seed
Salt and pepper to taste

Directions:

Select the Sauté setting on the Instant Pot, add the butter, and heat for 1 minute. Add onions and garlic powder and sauté for 2 minutes. Stir in the lentils and buckwheat. Add the broth, tomatoes, chili powder, cumin seed, and salt and pepper to taste.

Select Pressure Cook or Manual, and adjust the pressure to High and the time to 20 minutes. After cooking, let the pressure release naturally for 10 minutes, then quickly release any remaining pressure.

Adjust the salt and pepper and serve.

Nutrition:

Calories 453, Total Fat 9. 8g, Saturated Fat 4. 5g, Cholesterol 15mg, Sodium 829mg, Total Carbohydrate 70. 5g, Dietary Fiber 21. 8g, Total Sugars 6. 7g, Protein 24. 8g

326. Lemony Lentils with Spinach

Preparation Time: 10 minutes | **Cooking Time:** 20 minutes | **Servings:** 2

Ingredients:

1 tablespoon coconut oil

1 small onion, diced

½ carrot, diced

½ cup broccoli

1 teaspoon garlic powder

½ teaspoon kosher salt

Ground black pepper to taste

½ teaspoon crushed red pepper flakes, or to taste

½ cup green lentils

½ cup diced tomatoes

1 cup vegetable broth

½ cup spinach, chopped

1 lemon, zest, and juice

Directions:

Select the Sauté setting on the Instant Pot, add coconut oil and stir onions and carrots, and broccoli in the hot oil until softened, about 2 minutes. Add garlic powder, kosher salt, black pepper, and red pepper flakes; cook and stir to coat for 1 minute.

Stir lentils, tomatoes, and their juice, and vegetable broth into onion mixture. Lock the lid into place. Select Pressure Cook or Manual, and adjust the pressure to High and the time to 12 minutes. After cooking, let the pressure release naturally for 10 minutes, then quickly release any remaining pressure.

Add spinach, lemon zest, and lemon juice; cook until spinach is wilted, about 5 minutes. Season with salt and black pepper.

Nutrition:

Calories291, Total Fat 8. 3g, Saturated Fat 6. 2g, Cholesterol 0mg, Sodium 987mg, Total Carbohydrate 39. 8g, Dietary Fiber 17. 4g, Total Sugars 5. 8g, Protein 16. 5g

327. Garlic Lentil Curry

Preparation Time: 10 minutes | **Cooking Time:** 15min | **Servings:** 2

Ingredients:

¼ cup dry brown lentils

1/4 cup dry red lentils

2 cups of water

5 whole garlic cloves

¼ teaspoon salt

¼ teaspoon ground coriander

¼ teaspoon cayenne pepper, or to taste

1/8 teaspoon turmeric powder

1 tablespoon butter

1 small onion, sliced

½ teaspoon cumin seeds

1/8 cup soy milk

Directions:

Soak brown and red lentils in ample cool water for 1 hour to overnight. Drain and rinse.

Select the Sauté setting on the Instant Pot, add butter and stir onions, and cook, stirring often, until they turn golden brown. Stir in the cumin seeds, and cook until fragrant, about 1 minute. Pour in the water, then add garlic, salt, ground coriander, turmeric powder, and cayenne pepper.

Add both lentils.

Select Pressure Cook or Manual, and adjust the pressure to High and the time to 12 minutes. After cooking, let the pressure release naturally for 10 minutes, then quickly release any remaining pressure.

Stir soy milk into the lentils.

Nutrition:

Calories 171, Total Fat 6. 5g, Saturated Fat 3. 8g, Cholesterol 15mg, Sodium 700mg, Total Carbohydrate 20. 3g, Dietary Fiber 8. 8g, Total Sugars 2. 7g, Protein 7. 9g

328. Moroccan Black-Eyed Peas

Preparation Time: 15 minutes | **Cooking Time:** 30 minutes | **Servings:** 2

Ingredients:

½ cup dried black-eyed peas (cowpeas)

1 small onion, chopped

1 cup tomato paste

1 tablespoon coconut oil

1/8 cup chopped fresh cilantro

½ teaspoon garlic powder

½ teaspoons salt

½ teaspoon cumin powder

½ teaspoon paprika

1 teaspoon ginger powder

2 cups of water

Directions:

Place black-eyed peas into a large container and cover with several inches of cool water; let it stand for 8 hours to overnight. Drain and rinse peas.

Combine black-eyed peas, onions, tomato paste, coconut oil, cilantro, garlic powder, salt, cumin, paprika, and ginger powder in an Instant Pot; pour 2 cups of water over the pea mixture.

Select Pressure Cook or Manual, and adjust the pressure to High and the time to 12 minutes. After cooking, let the pressure release naturally for 10 minutes, then quickly release any remaining pressure.

Serve and enjoy.

Nutrition:

Calories 233, Total Fat 8. 1g, Saturated Fat 6g, Cholesterol 0mg, Sodium 733mg, Total Carbohydrate 37. 5g, Dietary Fiber 8. 4g, Total Sugars 17. 7g, Protein 9. 3g

329. Black-Eyed Pea Chowder

Preparation Time: 15 minutes | **Cooking Time:** 30 minutes | **Servings:** 2

Ingredients:

½ cup chopped leeks	1 tablespoon olive oil
½ cup chopped onions	1 cup chopped green bell pepper
½ cup black-eyed peas	1 cup diced tomatoes
½ cup of corn	1 cup vegetable broth
½ cup kale	

Directions:

Select the Sauté setting on the Instant Pot, add olive oil and onions in the Instant Pot, and cook until tender. Add the green bell pepper, chopped leek, black-eyed peas, tomatoes, corn, and kale. Mix well.

Pour vegetable broth. Select Pressure Cook or Manual, and adjust the pressure to High and the time to 12 minutes. After cooking, let the pressure release naturally for 10 minutes, then quickly release any remaining pressure.

Open lid. Serve and enjoy.

Nutrition:

Calories 147, Total Fat 1. 4g, Saturated Fat 0. 1g, Cholesterol 0mg, Sodium 37mg, Total Carbohydrate 30. 9g, Dietary Fiber 6. 2g, Total Sugars 8. 7g, Protein 6. 8g

330. Baked Barbeque Beans

Preparation Time: 15 minutes | **Cooking Time:** 40 minutes | **Servings:** 2

Ingredients:

½ cup dry navy beans	2 cups of water
¼ teaspoon salt	1 small onion, finely chopped
¼ red or green bell pepper, cored, seeded, and finely chopped	¼ cup barbecue sauce
½ teaspoon mustard	¼ cup lemon juice
½ cup honey	Enough water

Directions:

Add navy beans, water, and salt into Instant Pot. Cook on Manual (High Pressure) for 25 minutes. Allow the pressure to naturally release.

Remove the lid and pour beans into a colander/strainer. Rinse with cold water. Set aside.

Set Instant Pot to Sauté setting. Add bell pepper and onions and cook until tender. Turn IP off. Add barbecue sauce, mustard, lemon juice to the Instant pot and stir well to combine. Add honey, water, and beans and stir to combine.

Secure IP lid, close steam valve, and cook on Manual (High pressure) for 15 minutes. Allow the pressure to naturally release.

Carefully open the lid, and gently stir the mixture to combine. Enjoy!

Nutrition:

Calories 510, Total Fat 1. 4g, Saturated Fat 0. 3g, Cholesterol 0mg, Sodium 661mg, Total Carbohydrate 118. 1g, Dietary Fiber 14. 2g, Total Sugars 82. 7g, Protein 12. 9g

331. Black Beans with Mint

Preparation Time: 15 minutes | **Cooking Time:** 40 minutes | **Servings:** 2

Ingredients:

½ cup dried black beans	1 tablespoon coconut oil
½ cup chopped onions	½ cup chopped red bell pepper
¼ medium jalapeno pepper, seeded and finely chopped	1 teaspoon garlic powder

½ teaspoons salt	½ teaspoon cumin seed
¼ teaspoon coriander powder	1/8 teaspoon dried basil
1 bay leaves	2 cups vegetable stock
½ cup halved cherry tomatoes	½ cup chopped mint leaves

Directions:

Set an Instant Pot to Sauté. Allow to heat for 3 minutes. Add coconut oil, onions, red bell peppers, jalapeno pepper, garlic powder, salt, cumin seed, coriander powder, and basil. Cook stirring often, about 5 minutes.

Add bay leaves, stock, and black beans. Stir to blend. Cover Instant Pot, and fasten the lid. Lock and seal steam valve. Set to High Pressure for 30 minutes.

When the cooking time has ended, allow Instant Pot to naturally release pressure for 20 minutes. Uncover and turn off Instant Pot.

To serve, spoon beans and cooking liquid into bowls and top evenly with cherry tomatoes and mint leaves.

Nutrition:

Calories 277, Total Fat 8. 1g, Saturated Fat 6. 1g, Cholesterol 0mg, Sodium 646mg, Total Carbohydrate 41. 3g, Dietary Fiber 11. 3g, Total Sugars 6g, Protein 13g

332. Curried Pinto Beans

Preparation Time: 15 minutes | **Cooking Time:** 30 minutes | **Servings:** 2

Ingredients:

¼ teaspoon of sea salt	½ tablespoon garlic powder
½ cup onion, chopped	½ teaspoon dried rosemary
1 cup dried pinto beans	2 cups vegetable broth

Directions:

Place all ingredients into the Instant Pot. Add 2 cups of vegetable broth. Stir to mix.

Cover with the lid and ensure the vent is in the "Sealing" position. Pressure Cook on High for 30 minutes. Allow the steam pressure to release naturally for 20 minutes.

Serve and enjoy.

Nutrition:

Calories 393, Total Fat 2. 7g, Saturated Fat 0. 6g, Cholesterol 0mg, Sodium 1011mg, Total Carbohydrate 65. 7g, Dietary Fiber 15. 9g, Total Sugars 4. 5g, Protein 26. 2g

333. Pinto Beans Curry

Preparation Time: 15 minutes | **Cooking Time:** 60 minutes | **Servings:** 2

Ingredients:

½ tablespoon butter	1 red onion
½ teaspoon garlic powder	1 1/2 cup dry pinto beans
1 bay leaf	Freshly cracked pepper
2 cups reduced-sodium vegetable broth	½ cup diced tomatoes

Directions:

Add butter, onion, garlic powder, pinto beans, bay leaves, pepper, and broth to the pot, stir briefly to combine, then place the lid on the Instant Pot. Close the steam valve, press the Manual button, select High pressure, then press the + button to increase the time to 35 minutes. Allow the pinto beans to cook through the 35-minute cycle, then let the pressure release naturally (you'll know the pressure has been released when the silver float valve has fallen back down and is no longer flush with the top of the lid).

Once the pressure has been released, open the steam valve, and then remove the lid. Discard the bay leaf. Add the diced tomatoes with all their juices, then stir to combine.

Press the Cancel button to Cancel the "keep warm" function, then press the Sauté button and use the Adjust button to select the "Normal" heat level. Let the mixture simmer, stirring often, until the beans are very tender and the liquid has thickened.

Serve and enjoy.

Nutrition:

Calories 409, Total Fat 4. 3g, Saturated Fat 2. 1g, Cholesterol 8mg, Sodium 567mg, Total Carbohydrate 71g, Dietary Fiber 17. 9g, Total Sugars 7. 7g, Protein 21. 9g

334. Tempeh White Bean Gravy

Preparation Time: 05 minutes | **Cooking Time:** 20 minutes | **Servings:** 2

Ingredients:

½ cup cups vegetable broth	¼ cup of soy sauce
¼ cup of coconut oil	1 teaspoon garlic powder
½ cup chopped onion	1 cup chopped tempeh
1/8 teaspoon dried basil	1/8 teaspoon dried parsley
1/8 teaspoon ground black pepper	1 cup white beans, drained and rinsed
Enough water	

Directions:

Add vegetable broth, soy sauce, coconut oil, garlic powder, onion, tempeh, basil, parsley, black pepper, and white beans to the Instant Pot. Pour the remaining ¼ cup water over everything.

Choose the soup function for 20 minutes.

Once done, remove the lid.

Serve and enjoy.

Nutrition:

Calories 376, Total Fat 29. 4g, Saturated Fat 23. 6g, Cholesterol 0mg, Sodium 2233mg, Total Carbohydrate 22. 4g, Dietary Fiber 4. 9g, Total Sugars 4. 2g, Protein 9. 2g

335. Three-Bean Chili

Preparation Time: 10 minutes | **Cooking Time:** 30 minutes | **Servings:** 2

Ingredients:

¼ cup dried pinto beans soaked 8 hours or overnight	¼ cup dried kidney beans soaked 8 hours or overnight
¼ cup dried black beans soaked 8 hours or overnight	½ tablespoon olive oil
1 small onion chopped	1 teaspoon salt
½ tablespoon tomato paste	½ teaspoon garlic powder
1 teaspoon paprika	1 teaspoon cumin powder
½ teaspoon coriander powder	½ cup crushed tomatoes 1 can

2 cups of water	Chopped fresh cilantro

Directions:

Drain and rinse beans. Press Sauté; to the Instant Pot. Cook for 3 to 4 minutes. Remove to a bowl. Heat olive oil in Instant Pot. Add onion, cook, and stir for 3 minutes or until softened. Add salt, tomato paste, garlic powder, paprika, cumin powder, and coriander powder; cook and stir for 1 minute. Stir in tomatoes, water, beans; mix well.

Secure lid and move pressure release valve to sealing position. Press Manual or Pressure Cook; cook at High pressure 20 minutes.

When cooking is complete, use Natural-release for 10 minutes, then release remaining pressure. Garnish with cilantro.

Nutrition:

Calories 120, Total Fat 4. 1g, Saturated Fat 0. 6g, Cholesterol 0mg, Sodium 1221mg, Total Carbohydrate 22. 4g, Dietary Fiber 10g, Total Sugars 2. 8g, Protein 7. 4g

336. Broccoli and Black Bean Chili

Preparation Time: 15 minutes | **Cooking Time:** 15 minutes | **Servings:** 2

Ingredients:

½ tablespoon coconut oil	1 cup broccoli
1 cup chopped red onions	½ tablespoon paprika
1/2 teaspoon salt	¼ cup tomatoes
1 cup black beans drained, rinsed	¼ chopped green chills
½ cup of water	

Directions:

In the Instant Pot, select Sauté; adjust to normal. Heat coconut oil in Instant Pot. Add broccoli, onions, paprika, and salt; cook 8 to 10 minutes, stirring occasionally, until thoroughly cooked. Select Cancel.

Stir in tomatoes, black beans, chills, and water. Secure lid set pressure valve to Sealing. Select Manual, cook on High pressure 5 minutes. Select Cancel. Keep the pressure valve in the Sealing position to release pressure naturally.

Nutrition:
Calories 408, Total Fat 5. 3g, Saturated Fat 3. 4g, Cholesterol 0mg, Sodium 607mg, Total Carbohydrate 70. 7g, Dietary Fiber 18. 1g, Total Sugars 6g, Protein 23. 3g

337. Potato and Chickpea Curry

Preparation Time: 05 minutes | **Cooking Time:** 10 minutes | **Servings:** 2

Ingredients:

½ tablespoon coconut oil	1 small onion chopped
2 teaspoons paprika	½ teaspoon garlic powder
¼ teaspoon salt	¼ teaspoon chipotle chili powder
¼ teaspoon ground cumin	1 cup vegetable broth
1 cup chickpea rinsed and drained	¼ cup potatoes peeled and cut into 1/2-inch pieces
½ cup diced tomatoes	

Directions:
Press Sauté, heat coconut oil in Instant Pot. Add chopped onions; cook 3 minutes or until softened. Add paprika, garlic powder, salt, chipotle chili powder, and ground cumin; cook and stir for 1 minute. Stir in broth, scraping up browned bits from the bottom of Instant Pot. Add chickpea, potatoes, and diced tomatoes; mix well.

Secure lid and move pressure release valve to the Sealing position. Press Manual or Pressure Cook; cook at High Pressure for 4 minutes.

When cooking is complete, press Cancel and use Quick-release.

Press Sauté; cook and stir for 3 to 5 minutes or until thickened to desired consistency. Serve with desired toppings.

Nutrition:
Calories 575, Total Fat 11. 3g, Saturated Fat 3. 8g, Cholesterol 0mg, Sodium 679mg, Total Carbohydrate 96. 2g, Dietary Fiber 25. 1g, Total Sugars 13. 8g, Protein 26. 7g

338. Vegetarian Chili

Preparation Time: 15 minutes | **Cooking Time:** 20 minutes | **Servings:** 2

Ingredients:

1 tablespoon avocado oil	½ teaspoon garlic powder
1 cup chopped onion	½ cup chopped carrots
¼ cup chopped green bell pepper	¼ cup chopped red bell pepper
1 tablespoon chili powder	½ cup chopped fresh mushrooms
½ cup whole peeled tomatoes with liquid, chopped	¼ cup black beans
¼ cup kidney beans	¼ cup pinto beans
¼ cup whole kernel corn	½ tablespoon cumin seed
1/2 tablespoons dried basil	1/2 tablespoon garlic minced

Directions:
Select the Sauté setting on the Instant Pot, add avocado oil, cook and stir the garlic minced, onions, and carrots in the Instant Pot until tender. Mix in the green bell pepper, red bell pepper, and chili powder. Season with chili powder. Continue cooking for 2 minutes, or until the peppers are tender.

Mix the mushrooms into the Instant pot. Stir in the tomatoes with liquid, black beans, kidney beans, pinto beans, and corn. Season with cumin seed, basil, and garlic powder.

Select Pressure Cook or Manual, and adjust the pressure to High and the time to 12 minutes. After cooking, let the pressure release naturally for 10 minutes, then quickly release any remaining pressure.

Nutrition:
Calories 348, Total Fat 3. 3g, Saturated Fat 0. 6g, Cholesterol 0mg, Sodium 77mg, Total Carbohydrate 65g, Dietary Fiber 16. 5g, Total Sugars 9. 5g, Protein 19. 1g

339. Coconut Curry Chili

Preparation Time: 15 minutes | **Cooking Time:** 30 minutes | **Servings:** 2

Ingredients:

1 cup tomatoes	2 cups of water
1 tablespoon minced garlic	½ cup garbanzo beans
½ cup red kidney beans	1/2 cup chopped zucchini
¼ cup mango	1 1/2 tablespoons curry powder
1cup onions, chopped	Salt and ground black pepper to taste
½ cup of coconut milk	

Directions:

In the Instant Pot, add all ingredients like tomatoes, water, garlic, garbanzo beans, kidney beans, zucchini, mango, curry powder, onions, salt, and black pepper.

Select Pressure Cook or Manual, and adjust the pressure to High and the time to 12 minutes. After cooking, let the pressure release naturally for 10 minutes, then quickly release any remaining pressure.

Stir coconut milk.

Serve.

Nutrition:

Calories 548, Total Fat 18. 6g, Saturated Fat 13. 2g, Cholesterol 0mg, Sodium 46mg, Total Carbohydrate 78g, Dietary Fiber 21. 1g, Total Sugars 16. 6g, Protein 24g

340. Spicy Butternut Squash Chili

Preparation Time: 15 minutes | **Cooking Time:** 30 minutes | **Servings:** 2

Ingredients:

½ teaspoon crushed red pepper flakes, or to taste	1 teaspoon garlic powder
½ large onion, diced	1 green bell pepper, chopped
1 red bell pepper, chopped	½ cup kidney beans
½ cup black beans	½ cup pinto beans,
1 cup tomato paste	2 tomatoes, diced
½ cup butter squash diced	½ cup green peas
½ teaspoons chili powder	1 teaspoon cumin
Salt and pepper	

Directions:

In the Instant Pot, combine red pepper flakes, garlic powder, onion, kidney beans, black beans, pinto beans, tomato paste, diced tomatoes, and butter squash.

Add the green and red bell pepper and water and cook for 5 minutes. Season with chili powder, cumin, and salt.

Stir the green peas, salt, and pepper into the Instant pot. Select Pressure Cook or Manual, and adjust the pressure to High and the time to 12 minutes. After cooking, let the pressure release naturally for 10 minutes, then quickly release any remaining pressure.

Serve and enjoy.

Nutrition:

Calories 620, Total Fat 2. 9g, Saturated Fat 0. 6g, Cholesterol 0mg, Sodium 37mg, Total Carbohydrate 117. 2g, Dietary Fiber 29. 3g, Total Sugars 16. 1g, Protein 37g

341. Creamy White Beans and Chickpeas Chili

Preparation Time: 05 minutes | **Cooking Time:** 35 minutes | **Servings:** 2

Ingredients:

1 teaspoon coconut oil	1 onion finely diced
½ teaspoon garlic powder	2 cups vegetable broth
½ cup chickpeas	½ cup navy beans
½ tablespoon chili powder	½ cumin powder
½ teaspoon kosher salt	¼ teaspoon black pepper
1/2 cup butter	3 tablespoon coconut flour
1 cup coconut milk warmed	¼ cup coconut cream
½ tablespoon lime juice	

Directions:

Add coconut oil to the Instant Pot. Using the display panel select the Sauté function.

When oil gets hot, add onion to the pot and sauté until soft, 3-4 minutes. Add garlic powder and cook for 1-2 minutes more.

Add broth to the pot and deglaze by using a wooden spoon to scrape the brown bits from the bottom of the pot.

Add chickpeas, beans, chili and cumin powder, salt, and pepper, and stir to combine.

Turn the pot off by selecting Cancel, then secure the lid, making sure the vent is closed.

Using the display panel select the Manual or Pressure Cook function. Use the + /- keys and program the Instant Pot for 15 minutes.

When the time is up, let the pressure naturally release for 10 minutes, then quickly release the remaining pressure.

In a medium bowl, melt butter, then whisk in flour until well combined. Stir into the pot and simmer 3-5 minutes until thickened, returning to Sauté mode as needed.

Stir in coconut milk, coconut cream, and lime juice. Adjust seasonings.

Nutrition:
Calories 1086, Total Fat 71. 3g, Saturated Fat 47. 6g, Cholesterol 122mg, Sodium 1764mg, Total Carbohydrate 86. 3g, Dietary Fiber 32. 3g, Total Sugars 14. 5g, Protein 32. 1g

342. Potato Chili

Preparation Time: 10 minutes | **Cooking Time:** 25 minutes | **Servings:** 2

Ingredients:

½ teaspoon olive oil	½ cup onion chopped
½ teaspoon garlic powder	½ teaspoon chili powder
½ teaspoon ground cumin	1 cup diced tomatoes
½ cup black beans rinsed and drained	1 medium red bell pepper seeded and diced
1 medium potato peeled and diced	1 teaspoon kosher salt
¼ cup frozen corn kernels	

Directions:
Select Sauté and add the olive oil to the Instant Pot. Add the onions and garlic powder. Sauté for

2 minutes, or until the garlic powder is fragrant and the onion is soft and translucent.

Add the chili powder and ground cumin, followed by the tomatoes, black beans, red bell pepper, potato, corn, and salt. Stir well.

Cover, lock the lid and flip the steam release handle to the Sealing position. Select Pressure Cook High and set the cooking time for 15 minutes. When the cooking time is complete, allow the pressure to release naturally for about 20 minutes.

Remove the lid and ladle the chili into serving bowls. Serve hot.

Nutrition:
Calories 207, Total Fat 2. 1g, Saturated Fat 0. 3g, Cholesterol 0mg, Sodium 1207mg, Total Carbohydrate 41. 4g, Dietary Fiber 8. 8g, Total Sugars 7. 7g, Protein 8. 2g

343. Beans Baby Potato Curry

Preparation Time: 10 minutes | **Cooking Time:** 30 minutes | **Servings:** 2

Ingredients:

1 small onion, chopped	½ teaspoon garlic, chopped finely
1 cup baby potatoes	½ tablespoon curry powder
2 cups of water	½ cup pinto beans
½ cup milk	½ tablespoon honey
Salt & pepper to taste	½ teaspoon chili pepper flakes
1 tablespoon arrowroot powder	

Directions:
Set your Instant Pot to Sauté. Once hot, add a few drops of water and cook the onions until translucent, then add the garlic and cook for one minute longer. Press the Keep Warm/Cancel button.

Add everything to the Instant Pot except the arrowroot powder.

Set the Instant Pot to 20 minutes on Manual High pressure and allow the pressure to release naturally after this time.

Press Keep Warm/Cancel, remove the lid, and press Sauté. Put the arrowroot into a small bowl or cup and mix into it a few tablespoons of water to make a thickness but pour slurry. Pour it into the Instant Pot stirring as you go.

Add salt and pepper to taste then cook for about 5 minutes until they are tender and the gravy has thickened.

Serve immediately.

Nutrition:

Calories342, Total Fat 2. 3g, Saturated Fat 1g, Cholesterol 5mg, Sodium 58mg, Total Carbohydrate 67. 2g, Dietary Fiber 12. 1g, Total Sugars 10g, Protein 14. 2g

344. Butter Tofu with Soy Bean and Chickpeas

Preparation Time: 10 minutes | **Cooking Time:** 30 minutes | **Servings:** 2

Ingredients:

2 large ripe tomatoes	½ teaspoon garlic powder
½ teaspoon ginger powder	½ tablespoon hot green chili
1 cup of water	¼ teaspoon garam masala
1/8 teaspoon paprika	¼ teaspoon salt
¼ cup of soybeans	½ cup chickpeas
½ teaspoon honey	½ cup coconut cream
Cilantro for garnish	

Directions:

Blend the tomatoes, garlic powder, ginger powder, hot green chili with water until smooth.

Add pureed tomato mixture to the Instant Pot.

Add soybeans, chickpeas, spices, and salt. Close the lid and cook on Manual for 8 to 10 minutes. Quick-release after 10 minutes.

Start the Instant Pot on Sauté. Add the coconut cream, Garam masala, honey, and mix in. Bring to a boil, taste, and adjust salt. Add more paprika and salt if needed.

Serve with cilantro garnishing

Nutrition:

Calories 242, Total Fat 1. 3g, Saturated Fat 1. 5g, Cholesterol 5mg, Sodium 38mg, Total Carbohydrate 47. 2g, Dietary Fiber 10. 1g, Total Sugars 10g, Protein 14. 2g.

345. Black Eyed Peas Curry with Jaggery

Preparation Time: 10 minutes | **Cooking Time:** 30 minutes | **Servings:** 2

Ingredients:

¼ cup dried black-eyed peas, soaked in water for about 1-2 hours	2 cups of water
1 dried curry leaves	1/8 teaspoon mustard seeds
½ teaspoon garlic powder	1/2 small onion, finely chopped
2 tablespoons tomato paste	½ teaspoon ground cumin
1 teaspoon ground coriander	¼ teaspoon ground turmeric
1 tablespoon jaggery	1 tablespoon fresh lemon juice
Chili powder, to taste (optional	1 tablespoon avocado oil
Salt	Fresh cilantro, finely chopped

Directions:

Select the Sauté button into the Instant Pot and add avocado oil.

Once the oil is hot, add the mustard seeds and curry leaves. Fry for a few seconds until fragrant. Add the onions and garlic powder. Sauté until fragrant and the onions start to become translucent. Be sure not to burn either. If you see this happening add more oil or turn down the sauté heat.

Quickly add the tomato paste, ground cumin, and ground coriander. Combine and cook for a minute mixing frequently.

Drain the soaked black-eyed peas and add them into the Instant Pot.

Mix in the water, turmeric powder, chili powder, jaggery, fresh lemon juice, and salt.

Close the Instant Pot lid, select the Pressure Cook button to cook on High. Set the timer for about 13-15 minutes.

When the time is up, allow the pressure to release naturally.

Once the pressure has been released, remove the lid, and press the Sauté (normally Low) button again on the Instant Pot. The black-eyed peas should be fully cooked.

Simmer for a few more minutes until the curry becomes thick.

Add salt to taste. Also, feel free to adjust the amount of lemon juice and jaggery as needed.

Turn the Instant Pot off. Add freshly chopped cilantro and serve hot.

Nutrition:
Calories79, Total Fat 0. 9g, Saturated Fat 0. 2g, Cholesterol 0mg, Sodium 75mg, Total Carbohydrate 18g, Dietary Fiber 4. 7g, Total Sugars 8. 2g, Protein 4g

346. Jackfruit with Beans Curry

Preparation Time: 10 minutes | **Cooking Time:** 20 minutes | **Servings:** 2

Ingredients:

½ tablespoon coconut oil	½ tablespoon curry powder
¼ teaspoon paprika	½ teaspoon cumin seeds
¼ teaspoon turmeric powder	1 sprigs fresh rosemary
½ cup onion, finely chopped	1 teaspoon garlic powder
1 teaspoon ginger powder	1 celery, chopped
1 cup jackfruit, drained and rinsed	½ cup pinto beans
½ medium zucchini, diced	½ cup full-fat milk
1 cups vegetable broth	1/4 cup parsley leaves, chopped
Salt, to taste	

Directions:
Plug your Instant Pot and press the Sauté mode button. Add coconut oil, once heated add dry spices, curry powder, paprika, cumin seeds, turmeric powder, rosemary, and cook for a minute stirring constantly.

Add onions, garlic powder, ginger powder, and celery, and cook for 2 minutes or until onions are soft. Add jackfruit, pinto beans, zucchini and stir to coat.

Add salt, milk, and vegetable broth.

Close the Instant Pot lid and press Manual mode for 10 minutes. When finished, allow Instant Pot to natural release for 10 minutes. Carefully release the knob to release the remaining

pressure. Remove lid, stir in parsley leaves, and check seasonings.

Serve.

Nutrition:
Calories320, Total Fat 5. 5g, Saturated Fat 3. 5g, Cholesterol 1mg, Sodium 582mg, Total Carbohydrate 50. 7g, Dietary Fiber 17. 6g, Total Sugars 7g, Protein 17. 5g

347. Smoky, Black Beans Chickpeas, and Corn

Preparation Time: 05 minutes | **Cooking Time:** 10 minutes | **Servings:** 2

Ingredients:

2 teaspoons ground cumin	½ cup onion, chopped
1 teaspoon garlic powder	¼ teaspoon salt
1 cup black beans	½ cup chickpea
½ cup dried corn	2 cups vegetable broth or water
Chopped fresh cilantro to serve	Lime juice to serve

Directions:
Place all ingredients into the Instant Pot. Add 2 cups of broth or water. Stir to mix. Cover with the lid and ensure the vent is in the "Sealing" position. Pressure Cook on High for 5 minutes. Allow the steam pressure to release naturally for 5 minutes, then release any remaining pressure manually.

Garnish with fresh cilantro and a squeeze of lime juice.

Nutrition:
Calories 616, Total Fat 6. 8g, Saturated Fat 1. 2g, Cholesterol 0mg, Sodium 1087mg, Total Carbohydrate 105. 8g, Dietary Fiber 25. 9g, Total Sugars 11. 4g, Protein 37. 9g

348. Coconut Salad

Preparation Time: 10 minutes | **Cooking Time:** 0 minutes | **Servings:** 6

Ingredients:

2 cups coconut flesh, unsweetened and shredded	½ cup walnuts, chopped

1 cup blackberries   1 tablespoon stevia
1 tablespoon coconut
oil, melted

Directions:
In a bowl, combine the coconut with the walnuts and the other ingredients, toss and serve.

Nutrition:
Calories 250, Fat 23.8, Fiber 5.8, Carbs 8.9, Protein 4.5

349. Avocado and Rhubarb Salad

Preparation Time: 10 minutes | **Cooking Time:** 0 minutes | **Servings:** 4

Ingredients:

1 tablespoon stevia	1 cup rhubarb, sliced and boiled
2 avocados, peeled, pitted, and sliced	1 teaspoon vanilla extract
Juice of 1 lime	

Directions:
In a bowl, combine the rhubarb with the avocado and the other ingredients, toss and serve.

Nutrition:
Calories 140, Fat 2, Fiber 2, Carbs 4, Protein 4

350. Vegetable Mushroom Side Dish

Preparation Time: 15-30 minutes | **Cooking Time:** 85 minutes | **Servings:** 4

Ingredients:

2 tbsp plant butter	1 large onion, diced
1 cup celery, diced	½ cup carrots, diced
½ tsp dried marjoram	1 tsp dried basil
2 cups chopped cremini mushrooms	1 cup vegetable broth
¼ cup chopped fresh parsley	1 medium whole-grain bread loaf, cubed

Directions:
Melt the butter in a large skillet and sauté the onion, celery, mushrooms, and carrots until softened, 5 minutes.

Mix in the marjoram, basil, and season with salt and black pepper.

Pour in the vegetable broth and mix in the parsley and bread. Cook until the broth reduces by half, 10 minutes.

Pour the mixture into a baking dish and cover with foil. Bake in the oven at 375 F for 30 minutes.

Uncover and bake further for 30 minutes or until golden brown on top and the liquid absorbs.

Remove the dish from the oven and serve the stuffing.

Nutrition:
Calories 575 kcal Fats 60. 9g Carbs 10. 3g Protein 3. 3g

351. Asian Dumplings

Preparation Time: 32 minutes | **Cooking Time:** 15-120 minutes | **Servings:** 12 Dumplings

Ingredients:

1 1/12 Tablespoons Sesame Oil	3 Cloves Garlic, minced
1 Tablespoon Fresh Ginger, minced	1 Cup Mushrooms, minced
1/2 cup Tamari Sauce, Soy Sauce, or Coconut Aminos(for soy-free)	1 Teaspoon Sriracha
1 Tablespoon Rice Vinegar	1 Tablespoon Sesame Seeds
12 Vegan Dumpling Wrappers	1 1/2 Cups Water(for steaming

Directions:
On saute mode, heat the sesame oil. When hot, add garlic and ginger. Cook for 1 minute.

Add mushrooms and saute until juices are released from mushrooms.

Add tamari, soy sauce, or coconut aminos, sriracha, rice vinegar, and sesame seeds. Saute until all liquid is cooked out.

Prepare a small bowl of water. Lay a wrapper and spread water around the edge with fingers.

Fill each dumpling with 1 tablespoon of filling in the middle of the wrapper and press edges together to seal. Place each dumpling onto the vegetable steamer that is lightly coated with oil. After all wrappers are made, remove the liner from the instant pot and add water.

Place the vegetable steamer filled with dumplings into the instant pot. Cover with lid and seal. Select the steam option and set it to 7 minutes.

When done, open the steam release valve manually.

Serve immediately with tamari sauce, soy sauce, coconut aminos, or sriracha for dipping.

Enjoy!

Nutrition:
Calories: 140 Cal Fat: 0.9 g Carbs: 27.1 g Protein: 6.3 g Fiber: 6.2 g

Chapter 4: Soups and Stews

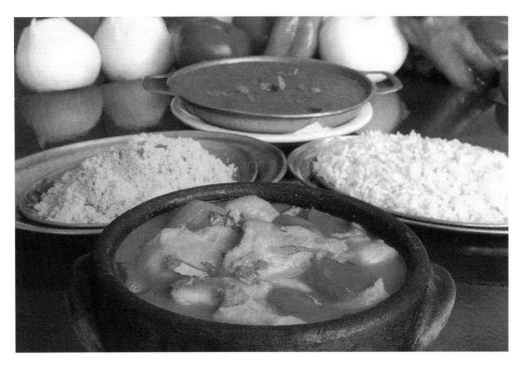

352. Chickpea And Black Olive Stew

Preparation Time: 15-30 minutes | **Cooking Time:** 15 minutes | **Servings:** 4

Ingredients:

2 tbsp olive oil	2 cups chopped onion
2 garlic cloves, minced	2 carrots, peeled and cut into thick slices
1/3 cup white wine	3 cups cherry tomatoes
2/3 cup vegetable stock	1 1/3 cups canned chickpeas, drained and rinsed
½ cup pitted black olives	1 tbsp chopped fresh oregano

Directions:

Heat the olive oil in a medium pot and sauté the onion, garlic, and carrots until softened, 5 minutes.

Mix in the white wine, allow reduction by one-third, and mix in the tomatoes, and vegetable stock. Cover the lid and cook until the tomatoes break, soften, and the liquid reduces by half.

Stir in the chickpeas, olives, oregano and season with salt and black pepper. Cook for 3 minutes to warm the chickpeas.

Dish the stew and serve warm.

Nutrition:

Calories 698 kcal Fats 51. 3g Carbs 54. 1g Protein 12. 1g

353. Lentil and Wild Rice Soup

Preparation Time: 10 minutes | **Cooking Time:** 40 minutes | **Servings:** 4

Ingredients:

1/2 cup cooked mixed beans	12 ounces cooked lentils
2 stalks of celery, sliced	1 1/2 cup mixed wild rice, cooked
1 large sweet potato, peeled, chopped	1/2 medium butternut, peeled, chopped
4 medium carrots, peeled, sliced	1 medium onion, peeled, diced
10 cherry tomatoes	1/2 red chili, deseeded, diced

1 ½ teaspoon minced garlic

1/2 teaspoon salt

2 teaspoons mixed dried herbs

1 teaspoon coconut oil

2 cups vegetable broth

Directions:

Take a large pot, place it over medium-high heat, add oil and when it melts, add onion and cook for 5 minutes.

Stir in garlic and chili, cook for 3 minutes, then add remaining vegetables, pour in the broth, stir and bring the mixture to a boil.

Switch heat to medium-low heat, cook the soup for 20 minutes, then stir in remaining ingredients and continue cooking for 10 minutes until soup has reached the desired thickness.

Serve straight away.

Nutrition:

Calories: 331 Cal Fat: 2 g Carbs: 54 g Protein: 13 g Fiber: 12 g

354. Garlic and White Bean Soup

Preparation Time: 10 minutes | **Cooking Time:** 10 minutes | **Servings:** 4

Ingredients:

45 ounces cooked cannellini beans

1/4 teaspoon dried thyme

2 teaspoons minced garlic

1/8 teaspoon crushed red pepper

1/2 teaspoon dried rosemary

1/8 teaspoon ground black pepper

2 tablespoons olive oil

4 cups vegetable broth

Directions:

Place one-third of white beans in a food processor, then pour in 2 cups of broth and pulse for 2 minutes until smooth.

Place a pot over medium heat, add oil and when hot, add garlic and cook for 1 minute until fragrant. Add pureed beans into the pan along with remaining beans, sprinkle with spices and herbs, pour in the broth, stir until combined, and bring the mixture to boil over medium-high heat. Switch heat to medium-low level, simmer the beans for 15 minutes, and then mash them with a fork. Taste the soup to adjust seasoning and then serve.

Nutrition:

Calories: 222 Cal Fat: 7 g Carbs: 13 g Protein: 11.2 g Fiber: 9. 1 g

355. Vegetarian Irish Stew

Preparation Time: 5 minutes | **Cooking Time:** 38 minutes | **Servings:** 6

Ingredients:

1 cup textured vegetable protein, chunks

½ cup split red lentils

2 medium onions, peeled, sliced

1 cup sliced parsnip

2 cups sliced mushrooms

1 cup diced celery,

1/4 cup flour

4 cups vegetable stock

1 cup rutabaga

1 bay leaf

½ cup fresh parsley

1 teaspoon sugar

¼ teaspoon ground black pepper

1/4 cup soy sauce

¼ teaspoon thyme

2 teaspoons marmite

¼ teaspoon rosemary

2/3 teaspoon salt

¼ teaspoon marjoram

Directions:

Take a large soup pot, place it over medium heat, add oil and when it gets hot, add onions and cook for 5 minutes until softened.

Then switch heat to the low level, sprinkle with flour, stir well, add remaining ingredients, stir until combined, and simmer for 30 minutes until vegetables have cooked.

When done, season the stew with salt and black pepper and then serve.

Nutrition:

Calories: 117.4 Cal Fat: 4 g Carbs: 22.8 g Protein: 6.5 g Fiber: 7.3 g

356. White Bean and Cabbage Stew

Preparation Time: 5 minutes | **Cooking Time:** 8 hours | **Servings:** 4

Ingredients:

3 cups cooked great northern beans

1.5 pounds potatoes, peeled, cut into large dice

1 large white onion, peeled, chopped

½ head of cabbage, chopped

3 ribs celery, chopped

4 medium carrots, peeled, sliced

14.5 ounces diced tomatoes

1/3 cup pearled barley

1 teaspoon minced garlic

½ teaspoon ground black pepper

1 bay leaf

1 teaspoon dried thyme

½ teaspoon crushed rosemary

1 teaspoon salt

½ teaspoon caraway seeds

1 tablespoon chopped parsley

8 cups vegetable broth

Directions:

Switch on the slow cooker, then add all the ingredients except for salt, parsley, tomatoes, and beans and stir until mixed.

Shut the slow cooker with a lid, and cook for 7 hours at a low heat setting until cooked.

Then stir in remaining ingredients, stir until combined, and continue cooking for 1 hour. Serve straight away

Nutrition:

Calories: 150 Cal Fat: 0.7 g Carbs: 27 g Protein: 7 g Fiber: 9.4 g

357. Spinach and Cannellini Bean Stew

Preparation Time: 10 minutes | **Cooking Time:** 15 minutes | **Servings:** 6

Ingredients:

28 ounces cooked cannellini beans

24 ounces tomato passata

17 ounces spinach chopped

¼ teaspoon ground black pepper

2/3 teaspoon salt

1 ¼ teaspoon curry powder

1 cup cashew butter

¼ teaspoon cardamom

2 tablespoons olive oil

1 teaspoon salt

¼ cup cashews

2 tablespoons chopped basil

2 tablespoons chopped parsley

Directions:

Take a large saucepan, place it over medium heat, add 1 tablespoon oil and when hot, add spinach and cook for 3 minutes until fried.

Then stir in butter and tomato passata until well mixed, bring the mixture to a near boil, add beans, and season with ¼ teaspoon curry powder, black pepper, and salt.

Take a small saucepan, place it over medium heat, add remaining oil, stir in cashew, stir in salt and curry powder and cook for 4 minutes until roasted, set aside until required.

Transfer cooked stew into a bowl, top with roasted cashews, basil, and parsley, and then serve.

Nutrition:

Calories: 242 Cal Fat: 10.2 g Carbs: 31 g Protein: 11 g Fiber: 8.5 g

358. Cabbage Stew

Preparation Time: 10 minutes | **Cooking Time:** 50 minutes | **Servings:** 6

Ingredients:

12 ounces cooked Cannellini beans

8 ounces smoked tofu, firm, sliced

1 medium cabbage, chopped

1 large white onion, peeled, julienned

2 ½ teaspoon minced garlic

1 tablespoon sweet paprika

5 tablespoons tomato paste

3 teaspoons smoked paprika

1/3 teaspoon ground black pepper

2 teaspoons dried thyme

2/3 teaspoon salt

½ tsp ground coriander

3 bay leaves

4 tablespoons olive oil

1 cup vegetable broth

Directions:

Take a large saucepan, place it over medium heat, add 3 tablespoons oil and when hot, add onion and garlic and cook for 3 minutes or until saute.

Add cabbage, pour in water, simmer for 10 minutes or until softened, then stir in all the spices and continue cooking for 30 minutes.

Add beans and tomato paste, pour in water, stir until mixed and cook for 15 minutes until thoroughly cooked.

Take a separate skillet pan, add 1 tablespoon oil and when hot, add tofu slices and cook for 5 minutes until golden brown on both sides.

Serve cooked cabbage stew with fried tofu.

Nutrition:
Calories: 182 Cal Fat: 8.3 g Carbs: 27 g Protein: 5.5 g Fiber: 9.4 g

359. Kimchi Stew

Preparation Time: 10 minutes | **Cooking Time:** 25 minutes | **Servings:** 4

Ingredients:

1 pound tofu, extra-firm, pressed, cut into 1-inch pieces	4 cups napa cabbage kimchi, vegan, chopped
1 small white onion, peeled, diced	2 cups sliced shiitake mushroom caps
1 ½ teaspoon minced garlic	2 tablespoons soy sauce
2 tablespoons olive oil, divided	4 cups vegetable broth
2 tablespoons chopped scallions	

Directions:
Take a large pot, place it over medium heat, add 1 tablespoon oil and when hot, add tofu pieces in a single layer and cook for 10 minutes until browned on all sides.

When cooked, transfer tofu pieces to a plate, add remaining oil to the pot and when hot, add onion and cook for 5 minutes until soft.

Stir in garlic, cook for 1 minute until fragrant, stir in kimchi, continue cooking for 2 minutes, then add mushrooms and pour in broth.

Switch heat to medium-high level, bring the mixture to boil, then switch heat to medium-low level, and simmer for 10 minutes until mushrooms are softened.

Stir in tofu, taste to adjust seasoning, and garnish with scallions.

Serve straight away.

Nutrition:
Calories: 153 Cal Fat: 8.2 g Carbs: 25 g Protein: 8.4 g Fiber: 2.6 g

360. African Peanut Lentil Soup

Preparation Time: 10 minutes | **Cooking Time:** 25 minutes | **Servings:** 3

Ingredients:

1/2 cup red lentils	1/2 medium white onion, sliced
2 medium tomatoes, chopped	1/2 cup baby spinach
1/2 cup sliced zucchini	1/2 cup sliced sweet potatoes
½ cup sliced potatoes	½ cup broccoli florets
2 teaspoons minced garlic	1 inch of ginger, grated
1 tablespoon tomato paste	1/4 teaspoon ground black pepper
1 teaspoon salt	1 ½ teaspoon ground cumin
2 teaspoons ground coriander	2 tablespoons peanuts
1 teaspoon Harissa Spice Blend	1 tablespoon sambal oelek
1/4 cup almond butter	1 teaspoon olive oil
1 teaspoon lemon juice	2 ½ cups vegetable stock

Directions:
Take a large saucepan, place it over medium heat, add oil, and when hot, add onion and cook for 5 minutes until translucent.

Meanwhile, place tomatoes in a blender, add garlic, ginger, and sambal oelek along with all the spices, and pulse until pureed.

Pour this mixture into the onions, cook for 5 minutes, then add remaining ingredients except for spinach, peanuts, and lemon juice and simmer for 15 minutes.

Taste to adjust the seasoning, stir in spinach, and cook for 5 minutes until cooked.

Ladle soup into bowls, garnish with lime juice and peanuts and serve.

Nutrition:
Calories: 411 Cal Fat: 17 g Carbs: 50 g Protein: 20 g Fiber: 18 g

361. Spicy Bean Stew

Preparation Time: 5 minutes | **Cooking Time:** 50 minutes | **Servings:** 4

Ingredients:

7 ounces cooked black eye beans	14 ounces chopped tomatoes
2 medium carrots, peeled, diced	7 ounces cooked kidney beans
1 leek, diced	½ a chili, chopped
1 teaspoon minced garlic	1/3 teaspoon ground black pepper

2/3 teaspoon salt	1 teaspoon red chili powder
1 lemon, juiced	3 tablespoons white wine
1 tablespoon olive oil	1 2/3 cups vegetable stock

Directions:

Take a large saucepan, place it over medium-high heat, add oil and when hot, add leeks and cook for 8 minutes or until softened.

Then add carrots, continue cooking for 4 minutes, stir in chili and garlic, pour in the wine, and continue cooking for 2 minutes.

Add tomatoes, stir in lemon juice, pour in the stock and bring the mixture to boil.

Switch heat to medium level, simmer for 35 minutes until stew has thickened, then add both beans along with remaining ingredients and cook for 5 minutes until hot.

Serve straight away.

Nutrition:

Calories: 114 Cal Fat: 1.6 g Carbs: 19 g Protein: 6 g Fiber: 8.4 g

362. Eggplant, Onion, and Tomato Stew

Preparation Time: 5 minutes | **Cooking Time:** 5 minutes | **Servings:** 4

Ingredients:

3 1/2 cups cubed eggplant	1 cup diced white onion
2 cups diced tomatoes	1 teaspoon ground cumin
1/8 teaspoon ground cayenne pepper	1 teaspoon salt
1 cup tomato sauce	1/2 cup water

Directions:

Switch on the instant pot, place all the ingredients in it, stir until mixed, and seal the pot.

Press the 'manual' button and cook for 5 minutes at a high-pressure setting until cooked.

When done, do quick pressure release, open the instant pot, and stir the stew.

Serve straight away.

Nutrition:

Calories: 88 Cal Fat: 1 g Carbs: 21 g Protein: 3 g Fiber: 6 g

363. White Bean Stew

Preparation Time: 5 minutes | **Cooking Time:** 10 hours and 10 minutes | **Servings:** 10

Ingredients:

2 cups chopped spinach	28 ounces diced tomatoes
2 pounds white beans, dried	2 cups chopped chard
2 large carrots, peeled, diced	2 cups chopped kale
3 large celery stalks, diced	1 medium white onion, peeled, diced
1 ½ teaspoon minced garlic	2 tablespoons salt
1 teaspoon dried rosemary	½ teaspoon Ground black pepper, to taste
1 teaspoon dried thyme	1 teaspoon dried oregano
1 bay leaf	10 cups water

Directions:

Switch on the slow cooker, add all the ingredients in it, except for kale, chard, and spinach and stir until combined.

Shut the cooker with a lid and cook for 10 hours at a low heat setting until thoroughly cooked.

When done, stir in kale, chard, and spinach, and cook for 10 minutes until leaves wilt.

Serve straight away.

Nutrition:

Calories: 109 Cal Fat: 2.4 g Carbs: 17.8 g Protein: 5.3 g Fiber: 6 g

364. Brussel Sprouts Stew

Preparation Time: 10 minutes | **Cooking Time:** 55 minutes | **Servings:** 4

Ingredients:

35 ounces Brussels sprouts	5 medium potato, peeled, chopped
1 medium onion, peeled, chopped	2 carrot, peeled, cubed
2 teaspoon smoked paprika	1/8 teaspoon ground black pepper

1/8 teaspoon salt	3 tablespoons caraway seeds
1/2 teaspoon red chili powder	1 tablespoon nutmeg
1 tablespoon olive oil	4 ½ cups hot vegetable stock

Directions:

Take a large pot, place it over medium-high heat, add oil, and when hot, add onion and cook for 1 minute.

Then add carrot and potato, cook for 2 minutes, then add Brussel sprouts and cook for 5 minutes. Stir in all the spices, pour in vegetable stock, bring the mixture to boil, switch heat to medium-low and simmer for 45 minutes until cooked and stew reaches the desired thickness. Serve straight away.

Nutrition:

Calories: 156 Cal Fat: 3 g Carbs: 22 g Protein: 12 g Fiber: 5.1100 g

365. Vegetarian Gumbo

Preparation Time: 10 minutes | **Cooking Time:** 45 minutes | **Servings:** 4

Ingredients:

1 1/2 cups diced zucchini	16-ounces cooked red beans
4 cups sliced okra	1 1/2 cups diced green pepper
1 1/2 cups chopped white onion	1 1/2 cups diced red bell pepper
8 cremini mushrooms, quartered	1 cup sliced celery
3 teaspoons minced garlic	1 medium tomato, chopped
1 teaspoon red pepper flakes	1 teaspoon dried thyme
3 tablespoons all-purpose flour	1 tablespoon smoked paprika
1 teaspoon dried oregano	1/4 teaspoon nutmeg
1 teaspoon soy sauce	1 1/2 teaspoons liquid smoke
2 tablespoons mustard	1 tablespoon apple cider vinegar

1 tablespoon Worcestershire sauce, vegetarian	1/2 teaspoon hot sauce
3 tablespoons olive oil	4 cups vegetable stock
1/2 cups sliced green onion	4 cups cooked jasmine rice

Directions:

Take a Dutch oven, place it over medium heat, add oil and flour and cook for 5 minutes until fragrant.

Switch heat to the medium low level, and continue cooking for 20 minutes until the roux becomes dark brown, whisking constantly.

Meanwhile, place the tomato in a food processor, add garlic and onion along with remaining ingredients, except for stock, zucchini, celery, mushroom, green and red bell pepper, and pulse for 2 minutes until smooth.

Pour the mixture into the pan, return pan over medium-high heat, stir until mixed, and cook for 5 minutes until all the liquid has evaporated. Stir in stock, bring it to simmer, then add remaining vegetables and simmer for 20 minutes until tender.

Garnish gumbo with green onions and serve with rice.

Nutrition:

Calories: 160 Cal Fat: 7.3 g Carbs: 20 g Protein: 7 g Fiber: 5.7 g

366. Black Bean and Quinoa Stew

Preparation Time: 10 minutes | **Cooking Time:** 6 hours | **Servings:** 6

Ingredients:

1 pound black beans, dried, soaked overnight	3/4 cup quinoa, uncooked
1 medium red bell pepper, cored, chopped	1 medium red onion, peeled, diced
1 medium green bell pepper, cored, chopped	28-ounce diced tomatoes
2 dried chipotle peppers	1 ½ teaspoon minced garlic
2/3 teaspoon sea salt	2 teaspoons red chili powder

1/3 teaspoon ground black pepper

1 teaspoon coriander powder

1 dried cinnamon stick

1/4 cup cilantro

7 cups of water

Directions:

Switch on the slow cooker, add all the ingredients in it, except for salt, and stir until mixed.

Shut the cooker with a lid and cook for 6 hours at a high heat setting until cooked.

When done, stir salt into the stew until mixed, remove cinnamon sticks and serve.

Nutrition:

Calories: 308 Cal Fat: 2 g Carbs: 70 g Protein: 23 g Fiber: 32 g

367. Root Vegetable Stew

Preparation Time: 10 minutes | **Cooking Time:** 8 hours and 10 minutes | **Servings:** 6

Ingredients:

2 cups chopped kale

1 large white onion, peeled, chopped

1 pound parsnips, peeled, chopped

1 pound potatoes, peeled, chopped

2 celery ribs, chopped

1 pound butternut squash, peeled, deseeded, chopped

1 pound carrots, peeled, chopped

3 teaspoons minced garlic

1 pound sweet potatoes, peeled, chopped

1 bay leaf

1 teaspoon ground black pepper

1/2 teaspoon sea salt

1 tablespoon chopped sage

3 cups vegetable broth

Directions:

Switch on the slow cooker, add all the ingredients in it, except for the kale, and stir until mixed.

Shut the cooker with a lid and cook for 8 hours at a low heat setting until cooked.

When done, add kale into the stew, stir until mixed, and cook for 10 minutes until leaves have wilted.

Serve straight away.

Nutrition:

Calories: 120 Cal Fat: 1 g Carbs: 28 g Protein: 4 g Fiber: 6 g

368. Portobello Mushroom Stew

Preparation Time: 10 minutes | **Cooking Time:** 8 hours | **Servings:** 4

Ingredients:

8 cups vegetable broth

1 cup dried wild mushrooms

1 cup dried chickpeas

3 cups chopped potato

2 cups chopped carrots

1 cup corn kernels

2 cups diced white onions

1 tablespoon minced parsley

3 cups chopped zucchini

1 tablespoon minced rosemary

1 1/2 teaspoon ground black pepper

1 teaspoon dried sage

2/3 teaspoon salt

1 teaspoon dried oregano

3 tablespoons soy sauce

1 1/2 teaspoons liquid smoke

8 ounces tomato paste

Directions:

Switch on the slow cooker, add all the ingredients in it, and stir until mixed.

Shut the cooker with a lid and cook for 10 hours at a high heat setting until cooked.

Serve straight away.

Nutrition:

Calories: 447 Cal Fat: 36 g Carbs: 24 g Protein: 11 g Fiber: 2 g

369. Fresh Bean Soup

Preparation Time: 05 minutes | **Cooking Time:** 15 minutes | **Servings:** 4

Ingredients:

2 tablespoons olive oil

2 medium onions, finely chopped

2 cups of water

3 cups fresh shelled green beans

Salt and pepper to taste

Directions:

Heat the olive oil in a heavy-bottomed saucepan over medium heat. Cook the onions until soft and translucent, about 3 minutes. Pour in the water and beans, season to taste with salt and pepper. Increase the heat to medium-high, bring to a boil, then reduce heat to low, cover, and simmer until the peas are tender, 12 to 18 minutes.

Puree the peas in a blender or food processor in batches. Strain back into the saucepan. Season to taste with salt and pepper before serving.

Nutrition:

Calories 111, Total Fat 7.2g, Saturated Fat 1g, Cholesterol 0mg, Sodium 8mg, Total Carbohydrate 10.4g, Dietary Fiber 3g, Total Sugars 4.4g, Protein 2.6g, Calcium 25mg, Iron 1mg, Potassium 170mg, Phosphorus 104mg

370. Macaroni Soup

Preparation Time: 15 minutes | **Cooking Time:** 55 minutes | **Servings:** 4

Ingredients:

2 tablespoons olive oil	2 large cloves garlic, minced
1 large onion finely chopped	1 cup of water
1/4 teaspoon Italian seasoning 1 tablespoon chopped fresh parsley	1/4 teaspoon garlic powder
Black pepper to taste	1 cup macaroni

Directions:

Heat the olive oil in a soup pot over medium-low heat. Stir in the minced garlic and onion; cook and stir until soft, about 5 minutes. Turn heat to medium; stir in water, Italian seasoning, parsley, garlic powder, and pepper. Bring to a simmer. Cook for 40 minutes with the lid slightly ajar. Stir macaroni into soup; cook at a strong simmer until macaroni is tender, about 12 minutes.

Nutrition:

Calories 116, Total Fat 5.1g, Saturated Fat 0.7g, Cholesterol 0mg, Sodium 4mg, Total Carbohydrate 14.7g, Dietary Fiber 1.7g, Total Sugars 1.9g, Protein 3.2g, Calcium 13mg, Iron 1mg, Potassium 100mg, Phosphorus 105 mg

371. Carrot, cauliflower, and Cabbage Soup

Preparation Time: 30 minutes | **Cooking Time:** 20 minutes | **Servings:** 4

Ingredients:

4 large carrots, thinly sliced	1 cup cauliflower, thinly sliced
1 large onion, thinly sliced	1/4 medium head green cabbage, thinly sliced
2 cloves garlic, smashed	6 cups of water
1 tablespoon olive oil	1/4 teaspoon dried thyme
1/4 teaspoon dried basil	1 teaspoon dried parsley
1/8 teaspoon salt	Ground black pepper to taste

Directions:

Combine the carrots, cauliflower, onion, cabbage, garlic, water, olive oil, thyme, basil, parsley, salt, and pepper in a pot over medium-high heat; bring to a simmer and cook until the carrots are tender for about 20 minutes. Transfer to a blender in small batches and blend until smooth.

Nutrition:

Calories 57, Total Fat 2.4g, Saturated Fat 0.3g, Cholesterol 0mg, Sodium 98mg, Total Carbohydrate 8.5g, Dietary Fiber 2.3g, Total Sugars 4g, Protein 1.1g, Calcium 37mg, Iron 0mg, Potassium 249mg, Phosphorus 150 mg

372. Carrot Soup

Preparation Time: 15 minutes | **Cooking Time:** 20 minutes | **Servings:** 4

Ingredients:

3 cups carrots, chopped	6 cups of water
3 cloves garlic, chopped	2 tablespoons dried dill weed
1/4 pound olive oil	1/8 teaspoons salt

Directions:

In a medium-sized pot, over high heat, combine the water, carrots, garlic, dill weed, salt, and olive oil. Bring to a boil, reduce heat and simmer for 30 minutes or until carrots are soft.

In a blender, puree the soup, return to the pot and simmer for an additional 30 to 45 minutes. Season with additional dill or garlic if needed.

Nutrition:

Calories 169, Total Fat 17.7g, Saturated Fat 2.5g, Cholesterol 0mg, Sodium 81mg, Total Carbohydrate 4.1g, Dietary Fiber 0.9g, Total Sugars 1.5g, Protein 0.6g, Calcium 38mg, Iron 1mg, Potassium 140mg, Phosphorus 90 mg

373. Vegetable Barley Soup

Preparation Time: 5 minutes | **Cooking Time:** 15 minutes | **Servings:** 8

Ingredients:

1 cup barley	14.5 ounces diced tomatoes with juice
2 large carrots, chopped	15 ounces cooked chickpeas
2 stalks celery, chopped	1 zucchini, chopped
1 medium white onion, peeled, chopped	1/2 teaspoon ground black pepper
1 teaspoon garlic powder	1 teaspoon curry powder
1 teaspoon salt	1 teaspoon paprika
1 teaspoon white sugar	1 teaspoon dried parsley
1 teaspoon Worcestershire sauce	3 bay leaves
2 quarts vegetable broth	

Directions:

Place all the ingredients in a pot, stir until mixed, place it over medium-high heat and bring the mixture to a boil.

Switch heat to medium level, simmer the soup for 90 minutes until cooked, and when done, remove bay leaf from it.

Serve straight away.

Nutrition:

Calories: 188 Cal Fat: 1.6 g Carbs: 37 g Protein: 7 g Fiber: 8.4 g

374. Mushroom, Lentil, and Barley Stew

Preparation Time: 10 minutes | **Cooking Time:** 6 hours | **Servings:** 8

Ingredients:

3/4 cup pearl barley	2 cups sliced button mushrooms
3/4 cup dry lentils	1 ounce dried shiitake mushrooms
2 teaspoons minced garlic	1/4 cup dried onion flakes
2 teaspoons ground black pepper	1 teaspoon dried basil
2 ½ teaspoons salt	2 teaspoons dried savory
3 bay leaves	2 quarts vegetable broth

Directions:

Switch on the slow cooker, place all the ingredients in it, and stir until combined.

Shut with lid and cook the stew for 6 hours at a high heat setting until cooked.

Serve straight away.

Nutrition:

Calories: 213 Cal Fat: 1.2 g Carbs: 44 g Protein: 8.4 g Fiber: 9 g

375. Tomato Barley Soup

Preparation Time: 10 minutes | **Cooking Time:** 40 minutes | **Servings:** 6

Ingredients:

1/4 cup barley	1 cup chopped celery
14.5 ounces peeled and diced tomatoes	1 cup chopped white onions
2 tomatoes, diced	1 cup chopped carrots
2 teaspoons minced garlic	1/8 teaspoon ground black pepper
1 teaspoon salt	2 tablespoons olive oil
2 1/2 cups water	10.75 ounces chicken broth

Directions:

Take a large saucepan, place it over medium heat, add onion, carrot, and celery, stir in garlic and cook for 10 minutes until tender.

Then add remaining ingredients, stir until combined, and bring the mixture to a boil.

Switch heat to the level, simmer the soup for 40 minutes and then serve straight away.

Nutrition:
Calories: 129 Cal Fat: 5.5 g Carbs: 15.3 g Protein: 4.6 g Fiber: 3.7 g

376. Sweet Potato, Kale, and Peanut Stew

Preparation Time: 10 minutes | **Cooking Time:** 45 minutes | **Servings:** 3

Ingredients:

1/4 cup red lentils	2 medium sweet potatoes, peeled, cubed
1 medium white onion, peeled, diced	1 cup kale, chopped
2 tomatoes, diced	1/4 cup chopped green onion
1 teaspoon minced garlic	1 inch of ginger, grated
2 tablespoons toasted peanuts	1/4 teaspoon ground black pepper
1 teaspoon ground cumin	1/2 teaspoon turmeric
1/8 teaspoon cayenne pepper	1 tablespoon peanut butter
1 1/2 cups vegetable broth	2 teaspoons coconut oil

Directions:
Take a medium pot, place it on medium heat, add oil and when it melts, add onions and cook for 5 minutes.

Then stir in ginger and garlic, cook for 2 minutes until fragrant, add lentils and potatoes along with all the spices, and stir until mixed.

Stir in tomatoes, pour in the broth, bring the mixture to boil, then switch heat to the low level and simmer for 30 minutes until cooked.

Then stir in peanut butter until incorporated and then puree by using an immersion blender until half-pureed.

Return stew over low heat, stir in kale, cook for 5 minutes until its leaves wilts, and then season with black pepper and salt.

Garnish the stew with peanuts and green onions and then serve.

Nutrition:
Calories: 401 Cal Fat: 6.7 g Carbs: 77.3 g Protein: 10.8 g Fiber: 16 g

377. Lentil Stew

Preparation Time: 35 minutes | **Cooking Time:** 30-120 minutes | **Servings:** 4

Ingredients:

1 cup red lentils, soaked	1 medium-sized onion, peeled and finely chopped
½ cup sweet carrot puree	1 tbsp all-purpose flour
½ tsp freshly ground black pepper	½ tsp cumin, ground
½ tsp salt	2 tbsp olive oil

Directions:
Soak the lentils overnight.

Rinse well the lentils under cold running water using a large colander. Drain well and set aside.

Plug your instant pot and grease the stainless steel insert with olive oil. Press the "Saute" button and heat it. Add onions and flour. Cook for 10 minutes, stirring constantly.

Now, add the remaining ingredients and pour in about 4 cups of water. Close the lid and set the release steam handle. Press the "Manual" button and cook for 30 minutes on high pressure.

Press the "Cancel" button and release the steam handle. Turn off the pot and set it aside to chill for a while before serving.

Optionally, sprinkle with cayenne pepper and parsley.

Nutrition:
Calories: 140 Cal Fat: 0.9 g Carbs: 27.1 g Protein: 6.3 g Fiber: 6.2 g

378. Ginger Stew

Preparation Time: 35 minutes | **Cooking Time:** 30-120 minutes | **Servings:** 4

Ingredients:

2 cups green peas	1 large onion, chopped
4 cloves of garlic, finely chopped	3 ½ oz of olives, pitted
1 tbsp of ginger, ground	1 tbsp of turmeric, ground

1 tbsp of salt

4 cups of vegetable stock

3 tbsp olive oil

Directions:

Rinse well the green peas using a large colander. Drain and set aside.

Plug your instant pot and press the "Saute" button. Heat the olive oil in the stainless steel insert and add onions and garlic. Stir-fry for 2-3 minutes, or until translucent.

Now, add the remaining ingredients and close the lid. Set the steam release handle and press the "Stew" button.

When you hear the cooker's end signal, perform a quick release.

Open the pot and serve immediately.

Nutrition:

Calories: 140 Cal Fat: 0.9 g Carbs: 27.1 g Protein: 6.3 g Fiber: 6.2 g

379. Ziti Mushroom Stew

Preparation Time: 6 minutes | **Cooking Time:** 30-120 minutes | **Servings:** 4

Ingredients:

1bell pepper, seeded and minced	1onion, minced
1 (14-ounce can crushed tomatoes	4garlic cloves, minced
2tablespoons tomato paste	½cup dry red wine
8ounces white mushrooms, coarsely chopped	1cup hot water
8ounces uncooked ziti	1teaspoon dried basil
Salt and black pepper	2teaspoons minced fresh oregano
1teaspoon natural sugar	2tablespoons chopped parsley

Directions:

Add the ziti, mushroom, red wine, tomato paste in an instant pot.

Add the sugar, herbs, spices, hot water, and the rest of the ingredients.

Mix well and cook for 5 minutes with the lid on. Serve hot.

Nutrition:

Calories:680, Total Fat:71.8g, Saturated Fat:20.9g, Total Carbs:10g, Dietary Fiber:7g, Sugar:2g, Protein:3g, Sodium:525mg

380. Spiced Red Lentil Vegetable Stew

Preparation Time: 25 minutes | **Cooking Time:** 30 minutes | **Servings:** 2

Ingredients:

1 1/2 tablespoon olive oil	½ zucchini, thinly sliced
1 small onion, diced	1 leek, diced
½ teaspoon garlic powder	¼ teaspoon salt
¼ teaspoon turmeric powder	¼ teaspoon paprika
2 cups vegetable broth	½ cup diced tomatoes
½ cup chickpeas drained and rinsed	½ cup sweet potatoes, quartered
½ cup dried red lentils	½ tablespoon fresh basil, chopped
½ cup goat cheese, shredded (optional	

Directions:

Set Instant Pot to Sauté and heat olive oil; cook zucchini, onions, leeks, and garlic powder, stirring occasionally until softened, about 6 minutes. Add salt, turmeric powder, and paprika; cook, stirring, for 1 minute.

Stir in vegetable broth, tomatoes, chickpeas, sweet potatoes, red lentils, and water; Close the steam valve, press the Manual button, select High pressure, then press the + button to increase the time to 20 minutes.

Once the pressure has been released, open the steam valve, and then remove the lid. Stir in basil and goat cheese.

Nutrition:

Calories 569, Total Fat 14. 9g, Saturated Fat 3. 6g, Cholesterol 7mg, Sodium 1113mg, Total Carbohydrate 79. 9g, Dietary Fiber 27. 1g, Total Sugars 13. 1g, Protein 31. 9g

381. Pinto Bean Stew with Cauliflower

Preparation Time: 10 minutes | **Cooking Time:** 25 minutes | **Servings:** 2

Ingredients:

1 cup of water	1 teaspoon salt
¼ cup pinto beans	2 tablespoons coconut oil
½ small onion chopped	1 small zucchini chopped
½ teaspoon garlic powder	1 bay leaf
1 1/2 cups low sodium vegetable stock	½ cup steamed cauliflower
¼ cup grated mozzarella	1 tablespoon chopped fresh cilantro

Directions:

In a large bowl, dissolve 1 tablespoon of salt in the water. Add the pinto beans and soak at room temperature for 8 to 24 hours. Drain and rinse. Select Sauté and adjust to Normal or Medium heat. Add the coconut oil to the Instant Pot and heat until shimmering. Add the onion and zucchini, and sprinkle with salt. Cook, stirring often until the onion pieces separate and soften. Add the garlic powder and cook for about 1 minute, or until fragrant. Add the drained pinto beans, remaining ¼ teaspoon of salt, bay leaf, and vegetable stock.

Lock the lid into place. Select Pressure Cook or Manual, and adjust the pressure to High and the time to 15 minutes. After cooking, let the pressure release naturally for 10 minutes, then quickly release any remaining pressure.

Unlock the lid. Stir in the cauliflower and bring to a simmer to heat it through and thicken the sauce slightly. Taste the beans and adjust the seasoning. Ladle into bowls and sprinkle with the mozzarella cheese and cilantro.

Nutrition:

Calories 245, Total Fat 16. 2g, Saturated Fat 13. 7g, Cholesterol 2mg, Sodium 1745mg, Total Carbohydrate 22. 4g, Dietary Fiber 5. 6g, Total Sugars 4. 5g, Protein 7. 7g

382. Pumpkin Stew

Preparation Time: 10 minutes | **Cooking Time:** 15 minutes | **Servings:** 2

Ingredients:

1 cup vegetable broth	1 1/2 cups pumpkin cut into small cubes
1 cup kidney beans cooked, rinsed, and drained	1 cup onion chopped
½ cup green peas	1 teaspoon garlic powder
½ cup diced tomatoes	1 teaspoon red chili
¼ teaspoon ground cumin	

Directions:

Place all the ingredients in the inner pot. Cover with a lid, turn the lid clockwise to lock into place. Align the pointed end of the steam release handle to point to "Sealing". Press "Manual", use the [-] button to adjust cooking time to 5 minutes.

When cooking time is complete, press "Keep Warm/Cancel" once to Cancel the keep warm mode then wait 10 minutes for the pressure to go down.

Slide the steam release handle to the "Venting" position to release the remaining pressure until the float valve drops down.

Remove the lid. Allow to cool for 10 minutes before serving. Enjoy!

Nutrition:

Calories245, Total Fat 2. 4g, Saturated Fat 0. 4g, Cholesterol 0mg, Sodium 805mg, Total Carbohydrate 43. 2g, Dietary Fiber 13. 6g, Total Sugars 11. 4g, Protein 14. 5g

383. Cauliflower and Bean Stew

Preparation Time: 10 minutes | **Cooking Time:** 10 minutes | **Servings:** 2

Ingredients:

1 cup cauliflower cut into 1-inch pieces	1 cup chickpea rinsed and drained
1 cup black beans, rinsed and drained	½ cup crushed tomatoes preferably fire-roasted
1 small onion chopped	¼ cup vegetable broth

1 orange juice	1 canned chipotle pepper in adobo sauce minced
1 teaspoon salt	1 teaspoon ground cumin
1 bay leaf	Fresh cilantro sprigs

Directions:

Combine cauliflower, chickpea, black beans, tomatoes, onions, broth, orange juice, chipotle pepper, salt, cumin, and bay leaf in Instant Pot; mix well.

Secure lid and move pressure release valve to sealing position. Press Manual or Pressure Cook; cook at High pressure 6 minutes.

When cooking is complete, use Natural-release for 5 minutes, then release remaining pressure. Press Sauté; cook 3 to 5 minutes or until the stew thickens slightly, stirring frequently. Remove and discard bay leaf. Garnish with cilantro.

Nutrition:

Calories 614, Total Fat 4. 6g, Saturated Fat 0. 9g, Cholesterol 0mg, Sodium 1816mg, Total Carbohydrate 115. 3g, Dietary Fiber 24. 8g, Total Sugars 12g, Protein 32. 9g

384. Cabbage Soup

Preparation Time: 10 minutes | **Cooking Time:** 20 minutes | **Servings:** 2

Ingredients:

1 head cabbage	½ tablespoon dried basil
2 Oz Cheddar cheese chunks	½ tablespoon coconut cream
½ teaspoon garlic powder	Salt to taste

Directions:

Add all ingredients to the blender pitcher and lock the lid.

Select the "Soup" setting for 20:00 minutes.

Garnish with shredded cheddar cheese and serve.

Nutrition:

Calories 213, Total Fat 10. 5g, Saturated Fat 6. 8g, Cholesterol 29mg, Sodium 316mg, Total Carbohydrate 21. 8g, Dietary Fiber 9. 1g, Total Sugars 11. 9g, Protein 11. 8g

385. Vegetable Stew

Preparation Time: 15 minutes | **Cooking Time:** 20 minutes | **Servings:** 2

Ingredients:

1 small onion, minced	1 teaspoon garlic powder
1 leek, minced	½ zucchini, minced
1/4 cup vegetable broth	2 oz. button mushrooms, sliced
1 teaspoon dried basil	½ teaspoon Italian seasoning
1/2 teaspoon salt	1/4 teaspoon ground pepper
2 tomatoes, chopped	1 medium parsnip, chopped
½ yum, chopped	¼ tablespoon balsamic vinegar
1 tablespoon cornstarch	¼ cup green beans
Enough water	

Directions:

Add onion and mushrooms to the Instant Pot. Press the Sauté button and sauté until mushrooms have released their liquid and shrunk in size, about 8 minutes. Stir every couple of minutes.

Add garlic powder and sauté for 2 more minutes. Add salt, basil, pepper. Stir.

Press Cancel to stop Sauté function. Lock lid in place.

Add the remaining ingredients to the pot with broth. Press Manual and adjust the time to 10 minutes of pressure cooking.

Meanwhile add water and cornstarch and make a mixer.

When the time has lapsed, quickly release the pressure from the Instant Pot. Remove the lid from you.

Add a cornstarch mixer into the pot and make a thick soup.

Carefully transfer soup into a bowl, serve, and enjoy.

Nutrition:

Calories 158, Total Fat 1. 2g, Saturated Fat 0. 2g, Cholesterol 1mg, Sodium 714mg, Total Carbohydrate 35. 1g, Dietary Fiber 6. 4g, Total Sugars 11. 1g, Protein 5. 5g

386. Cauliflower Soup

Preparation Time: 10 minutes | **Cooking Time:** 5 minutes | **Servings:** 2

Ingredients:

5 cups vegetable broth or water

1 medium onion chopped

1 - 2 stalks leek thinly sliced

2 cloves garlic crushed

1 lb. cauliflower cut in big chunks

1 teaspoon salt

1/2 teaspoon pepper

1 teaspoon fresh basil

1/4 cup almond flour

2/3 cup water

1 cup grated goat cheese

1/2 cup milk

Salt and pepper to taste

Directions:

Add the first 8 ingredients (including basil) to the Instant Pot and lock lid. Make sure the valve is set to Sealing and press Pressure Cooker (or Manual). Set the time with the + /- button for 5 minutes.

While cooking, stir in flour and water until smooth. When the IP beeps, flip the valve from Sealing to Venting and when the pin drops, press Cancel and remove the lid.

Press the Sauté button and cook again, stirring frequently. Whisk the flour-water mixture and add about half of it to the soup.

Use a hand blender to puree the soup. Or use a blender or food processor and put it back in the pan.

Press Cancel and add the cheese. Stir until melted. Do not cook after the cheese has gone in. Add the milk, salt, and pepper to your taste. Serve with a pinch of grated cheese.

Nutrition:

Calories 202, Total Fat 8. 4g, Saturated Fat 4. 4g, Cholesterol 20mg, Sodium 1345mg, Total Carbohydrate 23. 2g, Dietary Fiber 7. 8g, Total Sugars 11. 3g, Protein 12. 6g

387. Pumpkin Soup

Preparation Time: 10 minutes | **Cooking Time:** 20 minutes | **Servings:** 2

Ingredients:

1 lb pumpkin peeled and seeded 1/2-1inch cubes

1 cup vegetable broth or water

1 teaspoon dried rosemary

1/4 teaspoon grated cinnamon

1/2 teaspoon salt

1 cup of coconut milk

2 tablespoons butter

1 tablespoon almond flour

Directions:

Mix the pumpkin cubes, broth, rosemary, cinnamon, and salt in an Instant Pot. Lock the lid onto the pot.

Press Soup/Broth, Pressure Cooker, or Manual on High Pressure for 5 minutes with the Keep Warm setting off. The valve must be closed.

Use the Quick-release mode to return the pot pressure to normal. Unlock the lid and open the pot. Add coconut milk.

Use an immersion blender to puree the soup right in the pot. Or work in halves to puree the soup in a covered blender. If necessary, pour all the soup back into the pan.

Press the Sauté button and set it for Low, 250°F. Set the timer for 5 minutes.

Bring the soup to a simmer, stirring often. In the meantime, place the butter in a small bowl or measuring container and place it in the microwave in 5-second increments. Use a fork to mix the flour and make a thin paste.

When the soup is boiling, Whisk the butter mixture in the pan. Continue whisking until the soup is a bit thick, about 1 minute. Turn off the Sauté function and allow it to cool for a few minutes before serving.

Nutrition:

Calories 415, Total Fat 41g, Saturated Fat 32. 9g, Cholesterol 31mg, Sodium 1064mg, Total Carbohydrate 11. 5g, Dietary Fiber 3. 3g, Total Sugars 5. 2g, Protein 5. 9g

388. Almond Broccoli Soup

Preparation Time: 05 minutes | **Cooking Time:** 20 minutes | **Servings:** 2

Ingredients:

1/2 cup roasted almond divided	2 1/2 cups vegetable broth divided
½ tablespoon fresh basil leaves chopped	½ tablespoon fresh oregano leaves chopped
1 teaspoon garlic powder	15 oz can chickpeas drained and rinsed
1 small onion roughly chopped	1 small head broccoli cut into florets

Directions:

Add an almond to the blender pitcher and lock the lid.

Touch Pulse, then touch Start.

When the Pulse program is complete, scrape down the sides and bottom of the Pitcher.

Add 1/2 cup broth and lock the lid.

Touch Pulse, then Start.

When the Pulse program is complete, add the remaining broth, herbs, garlic powder, chickpeas, onion, and broccoli--in that order--and lock the lid.

Touch Soup two times and use +/- to set the time to 14 minutes, then touch Start.

Adjust seasonings and Serve.

Nutrition:

Calories192, Total Fat 9. 7g, Saturated Fat 0. 7g, Cholesterol 0mg, Sodium 450mg, Total Carbohydrate 20. 4g, Dietary Fiber 4g, Total Sugars 6. 4g, Protein 7. 8g

389. Jackfruit Stew

Preparation Time: 10 minutes | **Cooking Time:** 25 minutes | **Servings:** 2

Ingredients:

1 large onion chopped	3 cloves garlic minced
1 1/2 cup vegetable broth	1 teaspoon salt
1/2 teaspoon pepper	1 cup jackfruit
1 sweet potato cut into 1-inch pieces	1 carrot cut into 1-inch pieces
½ cup frozen peas	1 tablespoon cornstarch
3 tablespoons water	2 tablespoons chopped fresh parsley

Directions:

Mix the first six ingredients, including the jackfruit, in the Instant Pot. Lock lid in place and turn the valve to Sealing. Press the Pressure Cooker button and set the cooking time for 20 minutes at High Pressure.

During cooking, cut sweet potatoes and carrots with or without peel into 1-inch pieces. Make a mixture by stirring the corn-starch in the water until smooth.

When the Instant Pot beeps, let it go for 10 minutes. Release the remaining pressure naturally and open the pot when the pin drops. Add the sweet potatoes and carrots (not the peas) and gently squeeze them into the liquid. Lock lid and press hit pressure (or Manual). Set the cooking time to 4 minutes. When it's done, take a quick release (pin drop), open the pot.

Tap Cancel then Sauté. Stir in the corn-starch and add about half of the mortar as the stew cooks. Boil to thicken it, and if you want thicker, add more.

Press Cancel and add frozen peas. The heat of the stew is enough to cook them without turning them into mush. Add salt and pepper if necessary. Add the parsley if you use it,

Nutrition:

Calories 267, Total Fat 1. 8g, Saturated Fat 0. 4g, Cholesterol 0mg, Sodium 1786mg, Total Carbohydrate 56g, Dietary Fiber 8. 1g, Total Sugars 7. 5g, Protein 10g

390. Ginger & Turmeric Carrot Soup

Preparation Time: 10 minutes | **Cooking Time:** 25 minutes | **Servings:** 2

Ingredients:

½ tablespoon butter	1 onion and sliced
1 1/2 cups chopped carrots	½ cup chopped pumpkin
¼ cup tomato, chopped	1 teaspoon garlic powder
1 tablespoon grated ginger	1 tablespoon turmeric powder
Salt & pepper to taste	3 cups vegetable broth
1 cup of coconut milk	

Directions:
Set on Sauté mode and pour in the butter.
Add in the diced onion, carrots, and mix until combined.
Sauté for about 5 minutes or until the vegetables become soft.
Stir in the garlic powder, ginger turmeric powder, salt, and pepper.
Add in the pumpkin, tomatoes, broth, coconut milk, and stir to combine.
Lock the lid in place and close the steam vent.
Set on Manual or Pressure Cooker on High Pressure for 4 minutes.
Allow the Instant Pot to Natural-release for 5 minutes once the timer goes off.
Remove the lid and stir to combine.
Enjoy!

Nutrition:
Calories 435, Total Fat 34. 3g, Saturated Fat 28g, Cholesterol 8mg, Sodium 1228mg, Total Carbohydrate 25. 1g, Dietary Fiber 7. 4g, Total Sugars 11. 2g, Protein 12. 2g

391. Coconut Tofu Soup

Preparation Time: 10 minutes | **Cooking Time:** 10 minutes | **Servings:** 2

Ingredients:

2 cups vegetable broth or water	1/2 pound tofu
½ cup full fat coconut milk	1 tablespoon ginger
2 whole red chills	½ tablespoon lemon zest
1 teaspoon maple syrup	1/2 teaspoon salt
1/4 cup fresh lime juice from 2 or 3 limes	Chopped fresh parsley for garnish
Lime wedges for serving	

Directions:
In the Instant Pot, combine the broth, tofu, half the coconut milk, the ginger, chills (if using), lemon zest, maple syrup, and salt.
Lock lid on the Instant Pot. Close the Pressure-release valve. Select Manual or Pressure Cooker and set the pot at Low Pressure for 1 minute. At the end of the cooking time, quickly release the pressure.

Stir in the remaining coconut milk, and lime juice.
Divide the soup among two serving bowls. Garnish with parsley and serve with lime wedges alongside for squeezing.

Nutrition:
Calories 238, Total Fat 19. 2g, Saturated Fat 13. 7g, Cholesterol 0mg, Sodium 31mg, Total Carbohydrate 10. 3g, Dietary Fiber 2. 9g, Total Sugars 5g, Protein 11g

392. Millet Soup

Preparation Time: 10 minutes | **Cooking Time:** 30 minutes | **Servings:** 2

Ingredients:

½ tablespoon butter	1/4 cup onion
½ cup chopped parsnips	½ cup sliced leeks,
1 teaspoon garlic powder	½ tablespoon lemon zest
Pinch of salt & pepper	¼ cup millet
2 cups vegetable broth	½ cup of soy milk
1/8 cup lemon juice	1 cup fresh Swiss chard

Directions:
Heat the butter in an Instant Pot and select the Sauté function. When butter melts add the onion, parsnips, leeks, and garlic powder and sauté until soft, about 5 minutes.
Add lemon zest, broth, and millet, salt, and pepper, and stir to combine. Lock lid in place and turn the valve to Sealing. Press the Pressure Cooker button and set the cooking time for 20 minutes at High Pressure.
When the Instant Pot beeps, let it go for 10 minutes. Release the remaining pressure naturally and open the pot when the pin drops. Once the Millet is cooked and soft, stir in the soy milk, lemon juice, and Swiss chard. Stir until Swiss chard is wilted.
Lock lid and press hit pressure (or Manual). Set the cooking time to 4 minutes. When it's done, take a quick release (pin drop), open the Instant Pot. Serve immediately and enjoy! Soup can be frozen and reheated as desired.

Nutrition:
Calories 249, Total Fat 6. 8g, Saturated Fat 2. 7g, Cholesterol 8mg, Sodium 867mg, Total

Carbohydrate 35. 8g, Dietary Fiber 5. 4g, Total Sugars 7. 2g, Protein 11. 3g

393. White Lima beans Stew

Preparation Time:15 minutes | **Cooking Time:** 40 minutes | **Servings:** 2

Ingredients:

½ cup kale	½ tablespoons coconut oil
1 medium onion, chopped	½ teaspoon ginger powder
½ small bell pepper, seeded and finely chopped	½ teaspoon garlic powder
¼ tablespoon curry powder	1 medium zucchini, peeled and thinly sliced
¼ medium head broccoli, broken into bite-size florets	½ can white lima beans, rinsed
1 small diced tomato	¼ cup almond milk
2 cups vegetable broth or water	Salt to taste

Directions:

In a large bowl, add the white lima beans and soak at room temperature for 8 to 24 hours. Drain and rinse.

Select Sauté and adjust to Normal or Medium heat. Add the coconut oil to the inner pot of Instant Pot and heat. Add the onion and zucchini and sprinkle with 1/4 teaspoon of salt. Cook, stirring often until the onion pieces separate and soften. Add the garlic powder and ginger powder and cook for about 1 minute, or until fragrant. Add the drained white lima beans, remaining 1/4 teaspoon of salt tomatoes, and broth.

Lock lid in place and turn the valve to Sealing. Press the Pressure Cooker button and set the cooking time for 5 minutes at High Pressure. After cooking, let the pressure release naturally for 10 minutes, then quickly release any remaining pressure.

Unlock the lid. Stir in the broccoli, kale bell pepper, and almond milk and bring to a simmer to heat it through and thicken the sauce slightly. Serve.

Nutrition:
Calories 205, Total Fat 11. 4g, Saturated Fat 9. 4g, Cholesterol 0mg, Sodium 121mg, Total Carbohydrate 23. 4g, Dietary Fiber 6. 3g, Total Sugars 8. 4g, Protein 6. 3g

394. Lentil Soup with Spinach

Preparation Time:10 minutes | **Cooking Time:** 40 minutes | **Servings:** 2

Ingredients:

¼ cup lentils	4 cups water, divided
1 tablespoon butter	1 small onion, diced
1 small beetroot, diced	½ teaspoon salt, divided
1/8 teaspoon ground pepper	½ teaspoon garlic powder,
¼ teaspoon ground coriander	½ cup chopped spinach
½ cup small sweet potatoes, quartered	

Directions:

Wash the lentils very well and pick out any stones.

Add lentils and water to the Instant Pot and stir well.

Cover the Instant Pot and lock it in.

Make sure the vent on top is set to "Sealing". Set Manual or Pressure Cooker Timer for 25 minutes. Once the timer reaches zero, quickly release the pressure. Keep aside.

Then Select Sauté and adjust to medium heat. Add the butter to the Instant Pot and heat until melted. Add the onions and beetroot, sweet potato, and sprinkle salt and pepper. Cook, stirring often until the onion softens. Add the garlic powder and ground coriander cook for about 1 minute, or until fragrant. Add water and lock the lid into place. Select Pressure Cooker or Manual, and adjust the pressure to High and the time to 5 minutes. After cooking, let the pressure release naturally for 5minutes, then quickly release any remaining pressure.

Unlock the lid. Stir in the spinach and bring to a simmer to heat it through spinach wilt. Then add cooked lentils and adjust it tasty to add salt and pepper.

Serve and enjoy.

Nutrition:
Calories 211, Total Fat 6. 2g, Saturated Fat 3. 7g, Cholesterol 15mg, Sodium 689mg, Total Carbohydrate 31. 7g, Dietary Fiber 9. 4g, Total Sugars 6. 2g, Protein 8. 4g

395. Chickpea and Mushroom Soup

Preparation Time:05 minutes | **Cooking Time:** 30 minutes | **Servings:** 2

Ingredients:

½ tablespoon avocado oil	8 ounces mushrooms, sliced/chopped
¼ onion chopped	½ teaspoon garlic powder
½ can chickpeas, drained & rinsed	2 cups vegetable broth
½ tablespoon dried Italian seasoning	½ teaspoon dried basil
Pinch of hot pepper flakes	Salt & pepper to taste

Directions:
Select Sauté and adjust to Normal heat. Add the avocado oil to the Instant Pot and heat. Add garlic powder and onion and cook until the onions are slightly opaque and beginning to brown. Add mushrooms, when the mushrooms start to soften, add the spices, seasonings, and the chickpeas. Season with salt and pepper. Add broth and lock the lid into place. Select Pressure Cooker or Manual, and adjust the pressure to High and the time to 20minutes. After cooking, let the pressure release naturally for 5 minutes, then quickly release any remaining pressure. Unlock the lid.
Adjust the seasoning and serve.

Nutrition:
Calories163, Total Fat 4g, Cholesterol 2mg, Sodium 955mg, Total Carbohydrate 21. 5g, Dietary Fiber 4. 6g, Total Sugars 4. 2g, Protein 12. 6g

396. Corn Potato Stew

Preparation Time:10 minutes | **Cooking Time:** 25 minutes | **Servings:** 2

Ingredients:

1 cup vegetable broth	1 cup of water
½ pounds potatoes, peeled, and cut into 2-inch pieces	1 medium onion
¼ teaspoon garlic powder,	½ teaspoons dried basil, crushed
½ teaspoon chili powder	½ teaspoon ground cumin
¼ teaspoon salt	1 cup sweet corns, rinsed and drained
½ cup pinto beans, rinsed and drained	½ tablespoon fresh cilantro

Directions:
Add all of the ingredients to the Instant Pot and stir well.
Cover the Instant Pot and lock it in.
Lock the lid in place and close the steam vent.
Set on Manual or Pressure Cooker on High Pressure for 20 minutes.
Allow the IP to Natural-release for 5 minutes once the timer goes off.
Remove the lid and stir to combine.
Enjoy!

Nutrition:
Calories358, Total Fat 2. 6g, Saturated Fat 0. 5g, Cholesterol 0mg, Sodium 710mg, Total Carbohydrate 69g, Dietary Fiber 13. 8g, Total Sugars 7. 7g, Protein 18g

397. Tempeh wild Rice Soup

Preparation Time:05 minutes | **Cooking Time:** 20 minutes | **Servings:** 2

Ingredients:

1 tablespoon olive oil	1 tablespoon coconut flour
2 cups vegetable broth or water	1cup tempeh
¼ cup zucchini diced	¼ carrot shredded
¼ cup uncooked wild rice	¼ tablespoon maple syrup
1 teaspoon dried mint	1 teaspoon kosher salt
½ teaspoon pepper	1 clove garlic minced
1 teaspoon cilantro chopped for garnish	

Directions:
Add broth, tempeh, zucchini, carrot, wild rice, maple syrup, mint, salt, pepper, and minced garlic to the Instant Pot and stir to combine. Lock lid, making sure the vent is closed.

Using the display panel select the Manual or Pressure Cooker function. Use +/- keys and program the Instant Pot for 15 minutes.

When the time is up, let the pressure naturally release for 10 minutes, then quickly release the remaining pressure.

In a medium bowl, add coconut flour in olive oil until it makes a paste. Ladle 1 cup of the hot soup broth into the paste and stir to incorporate, then pour flour mixture into the Instant Pot.

Using the display panel select Cancel and then Sauté. Cook and stir until thickened, then stir in the half and half.

Serve warm topped with chopped cilantro.

Nutrition:
Calories 356, Total Fat 17. 8g, Saturated Fat 3. 4g, Cholesterol 0mg, Sodium 1957mg, Total Carbohydrate 29. 2g, Dietary Fiber 2. 7g, Total Sugars 3. 9g, Protein 24. 3g

398. Pear Pumpkin Soup

Preparation Time:05 minutes | **Cooking Time:** 10 minutes | **Servings:** 2

Ingredients:

½ teaspoon butter	¼ onion finely diced
1 cup pumpkin, peeled and cubed	1 pear peeled and cubed
½ teaspoon salt	¼ teaspoon cumin
¼ teaspoon ground coriander	1 cup vegetable broth or water
½ tablespoon coconut cream	½ teaspoon honey

Directions:
Add butter to the Instant Pot. Using the display panel select the Sauté function.

When butter gets melted, add onions to the Instant Pot and sauté until soft, 2-3 minutes. Add pear, salt, cumin, and spices and stir to combine.

Add broth to the Instant Pot then add pumpkin and stir. Turn the Instant Pot off by selecting Cancel, then lock the lid, making sure the vent is closed.

Using the display panel select the Manual or Pressure Cooker function. Use the + /- keys and program the Instant Pot for 5 minutes.

When the time is up, quickly release the remaining pressure, then select Cancel to turn off the pot.

Use an immersion blender to blend the soup until smooth.

Cool slightly, then stir in coconut cream and honey.

Serve warm.

Nutrition:
Calories 87, Total Fat 2. 8g, Saturated Fat 1. 6g, Cholesterol 3mg, Sodium 972mg, Total Carbohydrate 13. 3g, Dietary Fiber 2. 8g, Total Sugars 7. 4g, Protein 3. 6g

399. Zucchini Coconut Thai Soup

Preparation Time:15 minutes | **Cooking Time:** 20 minutes | **Servings:** 2

Ingredients:

½ tablespoon olive oil	½ onion, peeled and diced
½ pound zucchini, peeled and diced	1 cup spinach
1 small carrot	1 teaspoon ginger garlic paste
½ tablespoon red curry paste	2 cups vegetable broth or water
½ teaspoon maple syrup	½ cup coconut milk canned
1 tablespoon lime juice	1/4 teaspoon red pepper flakes
1 teaspoon of sea salt	1/2 teaspoon black pepper ground
1/4 cup basil	

Directions:
Press the Sauté button on the Instant Pot. When the display shows "Hot", add olive oil and heat it. Add the onions and carrots, zucchinis, spinach. Sauté for 3–5 minutes until onions are translucent.

Add the ginger-garlic paste and curry paste. Continue to sauté for 1 minute.

Add remaining ingredients, except basil. Lock lid.

Press the Soup button and set the time to 20 minutes. When the timer beeps, let the pressure release naturally for 10 minutes. Quickly release any additional pressure until the float valve drops and then unlock the lid.

In the Instant Pot, puree soup with a hand blender, or use a stand blender and puree in batches.

Ladle into bowls, garnish each bowl with basil, and serve hot.

Have fun!

Nutrition:
Calories 136, Total Fat 7. 2g, Saturated Fat 2. 1g, Cholesterol 0mg, Sodium 1930mg, Total Carbohydrate 11. 8g, Dietary Fiber 2. 3g, Total Sugars 5. 7g, Protein 7g

400. Vegetable and Cottage Cheese Soup

Preparation Time: 35 minutes | **Cooking Time:** 15 minutes | **Servings:** 2

Ingredients:

½ package cottage cheese, drained and cut into ¾-inch cubes	1 tablespoon coconut oil
½ teaspoon dried Italian seasoning	1 diced tomatoes
1 cup vegetable broth	½ cup fresh peas
½ cup kale	¼ cup cauliflower
½ cup 1-inch pieces green beans	½ cup chopped green sweet pepper
¼ cup sliced green olives	

Directions:

Put the cottage cheese in a plastic bag within a flat plate. Add the oil and Italian seasoning; Turn to cover the cottage cheese. Marinate in the refrigerator for 2 to 4 hours.

Press the Sauté button on the Instant Pot. When the display shows "Hot", add coconut oil and heat it. Press Sauté function and add cottage cheese and set timer for 5 minutes until cottage cheese browns.

Add broth and tomato into IP. Then Add peas, kale, cauliflower, green beans, green sweet pepper, and green olives and again set the timer for 10 minutes and lock the lid of Instant Pot.

When time is up, let the pressure release naturally for 10 minutes. Quickly release any additional pressure until the float valve drops and then unlock the lid.

Serve the soup and enjoy.

Nutrition:
Calories229, Total Fat 12. 3g, Saturated Fat 8. 6g, Cholesterol 13mg, Sodium 765mg, Total Carbohydrate 16. 9g, Dietary Fiber 4. 5g, Total Sugars 6. 4g, Protein 15g

401. Zucchini Tomato Soup

Preparation Time: 15 minutes | **Cooking Time:** 15 minutes | **Servings:** 2

Ingredients:

1 pound large tomatoes, cored and cut into pieces	¼ zucchini, cut into chunks
¼ cup broccoli	1 medium bell pepper, seeded and cut into pieces
1 teaspoon garlic powder	2 tablespoons butter, divided
1 tablespoon vinegar, divided	1 teaspoon plus a pinch of salt, divided
½ teaspoon plus a pinch of ground pepper, divided	¼ avocado
¼ tablespoon chopped fresh basil	Enough water

Directions:

Cut all the vegetables and set them aside.

Press the Sauté mode and pour in the butter. When it melts, add zucchini, broccoli, and bell pepper and mix them. Sauté for a few minutes or until the vegetables are tender, about 5 minutes. Add garlic powder, water, and spices and mix.

lock lid. Set Manual cook or Pressure for 4 minutes on High Pressure.

Allow the IP to Natural-release for 5 minutes once the timer goes off.

Remove the lid and mix well. Serve soup with a topping of avocado and fresh basil.

Have fun!

Nutrition:
Calories 228, Total Fat 17. 1g, Saturated Fat 8. 4g, Cholesterol 31mg, Sodium 1266mg, Total Carbohydrate 18. 5g, Dietary Fiber 6. 1g, Total Sugars 10. 1g, Protein 4. 1g

402. Vegetarian Spinach Soup

Preparation Time: 15 minutes | **Cooking Time:** 20 minutes | **Servings:** 2

Ingredients:

½ tablespoon coconut oil	¼ onion, finely chopped
½ stalk leek, finely chopped	1 teaspoon garlic powder
1 teaspoon basil, freshly chopped	¼ teaspoon red pepper flakes (optional
Salt	Freshly ground black pepper
2 cups vegetable broth	Enough water
1 (15. 5oz.) can chickpea, drained and rinsed	Juice of 1 lemon
1 large bunch Spinach, removed from stems and torn into medium pieces	

Directions:

In an Instant Pot press the Sauté button and set it for Medium, heat oil. Add onion, leek, and cook until slightly soft, 6 minutes. Add garlic powder, basil, and red pepper flakes and cook until fragrant, 1 minute more. Season with salt and pepper.

Add broth, water, lemon juice, chickpea, and Spinach. Press Soup/Broth, Pressure Cooker, or Manual on High Pressure for 10 minutes with the Keep Warm setting off. The valve must be closed.

Use the Quick-release method to return the pot pressure to normal. Unlock the lid and open the pot.

Use an immersion blender to puree the soup right in the pot.

Press the Sauté button and set it for Low, 250°F. Set the timer for 5 minutes.

Bring the soup to a simmer, stirring often.

Serve.

Nutrition:

Calories 336, Total Fat 7. 8g, Saturated Fat 2. 7g, Cholesterol 0mg, Sodium 669mg, Total Carbohydrate 50. 7g, Dietary Fiber 15. 2g, Total Sugars 9. 8g, Protein 20. 1g

403. Green Soup

Preparation Time: 10 minutes | **Cooking Time:** 35 minutes | **Servings:** 2

Ingredients:

4 cups vegetable broth	1 small onion, cut into 3/4inch pieces
1/3 cup rice	1 tablespoon vegetable oil
1 teaspoon garlic powder	Salt
1/4 cup Greek yogurt	1 tsp minced fresh mint
1/4 tsp finely grated lime zest plus 1/2 tsp juice	6 oz. collard greens stemmed and chopped
4 oz spinach, stemmed and chopped	1 cup beet greens

Directions:

Add broth, onion, rice, oil, garlic powder, and 1/2 teaspoon salt to the blender. Lock lid in place, then select Soup program 2 (for creamy soups). In the meantime, combine Greek yogurt, mint, lime zest and juice, and remaining 1/4 teaspoon salt in a bowl; refrigerate until ready to serve.

Pause program 12 minutes before it has been completed. Carefully remove the lid and stir in collard greens and spinach until completely submerged.

Return lid and resume program. Pause the program 1 minute before it has been completed. Stir in beet greens. Return lid and resume program. Once the program has completed, adjust soup consistency with extra broth as needed and season with salt and pepper to taste. Drizzle individual portions with yogurt sauce before serving.

Nutrition:

Calories 306, Total Fat 9. 7g, Saturated Fat 1. 8g, Cholesterol 1mg 0%, Sodium 225mg, Total Carbohydrate 48. 7g, Dietary Fiber 12. 6g, Total Sugars 3. 4g, Protein 13. 6g

404. Tofu and Quinoa Soup

Preparation Time: 10 minutes | **Cooking Time:** 20 minutes | **Servings:** 2

Ingredients:

4 ounces mushrooms, trimmed and quartered	1 small onion, cut into 3/4-inch pieces
1 1/2 tablespoons tomato paste	1 tablespoon olive oil
1 teaspoon garlic powder	1 teaspoon minced fresh basil
1/4 teaspoon pepper	3 cups vegetable broth
1 carrot, peeled and cut into 3/4-inch pieces	2 oz tofu and cut into ¼-inch pieces
1/4 cup quinoa	2 tablespoons minced fresh coriander

Directions:

Microwave mushrooms, onion, tomato paste, oil, garlic powder, basil, and pepper in Instant Pot, stirring occasionally until vegetables are softened, about 5 minutes; transfer to a blender along with broth, carrot. Lock the lid in place, then select Soup Program.

Pause program once preheating ends. Carefully remove the lid and stir in tofu and quinoa. Return lid and resume program. Once the program has completed, season with salt and pepper to taste. Sprinkle individual portions with coriander and serve.

Nutrition:
Calories 236, Total Fat 12. 2g, Saturated Fat 1. 9g, Cholesterol 0mg, Sodium 1188mg, Total Carbohydrate 18. 6g, Dietary Fiber 3. 5g, Total Sugars 6. 7g, Protein 15. 3g

405. Jackfruit Beetroot Soup

Preparation Time: 10 minutes | **Cooking Time:** 20 minutes | **Servings:** 2

Ingredients:

1 beetroot roughly chopped	½ large green turnips roughly chopped
½ cup jackfruit	2 cup water cold running tap water
½ teaspoon ginger powder	2 dried dates
Sea salt to taste	2 cups of cold running tap water

Directions:

Place all the ingredients into the Instant Pot. Pour 2 cups of cold running tap water into the pot. Do not add any salt. lock lid and pressure cook on Manual at High Pressure for 20 minutes. Turn off the heat and release it naturally (roughly 20 – 25 minutes).

Carefully open the lid and heat the pressure cooker to bring the soup back to a full boil. Add sea salt to taste.

Nutrition:
Calories 86, Total Fat 0. 3g, Saturated Fat 0. 1g, Cholesterol 0mg, Sodium 214mg, Total Carbohydrate 21g, Dietary Fiber 2. 6g, Total Sugars 5. 5g, Protein 2g

406. Quinoa Stew with Celery, Mushrooms, and Kale

Preparation Time: 25 minutes | **Cooking Time:** 30 minutes | **Servings:** 2

Ingredients:

½ tablespoon coconut oil, divided	½ cup chopped celery
½ cup sliced mushrooms	½ teaspoon garlic powder
1 teaspoon minced fresh basil	2 tomatoes
½ cup quinoa	2 cups vegetable broth
½ cup kale	1 teaspoon chopped parsley
Salt and pepper to taste	

Directions:

Select Sauté and adjust to Normal heat. Add the coconut oil to the Instant Pot and heat it. Add the celery sprinkle with salt and pepper. Cook, stir often until the celery softens. Add mushrooms, garlic powder, and basil and cook for about 1 minute, or until mushrooms soften. Add tomatoes and quinoa, kale, and broth.

Lock lid in place and turn the valve to Sealing. Press the Pressure Cooker button and set the cooking time for 15 minutes at High Pressure. After cooking, let the pressure release naturally for 10 minutes, then quickly release any remaining pressure.

Unlock the lid. Stir in the kale and stir until wilted to heat it through and thicken the sauce slightly. Taste the soup and adjust the seasoning. Ladle into bowls and sprinkle with the parsley.

Nutrition:
Calories 263, Total Fat 7. 7g, Saturated Fat 3. 7g, Cholesterol 0mg, Sodium 800mg, Total Carbohydrate 36. 3g, Dietary Fiber 5. 3g, Total Sugars 4. 6g, Protein 13g

407. Butternut Squash Stew with Black Beans

Preparation Time:10 minutes | **Cooking Time:** 30 minutes | **Servings:** 2

Ingredients:

½ tablespoon butter	½ onion, chopped
1 teaspoon garlic powder	¼ cup butternut squash puree
¼ cup tomatoes	1 cup vegetable stock or water
¼ cup black beans	½ teaspoon cumin
½ teaspoon chili powder	Salt and pepper to taste

Directions:
Select Sauté and adjust to medium heat. Add the butter to the Instant Pot and heat until melted. Add the onion and cumin and cook, stirring often, until the onion pieces separate and soften. Add butternut squash puree, tomatoes, vegetable stock (or water), and black beans.
Lock lid in place and turn the valve to Sealing. Press the Pressure Cooker button and set the cooking time for 10 minutes at High Pressure. After cooking, let the pressure release naturally for 20 minutes, then quickly release any remaining pressure.
Unlock the lid. Stir in the garlic powder, chili powder, salt, and pepper and bring to a simmer, taste the beans and adjust the seasoning.

Nutrition:
Calories 145, Total Fat 3. 6g, Saturated Fat 2g, Cholesterol 8mg, Sodium 58mg, Total Carbohydrate 23. 4g, Dietary Fiber 6. 1g, Total Sugars 3. 5g, Protein 6. 6g

408. Spicy Sweet Potato Stew

Preparation Time:10 minutes | **Cooking Time:** 15 minutes | **Servings:** 2

Ingredients:

1 cup vegetable broth	½ cup sweet potato cut into small cubes
½ cup pinto beans cooked, rinsed, and drained	½ cup red onion chopped
¼ cup green peas fresh or frozen	1 bell pepper
¼ teaspoon garlic powder	1 tomato
1 teaspoon red chili	1 teaspoon ground nutmeg

Directions:
Place all the ingredients like sweet potato, broth, pinto beans, onion, green peas, bell pepper, garlic powder, tomato, and red chili, and nutmeg in the Instant Pot. Lock lid in place and turn the valve to Sealing. Press the Pressure Cooker button and set the cooking time for 10 minutes at High Pressure. After cooking, let the pressure release naturally for 5 minutes, then quickly release any remaining pressure.
Slide the steam release handle to the "Venting" position to release the remaining pressure until the float valve drops down.
Remove the lid. Allow to cool 10 minutes before serving. Enjoy!

Nutrition:
Calories 184, Total Fat 1. 7g, Saturated Fat 0. 6g, Cholesterol 0mg, Sodium 543mg, Total Carbohydrate 34. 2g, Dietary Fiber 8. 6g, Total Sugars 10. 5g, Protein 9. 7g

409. Broccoli Potato Soup

Preparation Time:05 minutes | **Cooking Time:** 10 minutes | **Servings:** 2

Ingredients:

½ pound broccoli	1 pound Yukon gold potatoes
2 cups vegetable broth or water	½ large onion
1 teaspoon garlic powder	½ tablespoons dried rosemary

1 cup coconut milk unsweetened

Directions:

Place all ingredients except the coconut milk in the Instant Pot.

Select Manual function and cook on High Pressure for 6 minutes. When time is up, release pressure.

Add the coconut milk.

Puree with an immersion blender right in the pot until smooth.

This soup is delicious served over black, red, or wild rice, or alone.

Nutrition:

Calories 148Total Fat 2. 7g, Saturated Fat 2. 1g, Cholesterol 0mg, Sodium 55mg, Total Carbohydrate 28. 8g, Dietary Fiber 5. 9g, Total Sugars 4. 4g, Protein 5. 6g

410. Minestrone Soup

Preparation Time:05 minutes | **Cooking Time:** 15 minutes | **Servings:** 2

Ingredients:

½ cup chickpeas cooked	½ cup jackfruit
1 sweet potato diced	1 zucchini diced
½ leek diced	¼ onion
1 teaspoon garlic, minced	2 cups vegetable broth
2 tomatoes	1 tablespoon Italian seasoning
1 teaspoon salt	

Directions:

Add all ingredients to the Instant Pot and stir.

Close Instant Pot lid, and on Manual at High Pressure, set cooking time for 15minutes.

When time is up, let the Instant Pot release naturally for 10 minutes. Quickly release any remaining pressure.

Serve and enjoy!

Nutrition:

Calories 273, Total Fat 5g, Saturated Fat 0. 9g, Cholesterol 5mg, Sodium 1969mg, Total Carbohydrate 48. 7g, Dietary Fiber 7. 9g, Total Sugars 10. 9g, Protein 12g

411. Lemon Coriander Soup

Preparation Time:05 minutes | **Cooking Time:** 15 minutes | **Servings:** 2

Ingredients:

½ tablespoon butter	¼ teaspoon mustard seeds
¼ teaspoon turmeric powder	½ teaspoon Pigeon peas
½ teaspoon red lentils	½ teaspoon black lentils
1 lemon juiced (or adjust to taste	Salt to taste
Water as needed for desired consistency	1 small bunch of cilantro or coriander
2 teaspoons cumin seeds	1 teaspoon black pepper
2 green chilies (or to taste	1 teaspoon Ginger-Garlic

Directions:

Paste all the ingredients under "Paste" into a coarse paste without using water and keep aside.

Put Instant Pot on Sauté mode High and add butter.

Once butter is melted add mustard seeds and turmeric powder. Fry for a minute.

Now add ground cilantro paste and fry for 2 minutes.

Now add all three lentils and water, along with salt. Mix them well.

Turn off Sauté mode and put the lid on. Set vent to the Sealing position.

Do Manual High 8 mins. Do Natural-release but you can do Quick-release after 5 minutes in Warm mode.

After opening the lid, check for consistency, if desired add water, and put on Sauté mode for 2 to 3 minutes.

Now add lemon juice and garnish with cilantro. Serve hot.

Nutrition:

Calories73, Total Fat 5. 1g, Saturated Fat 1. 9g, Cholesterol 8mg, Sodium 227mg, Total Carbohydrate 5. 8g, Dietary Fiber 1. 3g, Total Sugars 1. 2g, Protein 1. 3g

412. Root Vegetable Soup

Preparation Time: 05 minutes | **Cooking Time:** 15 minutes | **Servings:** 2

Ingredients:

1 medium zucchini, peeled and cut into 1-inch-thick pieces	½ medium beets, peeled and cut into 1-inch cubes
1 medium carrot, peeled and cut into 1-inch-thick pieces	½ medium red onion, cut into thin wedges
½ teaspoon garlic powder	½ tablespoon butter
½ teaspoon dried rosemary, crushed	⅛ teaspoon ground black pepper
1 cup of coconut milk	1 cup vegetable broth
1 tablespoon coconut flour	Water to taste

Directions:

In Instant Pot, press Sauté and use the Adjust function to select "More" mode. When the word "Hot" appears, put butter. Add sliced zucchini, beets, carrot to Instant Pot; cook, stirring constantly, 5 minutes or until browned. Turn the cooker off.

Stir, onion, garlic powder, vegetable broth, rosemary, and black pepper.

Lock lid in place and turn the valve to Sealing. Press the Pressure Cooker button and set the cooking time for 10 minutes at High Pressure. When time is up, turn the cooker off. Open the cooker using natural pressure release. Remove the inner pot from the cooker.

After opening the lid, mix coconut flour and coconut milk and make a thick paste. Add the paste into soup check for consistency, if desired add more water and put on Sauté mode for 2 to 3 mins.

Serve hot.

Nutrition:

Calories 377, Total Fat 32. 6g, Saturated Fat 27. 6g, Cholesterol 8mg, Sodium 473mg, Total Carbohydrate 19. 6g, Dietary Fiber 6g, Total Sugars 10. 9g, Protein 7. 6g

413. Pumpkin and Parsnip Soup

Preparation Time: 15 minutes | **Cooking Time:** 20 minutes | **Servings:** 2

Ingredients:

1 tablespoon butter	1 1/2 cups peeled, diced pumpkin
1 cup thinly sliced parsnips	¾ cup thinly sliced celery
1 cup vegetable broth	¼ teaspoon ground white pepper
¼ teaspoon cinnamon	1/8 cup coconut cream
Fresh basil leaves	

Directions:

Select the Sauté setting on the Instant Pot and heat the butter. Add the pumpkin, celery, parsnip, salt, and pepper, and sauté for about 5 minutes, until the celery has softened and is translucent.

Add the vegetable broth and cinnamon, stir well. Lock lid and set the Pressure Release to Sealing. Press the Cancel button to reset the cooking program, then select the Soup/Broth setting and set the cooking time for 15 minutes at High Pressure.

Let the pressure release naturally for at least 10 minutes, then move the Steam Release to Vent to release any remaining steam.

Open the pot and stir in the coconut cream, then taste and adjust the seasoning with salt if needed.

Garnish with basil and serve.

Nutrition:

Calories 188, Total Fat 10. 4g, Saturated Fat 7. 1g, Cholesterol 15mg, Sodium 462mg, Total Carbohydrate 21. 8g, Dietary Fiber 5. 1g, Total Sugars 10. 1g, Protein 4. 1g

414. Black Bean Soup

Preparation Time: 10 minutes | **Cooking Time:** 30 minutes | **Servings:** 2

Ingredients:

½ cup dried black beans	2 cups of water
¼ medium onion, chopped	¼ bell pepper, seeded and chopped

½ teaspoon garlic powder	2 cups vegetable broth
½ teaspoon ground cumin	½ tablespoon chili powder
½ teaspoon salt	½ cup chopped fresh cilantro or cilantro sprigs
Lime slices or wedges	Coconut cream

Directions:

Add all ingredients except fresh cilantro, coconut cream, and lime slices; mix them well.

Lock lid in place and turn the valve to Sealing. Press Manual, cook at High Pressure 20 minutes.

When cooking is complete, use Natural-release for 10 minutes, then release remaining pressure. Press Sauté, cook 2 to 3 minutes or until soup is thickened,

Stir in cream, cook until heated through.

Serve with fresh cilantro and lime slices.

Nutrition:

Calories 206, Total Fat 4. 2g, Saturated Fat 2g, Cholesterol 0mg, Sodium 1374mg, Total Carbohydrate 29. 5g, Dietary Fiber 7. 4g, Total Sugars 2. 6g, Protein 13. 8g

415. Cabbage & Beet Stew

Preparation Time: 30 minutes | **Cooking Time:** 15-60 minutes | **Servings:** 4

Ingredients:

2 Tablespoons Olive Oil	3 cups Vegetable Broth
2 Tablespoons Lemon Juice, Fresh	½ Teaspoon Garlic Powder
½ Cup Carrots, Shredded	2 Cups Cabbage, Shredded
1 Cup Beets, Shredded	Dill for Garnish
½ Teaspoon Onion Powder	Sea Salt & Black Pepper to Taste

Directions:

Heat oil in a pot, and then sauté your vegetables. Pour your broth in, mixing in your seasoning. Simmer until it's cooked through, and then top with dill.

Interesting Facts: This oil is the main source of dietary fat in a variety of diets. It contains many vitamins and minerals that play a part in reducing the risk of stroke and lowers cholesterol and high blood pressure and can also

aid in weight loss. It is best consumed cold, as when it is heated it can lose some of its nutritive properties (although it is still great to cook with – extra virgin is best), many recommend taking a shot of cold olive oil daily! Bonus: if you don't like the taste or texture add a shot to your smoothie.

Nutrition:

Calories 70; Fat 2.7 g; Carbohydrates 13.8 g; Sugar 6.3 g; Protein 1.9 g; Cholesterol 0 mg

416. Basil Tomato Soup

Preparation Time: 20 minutes | **Cooking Time:** 15-60 minutes | **Servings:** 6

Ingredients:

28 oz can tomatoes	¼ cup basil pesto
¼ tsp dried basil leaves	1 tsp apple cider vinegar
2 tbsp erythritol	¼ tsp garlic powder
½ tsp onion powder	2 cups of water
1 ½ tsp kosher salt	

Directions:

Add tomatoes, garlic powder, onion powder, water, and salt in a saucepan.

Bring to boil over medium heat. Reduce heat and simmer for 2 minutes.

Remove the saucepan from heat and puree the soup using a blender until smooth.

Stir in pesto, dried basil, vinegar, and erythritol. Stir well and serve warm.

Nutrition:

Calories 30; Fat 0 g; Carbohydrates 12.1 g; Sugar 9.6 g; Protein 1.3 g; Cholesterol 0 mg

417. Ginger Peanut Soup

Preparation Time: 30 mins. | **Cooking Time:** 15-60 minutes | **Servings:** 6

Ingredients:

1 and 1/2 cups chopped cauliflower	3 cups water or 3 cups vegetable stock
1 and 1/2 cups chopped broccoli	3 chopped cloves garlic
1 chopped onion, medium	5 tbsp. peanut butter, natural-style
1 tbsp. ginger, fresh & grated	1/4 tsp. cayenne pepper

1 can of tomatoes, diced (approximately 28 oz.)

½ tsp. pepper

2 tbsp. olive oil

½ tsp. salt

Directions:

On medium heat in a large soup pot, sauté the cauliflower, garlic, broccoli, ginger, onions, cayenne, pepper, and salt in oil until all of the vegetables are tender.

Add the peanut butter, stock, and tomatoes. Decrease the heat & simmer approximately 20 to 22 minutes, stirring occasionally.

Nutrition:

251.3 Calories, 17.5 g Total Fat, 0 mg Cholesterol, 19.7 g Total Carbohydrate, 5.9 g Dietary Fiber, 9 g Protein

418. African Vegetable Soup

Preparation Time: 50 mins. | **Cooking Time:** 15-60 minutes | **Servings:** 6

Ingredients:

1 cup chickpeas (cooked or canned)	3 tbsp. vegetable oil
1 cup finely chopped onion	2 diced celery ribs
1 potato, small & chopped	1/8 tsp. cayenne
4 tomatoes, small & chopped	1 carrot, small & diced
4 cups vegetable stock	1 tsp. ground coriander
½ tsp. cinnamon	1 cup tomato juice
1 finely chopped zucchini, small	½ cup crumbled curly vermicelli
1 tsp. turmeric	¼ cup lemon juice, fresh
Pepper and salt, to taste	

Directions:

Sauté the celery and onions in oil in a soup pot, until onions are translucent.

Add the potatoes, carrots, and spices. Cook for an additional 5 minutes, stirring over and over again.

Mix in the tomato juice, tomatoes, and stock. Simmer until the vegetables are just about tender.

Add the vermicelli and zucchini and simmer for approximately 5 more minutes.

Mix in the lemon juice, chickpeas, pepper, and salt.

Garnish with mint leaves, chopped parsley, and strips of pimiento or red bell pepper.

Nutrition:

172.3 Calories, 7.6 g Total Fat, 0 mg Cholesterol, 24.1 g Total Carbohydrate, 4.7 g Dietary Fiber, 4.2 g Protein

419. Mexican Barley Stew

Preparation Time: 10 minutes | **Cooking Time:** 25 minutes | **Servings:** 2

Ingredients:

½ teaspoon butter	½ medium onion, chopped
1 leek stalk, chopped	1 parsnip, chopped
½ teaspoon garlic powder	1 bell pepper, seeded and chopped
2 cups of water	1 tomato, diced
½ cup white beans	1 teaspoon cumin
1 teaspoons salt	¼ cup barley (dry/uncooked)
¼ cup chopped fresh parsley	Freshly ground black pepper

Directions:

In an Instant Pot, press Sauté and melt the butter. Add the onion, leek, parsnip, garlic powder, and bell pepper. Sauté until the vegetables are tender, about 8 minutes.

Add the water, tomatoes, white beans, cumin, salt, barley, parsley, and season with pepper and lock the lid in place and turn the valve to Sealing. Press Manual or Pressure Cooker; cook at High Pressure 15 minutes.

When cooking is complete, use Natural-release for 10 minutes, then release remaining pressure. Divide into bowls and serve with any garnishes.

Nutrition:

Calories 358, Total Fat 2. 7g, Saturated Fat 0. 9g, Cholesterol 3mg, Sodium 1206mg, Total Carbohydrate 70. 2g, Dietary Fiber 17. 5g, Total Sugars 10. 5g, Protein 17. 5g

420. Kidney Beans Corn Stew

Preparation Time: 15 minutes | **Cooking Time:** 25 minutes | **Servings:** 2

Ingredients:

1 green chili	1 tablespoon coconut oil
1 small onion, finely chopped	½ teaspoon garlic minced
½ teaspoon cumin	¼ cup tomato paste
1 bay leaf	1 cup kidney beans, rinsed and drained
½ cup sweet corn, rinsed and drained	2 cups vegetable broth
1 cups of water	½ teaspoon salt and pepper to taste
¼ cup chopped coriander leaves, divided	

Directions:

In an Instant Pot, press Sauté and heat the coconut oil. Add the onion, garlic, cumin, and green chili. Sauté until the onion tender, about 2 minutes.

Add the broth, water, tomato paste, kidney beans, sweet corn, bay leaf, and season with salt and pepper and lock the lid in place and turn the valve to Sealing. Press Manual or Pressure Cooker; cook at High Pressure 20 minutes.

When cooking is complete, use Natural-release for 10 minutes, then release remaining pressure. Divide into bowls and serve with chopped coriander.

Nutrition:

Calories 503, Total Fat 10. 1g, Saturated Fat 6. 5g, Cholesterol 0mg, Sodium 1409mg, Total Carbohydrate 79g, Dietary Fiber 18. 5g, Total Sugars 10. 8g, Protein 29. 5g

421. Pigeon Peas Soup

Preparation Time: 10 minutes | **Cooking Time:** 20 minutes | **Servings:** 2

Ingredients:

½ tablespoon butter	1 tablespoon fresh ginger, peeled and finely chopped
1 tablespoon garlic, minced	½ large onion, finely chopped
1 parsnip, peeled and finely diced	½ cup broccoli
½ teaspoon salt	½ cup unsweetened soy milk
2 cups of water	½ cup dried pigeon peas, picked over and rinsed
1 tablespoon finely chopped parsley leaves for garnish	

Directions:

In an Instant Pot, press Sauté and melt the butter. Add the onion, ginger, garlic, parsnip, and broccoli. Sauté until the vegetables are tender, about 5 minutes.

Add the water, soy milk, pigeon peas and season with salt and lock the lid in place and turn the valve to Sealing. Press Manual or Pressure Cooker; cook at High Pressure 15 minutes.

When cooking is complete, use Natural-release for 10 minutes, then release remaining pressure. Let the soup cool slightly, then puree the soup in a blender until smooth.

Ladle soup into 2 bowls and garnish with chopped parsley.

Nutrition:

Calories 159, Total Fat 4. 3g, Saturated Fat 2g, Cholesterol 8mg, Sodium 649mg, Total Carbohydrate 25. 3g, Dietary Fiber 5. 9g, Total Sugars 5. 7g, Protein 6. 1g

422. Chia Seeds Tomato Soup

Preparation Time: 05 minutes | **Cooking Time:** 10 minutes | **Servings:** 2

Ingredients:

4 tomatoes, chopped	½ cup chia seeds
½ tablespoon butter	½ teaspoon garlic powder
½ small onion, roughly chopped	½ small zucchini, roughly chopped
1 1/2 cups vegetable broth	Salt and black pepper to taste

Directions:

Put Instant Pot on Sauté mode High and when hot add the butter.

Now add garlic powder and onion to fry, sauté well till onions soften.

Now add zucchini and chia seeds and fry for a minute.

Add in the tomatoes and mix well. Fry for 3 mines.

Now add in broth, salt, and pepper. Mix them well.

Lock lid in place and turn the valve to Sealing. Do Manual Low Pressure for 2 minutes.

When cooking is complete, use Natural-release for 10 minutes, then release remaining pressure. Blend the chia seeds tomato mixture into a smooth puree.

If desired adjust the consistency of soup. Serve hot.

Nutrition:
Calories116, Total Fat 5. 8g, Saturated Fat 2. 2g, Cholesterol 8mg, Sodium 303mg, Total Carbohydrate 13. 5g, Dietary Fiber 5. 4g, Total Sugars 6. 4g, Protein 4. 7g

423. Sweet Potato and Zucchini Soup

Preparation Time:05 minutes | **Cooking Time:** 10 minutes | **Servings:** 2

Ingredients:

¼ medium onion diced	1 teaspoon coconut oil
1 teaspoon garlic powder	2 zucchini, peeled and cut into 4-inch chunks
1 cup sweet potato	½ cup almond milk
3 cups vegetable broth	1 teaspoon salt
½ teaspoon pepper	

Directions:
Select the Sauté function to heat the Instant Pot. When the pot displays "Hot", add the coconut oil, onion, and garlic powder. Sauté until the onion softens. Press Cancel to turn off the sauté function.

Add the zucchini, sweet potato, almond milk, broth, salt, and pepper. Stir well. Lock lid in place and turn the valve to Sealing. Press the Pressure Cooker button and set the time to 10 minutes.

Once cooking is complete, turn the valve to the Venting position to release the pressure. When all the pressure is released, carefully remove the lid.

Stir the soup. Blend with an immersion blender or in batches in a stand blender until smooth. Serve hot.

Nutrition:
Calories277, Total Fat 16. 5g, Saturated Fat 13. 2g, Cholesterol 0mg, Sodium 1986mg, Total Carbohydrate 26g, Dietary Fiber 7. 2g, Total Sugars 12. 3g, Protein 12. 1g

424. Anise Seed and Cabbage Soup

Preparation Time:10 minutes | **Cooking Time:** 15 minutes | **Servings:** 2

Ingredients:

½ tablespoon olive oil	½ onion
½ teaspoon garlic minced	½ tablespoon anise seed
½ pound cabbage	½ cup almond milk
2 cups vegetable broth	½ teaspoon salt and black pepper for serving

Directions:
Select the Sauté function to heat the Instant Pot. When the pot displays "Hot", add the olive oil, onion, and garlic. Sauté until the onion softens. Add the cabbage, anise seed, almond milk, broth, salt, and pepper. Stir well. Lock lid in place and turn the valve to Sealing. Press the Pressure Cooker button and set the time to10 minutes.

Once cooking is complete, turn the valve to the Venting position to release the pressure. When all the pressure is released, carefully remove the lid.

Use a standing blender or an immersion blender to puree the soup to a smooth, creamy consistency.

Serve.

Nutrition:
Calories253, Total Fat 19. 6g, Saturated Fat 13. 6g, Cholesterol 0mg, Sodium 1376mg, Total Carbohydrate 14. 5g, Dietary Fiber 5g, Total Sugars 7. 5g, Protein 8. 3g

425. Bok Choy Soup

Preparation Time: 05 minutes | **Cooking Time:** 10 minutes | **Servings:** 2

Ingredients:

2 cups of bok choy, diced	1 celery
1 bell pepper	1 potato, peeled and diced
1. 5 cups of vegetable stock	½ cup of soy milk
Salt and pepper to taste	

Directions:

Add diced bok choy, celery, potato, vegetable stock, and soy milk, and bell pepper into Instant Pot.

Add salt and pepper to the mixture.

Turn the Instant Pot to the "Soup" function and let it cook. Alternatively, put everything in a pot and bring to boil, and simmer until the celeriac and potato are soft.

When cool, puree it with an immersion blender like this one or put it in a high-speed blender. Enjoy!

Nutrition:

Calories 131, Total Fat 1. 6g, Saturated Fat 0. 2g, Cholesterol 0mg, Sodium 131mg, Total Carbohydrate 26g, Dietary Fiber 3. 6g, Total Sugars 7. 5g, Protein 5. 8g

426. Spicy Peanut Soup with Potato and Spinach

Preparation Time: 05 minutes | **Cooking Time:** 10 minutes | **Servings:** 2

Ingredients:

½ tablespoons butter	½ onion, diced
1 bell pepper, minced	1 teaspoon garlic, minced
1 potato, peeled and cubed	1 tomato
½ cup of coconut milk	2 cups vegetable broth
1 teaspoon salt	½ teaspoon turmeric
1/8 cup chopped peanuts	1 teaspoon peanut butter
1 cup spinach, chopped	

Directions:

Select the Sauté function to heat the Instant Pot inner pot. When the pot displays "Hot", add butter, onion, and garlic. Sauté until the onion softens.

Add the bell pepper, potato, tomatoes, coconut milk, broth, turmeric, peanuts, salt, and pepper. Stir them well. Lock lid in place and turn the valve to Sealing. Press the Pressure Cooker button and set the time to10 minutes.

Once cooking is complete, turn the valve to the Venting position to release the pressure. When all the pressure is released, carefully remove the lid.

Add spinach and peanut butter into the mixer.

Use a standing blender or an immersion blender to puree the soup to a smooth, creamy consistency.

Serve.

Nutrition:

Calories 386, Total Fat 24. 9g, Saturated Fat 15. 9g, Cholesterol 8mg, Sodium 1992mg, Total Carbohydrate 32. 6g, Dietary Fiber 7. 1g, Total Sugars 9. 6g, Protein 12. 8g

427. Parsnip Ginger Soup with Tofu and Kale

Preparation Time: 10 minutes | **Cooking Time:** 20 minutes | **Servings:** 2

Ingredients:

½ tablespoon butter	1 small onion, diced
1 teaspoon ginger powder	1 teaspoon garlic powder
½ pound parsnip, cut into small coins	½ teaspoon cumin
½ teaspoon ground coriander	¼ teaspoon ground turmeric
1 1/2 cups of vegetable broth	½ cup of soy milk
½ teaspoon honey	½ fresh lime
1 cup tofu, diced into cubes	1 handful of fresh kale

Directions:

Set the Instant Pot to Sauté and add butter, add tofu and cook it for 5 minutes. Keep aside.

After adding onions. Cook for 5-10 minutes until the onion begins to soften.

Add the garlic and ginger powder to the pot and stir until fragrant.

Combine the parsnip, cumin, coriander powder, and turmeric powder in the Instant Pot. Stir well. Pour in the broth and lock the lid. Turn the vent to seal, press Cancel, and manually cook on High Pressure for 5 minutes.

After the 5 minutes, do a manual release.

Add the soy milk and honey if using to the Instant Pot. Allow the mixture to cool slightly and then use an immersion blender or other mixer to puree until smooth. Season with salt, pepper, and a squeeze of lime.

Stir the fresh kale into the still slightly warm soup. The kale should wilt on its own, but you can also warm it up together for the right temperature. Add the tofu and enjoy!

Nutrition:
Calories 303, Total Fat 10. 5g, Saturated Fat 3. 3g, Cholesterol 8mg, Sodium 478mg, Total Carbohydrate 38. 9g, Dietary Fiber 9. 2g, Total Sugars 12. 6g, Protein 18. 1g

428. Mushroom Soup

Preparation Time: 10 minutes | **Cooking Time:** 25 minutes | **Servings:** 2

Ingredients:

1 teaspoon avocado oil	½ medium onion, chopped
½ large leek stalk, chopped	½ large zucchini peeled & chopped
1 teaspoon garlic powder	8 ounces of mushrooms sliced
½ teaspoon dried rosemary	¼ teaspoon ground pepper
1 1/2 cups vegetable broth	¼ teaspoon salt
½ cup almond milk	

Directions:

Set the Instant Pot to Sauté mode. Heat the avocado oil, then add the onion, leek, and zucchini. Sauté the vegetables, stirring occasionally, until starting to soften, 3 to 4 minutes.

Add the garlic powder, mushrooms, rosemary, and pepper. Cook until the mushrooms are starting to release their liquid, 2 to 3 minutes. Stir in the broth and salt.

Put the lid on the Instant Pot, close the steam vent, and set it to High Pressure using the Manual setting. Decrease the time to 10 minutes. It will take the Instant Pot about 10 minutes to reach pressure.

Once the time is up, carefully release the steam using the Quick-release valve.

Transfer half of the soup to the blender, add the almond milk, hold on the top and blend until almost smooth, stopping the blender and opening the lid occasionally to release the steam. Transfer the pureed soup to a pot or bowl.

Nutrition:
Calories228, Total Fat 15. 9g, Saturated Fat 13g, Cholesterol 0mg, Sodium 702mg, Total Carbohydrate 17. 5g, Dietary Fiber 4. 8g, Total Sugars 8. 1g, Protein 9. 3g

429. Seitan Stew with Barley

Preparation Time: 10 minutes | **Cooking Time:** 20 minutes | **Servings:** 2

Ingredients:

1 teaspoon coconut oil	½ onion chopped
1 parsnip cut into thin half-circles	1 leek stalks diced
1 teaspoon garlic minced	1 teaspoon dried basil
½ teaspoons dried parsley	1 1/2 tablespoons tomato paste
2 cups vegetable broth	1 cup seitan
1 cup dry barley	½ teaspoon salt
½ teaspoon ground pepper	

Directions:

Set the Instant Pot to Sauté mode. Heat the coconut oil, then add the onion, parsnips, and leek. Sauté the vegetables, stirring occasionally, until starting to soften, 3 to 4 minutes.

Add the garlic, basil, parsley, and tomato paste. Cook, stirring constantly, for 1 minute.

Pour in the vegetable broth and stir to combine. Add the seitan, barley, and salt and pepper to the Instant Pot.

Put the lid on the Instant Pot, close the steam vent, and set it to High Pressure using the Manual setting. Set the time to 20 minutes.

Once the time is expired, use Natural-release for 10 minutes, then quickly release.

Serve soup with salt and pepper to taste.

Nutrition:
Calories 376, Total Fat 5. 8g, Saturated Fat 2. 9g, Cholesterol 0mg, Sodium 1600mg, Total Carbohydrate 57. 9g, Dietary Fiber 13. 7g, Total Sugars 8. 2g, Protein 23. 5g

430. Cottage Cheese Soup

Preparation Time:10 minutes | **Cooking Time:** 35 minutes | **Servings:** 2

Ingredients:

1 stalks leek, diced	1 tablespoon bell pepper, diced
¼ cup Swiss chard, sliced into strips	1/8 cup fresh kale
1 eggplant	½ tablespoon avocado oil
1/8 cup button mushrooms, diced	1 small onion, diced
½ cup cottage cheese	2 cups vegetable broth
1 bay leaf	½ teaspoon salt
¼ teaspoon garlic, minced	1/8 teaspoon paprika

Directions:
Place leek, bell pepper, Swiss chard, eggplant, and kale into a medium bowl, set aside in a separate medium bowl.
Press the Sauté button and add the avocado oil to Instant Pot. Once the oil is hot, add mushrooms and onion. Sauté for 4–6 minutes until the onion is translucent and fragrant.
Add leek, bell pepper, Swiss chard, and kale to Instant Pot. Cook for an additional 4 minutes. Press the Cancel button.
Add diced cottage cheese, broth, bay leaf, and seasonings to Instant Pot. Click the lid closed. Press the Soup button and set the time for 20 minutes.
When the timer beeps, allow a 10-minute natural release and quickly release the remaining pressure. Add eggplant on Keep Warm mode and cook for additional 10 minutes or until tender. Serve warm.

Nutrition:
Calories 212, Total Fat 3. 6g, Saturated Fat 1. 2g, Cholesterol 5mg, Sodium 1603mg, Total Carbohydrate 30. 7g, Dietary Fiber 11. 9g, Total Sugars 12. 7g, Protein 17g

431. Fresh Corn & Red Pepper Stew

Preparation Time:15 minutes | **Cooking Time:** 30 minutes | **Servings:** 2

Ingredients:

1 teaspoon coconut oil	¼ cup sweet onion, chopped,
1 1/2 cups fresh corn kernels	1 teaspoon garlic, minced
2 cups vegetable broth,	¼ teaspoon salt
1/8 cup coconut cream	½ tablespoon cornmeal
½ small red bell pepper, diced	Enough water

Directions:
Select the Sauté setting on the Instant Pot and heat the coconut oil. Add the onion, garlic, and salt and sauté for about 5 minutes, until the onion has softened and is translucent.
Add the fresh corn, broth, water, bell pepper, and stir well.
Lock lid and set the Pressure Release to Sealing. Press the Cancel button to reset the cooking program, then select the Soup/Broth setting and set the cooking time for 15 minutes at High Pressure.
Meanwhile add water, coconut cream, and cornmeal.
Let the pressure release naturally for at least 10 minutes, then move the Steam Release to Vent to release any remaining steam.
Open the pot and stir in the cornmeal mixer into soup, then taste and adjust the seasoning with salt if needed.

Nutrition:
Calories 183, Total Fat 8. 3g, Saturated Fat 5. 7g, Cholesterol 0mg, Sodium 1070mg, Total Carbohydrate 21. 8g, Dietary Fiber 3. 3g, Total Sugars 5. 8g, Protein 8. 4g

432. Zucchini & White Bean Stew

Preparation Time:10 minutes | **Cooking Time:** 35 minutes | **Servings:** 2

Ingredients:

¼ ounce mushrooms	1 cup hot water

½ large zucchini

1 tablespoon coconut oil, divided

1 small onion, thinly sliced

½ teaspoon garlic powder

¼ teaspoons dried basil, crumbled

1 small (1-inch) cinnamon stick

¼ teaspoon salt

1/8 teaspoon freshly ground pepper

1 bay leaf

2 cups vegetable broth

¼ cup dried white beans, rinsed and soaked overnight and drained

1 tomato

¼ cup finely chopped fresh cilantro

Directions:

Select the Sauté setting on the Instant Pot and heat ¼ tablespoon coconut oil. Add zucchini and roast it and keep aside.

Add remaining coconut oil, add onion and sauté for about 5 minutes, until the onion has softened and is translucent. Add garlic powder, basil, cinnamon stick, salt, pepper, bay leaf, and the chopped mushrooms cook, stirring, for 1 minute add vegetable broth and add white beans and roast zucchini.

Lock lid and set the Pressure Release to Sealing. Press the Cancel button to reset the cooking program, then select the Soup/Broth setting and set the cooking time for 25 minutes at High Pressure.

Let the pressure release naturally for at least 10 minutes, then move the Steam Release to Vent to release any remaining steam.

Open the pot and remove the cinnamon stick and bay leaf. Stir in tomatoes and cilantro.

Nutrition:

Calories 210, Total Fat 7. 5g, Saturated Fat 6g, Cholesterol 0mg, Sodium 307mg, Total Carbohydrate 30. 9g, Dietary Fiber 11. 1g, Total Sugars 8g, Protein 8. 5g

433. Potato Tofu Soup

Preparation Time:10 minutes | **Cooking Time:** 35 minutes | **Servings:** 2

Ingredients:

½ tablespoon olive oil

½ celery cleaned and sliced

½ teaspoon garlic powder

1 sweet potato peeled and cut into 2-inch cubes

½ large potato peeled and cut into 2-inch cubes

½ cup tofu

2 cups vegetable broth

Juice from one lemon

A handful of chopped parsley

Salt and pepper

Directions:

Hit the Sauté button and when it's hot, heat the olive oil in your Instant Pot and sauté the celery and garlic powder until they soften down, stirring often.

Add in the potatoes, sweet potatoes, tofu, broth, salt, and pepper, and stir well.

Lock lid, make sure the vent is sealed, and program for 6 minutes on High Pressure. You can do a Quick-release if you like or leave it to release on its own with soup like this it doesn't matter.

Once the pressure is released, open the lid and throw in the parsley and add the lemon juice.

Nutrition:

Calories 216, Total Fat 7. 6g, Saturated Fat 1. 5g, Cholesterol 0mg, Sodium 809mg, Total Carbohydrate 27. 2g, Dietary Fiber 3. 6g, Total Sugars 5. 2g, Protein 12. 2g

434. Tomato Gazpacho

Preparation Time: 2 Hours 25 minutes | **Cooking Time:** 15-60 minutes | **Servings:** 6

Ingredients:

2 Tablespoons + 1 Teaspoon Red Wine Vinegar, Divided

½ Teaspoon Pepper

1 Teaspoon Sea Salt

¼ Cup Basil, Fresh & Chopped

1 Avocado,

3 Tablespoons + 2 Teaspoons Olive Oil, Divided

1 Clove Garlic, crushed

1 Red Bell Pepper, Sliced & Seeded

1 Cucumber, Chunked

2 ½ lbs. Large Tomatoes, Cored & Chopped

Directions:

Place half of your cucumber, bell pepper, and ¼ cup of each tomato in a bowl, covering. Set it in the fridge.

Puree your remaining tomatoes, cucumber, and bell pepper with garlic, three tablespoons oil, two tablespoons of vinegar, sea salt, and black pepper into a blender, blending until smooth. Transfer it to a bowl, and chill for two hours.

Chop the avocado, adding it to your chopped vegetables, adding your remaining oil, vinegar, salt, pepper, and basil.

Ladle your tomato puree mixture into bowls, and serve with chopped vegetables as a salad.

Interesting Facts:

Avocados themselves are ranked within the top five of the healthiest foods on the planet, so you know that the oil that is produced from them is too. It is loaded with healthy fats and essential fatty acids. Like race bran oil it is perfect to cook with as well! Bonus: Helps in the prevention of diabetes and lowers cholesterol levels.

Nutrition:

Calories 70; Fat 2.7 g; Carbohydrates 13.8 g; Sugar 6.3 g; Protein 1.9 g; Cholesterol 0 mg

435. Tomato Pumpkin Soup

Preparation Time: 25 minutes | **Cooking Time:** 15-60 minutes | **Servings:** 4

Ingredients:

2 cups pumpkin, diced	1/2 cup tomato, chopped
1/2 cup onion, chopped	1 1/2 tsp curry powder
1/2 tsp paprika	2 cups vegetable stock
1 tsp olive oil	1/2 tsp garlic, minced

Directions:

In a saucepan, add oil, garlic, and onion and sauté for 3 minutes over medium heat.

Add remaining ingredients into the saucepan and bring to boil.

Reduce heat and cover and simmer for 10 minutes.

Puree the soup using a blender until smooth.

Stir well and serve warm.

Nutrition:

Calories 70; Fat 2.7 g; Carbohydrates 13.8 g; Sugar 6.3 g; Protein 1.9 g; Cholesterol 0 mg

436. Cauliflower Spinach Soup

Preparation Time: 45 minutes | **Cooking Time:** 15-60 minutes | **Servings:** 5

Ingredients:

1/2 cup unsweetened coconut milk	5 oz fresh spinach, chopped
5 watercress, chopped	8 cups vegetable stock
1 lb cauliflower, chopped	Salt

Directions:

Add stock and cauliflower in a large saucepan and bring to boil over medium heat for 15 minutes.

Add spinach and watercress and cook for another 10 minutes.

Remove from heat and puree the soup using a blender until smooth.

Add coconut milk and stir well. Season with salt. Stir well and serve hot.

Nutrition:

Calories 153; Fat 8.3 g; Carbohydrates 8.7 g; Sugar 4.3 g; Protein 11.9 g; Cholesterol 0 mg

437. Avocado Mint Soup

Preparation Time: 10 minutes | **Cooking Time:** 15-60 minutes | **Servings:** 2

Ingredients:

1 medium avocado, peeled, pitted, and cut into pieces	1 cup of coconut milk
2 romaine lettuce leaves	20 fresh mint leaves
1 tbsp fresh lime juice	1/8 tsp salt

Directions:

Add all ingredients into the blender and blend until smooth. The soup should be thick not as a puree.

Pour into the serving bowls and place in the refrigerator for 10 minutes.

Stir well and serve chilled.

Nutrition:

Calories 268; Fat 25.6 g; Carbohydrates 10.2 g; Sugar 0.6 g; Protein 2.7 g; Cholesterol 0 mg

438. Creamy Squash Soup

Preparation Time: 35 minutes | **Cooking Time:** 15-60 minutes | **Servings:** 8

Ingredients:

3 cups butternut squash, chopped	1 ½ cups unsweetened coconut milk
1 tbsp coconut oil	1 tsp dried onion flakes
1 tbsp curry powder	4 cups of water
1 garlic clove	1 tsp kosher salt

Directions:

Add squash, coconut oil, onion flakes, curry powder, water, garlic, and salt into a large saucepan. Bring to boil over high heat.

Turn heat to medium and simmer for 20 minutes.

Puree the soup using a blender until smooth. Return soup to the saucepan and stir in coconut milk and cook for 2 minutes.

Stir well and serve hot.

Nutrition:

Calories 146; Fat 12.6 g; Carbohydrates 9.4 g; Sugar 2.8 g; Protein 1.7 g; Cholesterol 0 mg

439. Zucchini Soup

Preparation Time: 20 minutes | **Cooking Time:** 15-60 minutes | **Servings:** 8

Ingredients:

2 ½ lbs zucchini, peeled and sliced	1/3 cup basil leaves
4 cups vegetable stock	4 garlic cloves, chopped
2 tbsp olive oil	1 medium onion, diced
Pepper	Salt

Directions:

Heat olive oil in a pan over medium-low heat.

Add zucchini and onion and sauté until softened.

Add garlic and sauté for a minute.

Add vegetable stock and simmer for 15 minutes.

Remove from heat. Stir in basil and puree the soup using a blender until smooth and creamy. Season with pepper and salt.

Stir well and serve.

Nutrition:

Calories 62; Fat 4 g; Carbohydrates 6.8 g; Sugar 3.3 g; Protein 2 g; Cholesterol 0 mg

440. Creamy Celery Soup

Preparation Time: 40 minutes | **Cooking Time:** 15-60 minutes | **Servings:** 4

Ingredients:

6 cups celery	½ tsp dill
2 cups of water	1 cup of coconut milk
1 onion, chopped	Pinch of salt

Directions:

Add all ingredients into the electric pot and stir well.

Cover the electric pot with the lid and select the soup setting.

Release pressure using a quick-release method than opening the lid.

Puree the soup using an immersion blender until smooth and creamy.

Stir well and serve warm.

Nutrition:

Calories 174; Fat 14.6 g; Carbohydrates 10.5 g; Sugar 5.2 g; Protein 2.8 g; Cholesterol 0 mg

441. Avocado Cucumber Soup

Preparation Time: 40 minutes | **Cooking Time:** 15-60 minutes | **Servings:** 3

Ingredients:

1 large cucumber, peeled and sliced	¾ cup of water
¼ cup lemon juice	2 garlic cloves
6 green onion	2 avocados, pitted
½ tsp black pepper	½ tsp pink salt

Directions:

Add all ingredients into the blender and blend until smooth and creamy.

Place in the refrigerator for 30 minutes.

Stir well and serve chilled.

Nutrition:

Calories 73; Fat 3.7 g; Carbohydrates 9.2 g; Sugar 2.8 g; Protein 2.2 g; Cholesterol 0 mg

442. Quick Jackfruit and Bean Stew

Preparation Time: 10 minutes | **Cooking Time:** 10 minutes | **Servings:** 2

Ingredients:

½ cup jackfruit cut into 1-inch pieces	½ cup kidney bean rinsed and drained
½ cup pinto beans rinsed and drained	1 tomato
½ onion chopped	2 cup vegetable broth or water
½ orange juiced	½ teaspoon salt and pepper
½ teaspoon cumin Fresh basil	1 bay leaf

Directions:

Combine kidney beans, jackfruit, pinto beans, tomato, onion, broth, orange juice, pepper, salt, cumin, and bay leaf in Instant Pot; mix them well.

Lock lid in place and turn the valve to Sealing. Press Manual or Pressure Cooker; cook at High Pressure 6 minutes.

When cooking is complete, use Natural-release for 5 minutes, then release remaining pressure. Press Sauté, cook for 3 to 5 minutes or until the stew thickens slightly, stirring frequently. Remove and discard bay leaf. Garnish with basil.

Nutrition:

Calories 222, Total Fat 2. 3g, Saturated Fat 0. 6g, Cholesterol 0mg, Sodium 1617mg, Total Carbohydrate 38. 5g, Dietary Fiber 9. 2g, Total Sugars 5. 9g, Protein 13. 6g

443. Split Pea Soup

Preparation Time: 15 minutes | **Cooking Time:** 15 minutes | **Servings:** 2

Ingredients:

½ onion chopped	1 zucchini chopped
¼ stalk leek chopped	1 teaspoon garlic powder
¼ teaspoon dried basil	2 cups vegetable broth
1 cup of water	1 cup dried split peas rinsed and sorted
½ teaspoon salt	½ teaspoon black pepper
1 bay leaf	

Directions:

Press Sauté, add onion, zucchini, and leek to Instant Pot; cook and stir 5 minutes or until vegetables are softened. Add garlic powder and basil; cook and stir for 1 minute. Stir in broth and water. Add split peas, salt, pepper, and bay leaf; mix well.

Lock lid and move pressure release valve to the Sealing position. Press Manual or Pressure Cooker; cook at High Pressure 8 minutes.

When cooking is complete, use Natural-release for 10 minutes, then release remaining pressure. Stir soup; remove and discard bay leaf.

Nutrition:

Calories 118, Total Fat 1. 7g, Saturated Fat 0. 4g, Cholesterol 0mg, Sodium 1358mg, Total Carbohydrate 16. 7g, Dietary Fiber 2. 3g, Total Sugars 3. 7g, Protein 9. 5g

444. Pasta Tofu Soup

Preparation Time: 10 minutes | **Cooking Time:** 10 minutes | **Servings:** 2

Ingredients:

½ tablespoon butter	½ teaspoon garlic ginger, crushed
¼ onion chopped	½ green chilies, finely chopped (or adjust to taste
½ big tomato, chopped	Salt to taste
¼ cup pasta	½ cup of tofu cubes
2 cups water or broth as needed	Cilantro to garnish

Directions:

Put Instant Pot on Sauté mode High and add butter. Once butter is hot, add garlic ginger and fry until aromatic.

Add onions and green chili, fry till edges of onions brown, then add tomatoes and fry for 2 to 3 minutes.

Add the pasta and tofu. Mix gently.

Add salt, and the water about 1/2 inch to 1 inch covering the pasta and mix well. Turn off the Sauté mode. Lock lid in place and turn the valve to Sealing.

Do Manual (Pressure Cooker) High 5 to 6 minutes. Let it naturally release or quick release after 10 minutes in Warm mode.

Garnish with cilantro if desired and serve hot.

Nutrition:
Calories 196, Total Fat 9. 2g, Saturated Fat 2. 7g, Cholesterol 19mg, Sodium 161mg, Total Carbohydrate 18g, Dietary Fiber 4g, Total Sugars 3. 3g, Protein 13. 3g

445. Creamy Garlic Onion Soup

Preparation Time: 45 minutes | **Cooking Time:** 15-60 minutes | **Servings:** 4

Ingredients:

1 onion, sliced	4 cups vegetable stock
1 1/2 tbsp olive oil	1 shallot, sliced
2 garlic clove, chopped	1 leek, sliced
Salt	

Directions:
Add stock and olive oil in a saucepan and bring to boil.
Add remaining ingredients and stir well.
Cover and simmer for 25 minutes.
Puree the soup using an immersion blender until smooth.
Stir well and serve warm.

Nutrition:
Calories 90; Fat 7.4 g; Carbohydrates 10.1 g; Sugar 4.1 g; Protein 1 g; Cholesterol 0 mg

446. Avocado Broccoli Soup

Preparation Time: 25 minutes | **Cooking Time:** 15-60 minutes | **Servings:** 4

Ingredients:

2 cups broccoli florets, chopped	5 cups vegetable broth
2 avocados, chopped	Pepper
Salt	

Directions:
Cook broccoli in boiling water for 5 minutes. Drain well.
Add broccoli, vegetable broth, avocados, pepper, and salt to the blender and blend until smooth.
Stir well and serve warm.

Nutrition:
Calories 269; Fat 21.5 g; Carbohydrates 12.8 g; Sugar 2.1 g; Protein 9.2 g; Cholesterol 0 mg

447. Green Spinach Kale Soup

Preparation Time: 15 minutes | **Cooking Time:** 15-60 minutes | **Servings:** 6

Ingredients:

2 avocados	8 oz spinach
8 oz kale	1 fresh lime juice
1 cup of water	3 1/3 cup coconut milk
3 oz olive oil	1/4 tsp pepper
1 tsp salt	

Directions:
Heat olive oil in a saucepan over medium heat.
Add kale and spinach to the saucepan and sauté for 2-3 minutes. Remove saucepan from heat.
Add coconut milk, spices, avocado, and water. Stir well.
Puree the soup using an immersion blender until smooth and creamy. Add fresh lime juice and stir well.
Serve and enjoy.

Nutrition:
Calories 233; Fat 20 g; Carbohydrates 12 g; Sugar 0.5 g; Protein 4.2 g; Cholesterol 0 mg

448. Cauliflower Asparagus Soup

Preparation Time: 30 minutes | **Cooking Time:** 15-60 minutes | **Servings:** 4

Ingredients:

20 asparagus spears, chopped	4 cups vegetable stock
½ cauliflower head, chopped	2 garlic cloves, chopped
1 tbsp coconut oil	Pepper
Salt	

Directions:
Heat coconut oil in a large saucepan over medium heat.
Add garlic and sauté until softened.
Add cauliflower, vegetable stock, pepper, and salt. Stir well and bring to boil.
Reduce heat to low and simmer for 20 minutes.
Add chopped asparagus and cook until softened.
Puree the soup using an immersion blender until smooth and creamy.
Stir well and serve warm.

Nutrition:
Calories 74; Fat 5.6 g; Carbohydrates 8.9 g; Sugar 5.1 g; Protein 3.4 g; Cholesterol 2 mg

449. African Pineapple Peanut Stew

Preparation Time: 30 mins. | **Cooking Time:** 15-60 minutes | **Servings:** 4

Ingredients:

4 cups sliced kale	1 cup chopped onion
1/2 cup peanut butter	1 tbsp. hot pepper sauce or 1 tbsp. Tabasco sauce
2 minced garlic cloves	1/2 cup chopped cilantro
2 cups pineapple, undrained, canned & crushed	1 tbsp. vegetable oil

Directions:
In a saucepan (preferably covered), sauté the garlic and onions in the oil until the onions are lightly browned, approximately 10 minutes, stirring often.

Wash the kale. Get rid of the stems. Mound the leaves on a cutting surface & slice crosswise into slices (preferably 1" thick).

Now put the pineapple and juice to the onions & bring to a simmer. Stir the kale in, cover, and simmer until just tender, stirring frequently for approximately 5 minutes.

Mix in the hot pepper sauce, peanut butter & simmer for another 5 minutes.

Add salt according to your taste.

Nutrition:
382 Calories, 20.3 g Total Fat, 0 mg Cholesterol, 27.6 g Total Carbohydrate, 5 g Dietary Fiber, 11.4 g Protein

450. Fuss-Free Cabbage and Tomatoes Stew

Preparation Time: 15-30 minutes | **Cooking Time:** 3 hours and 10 minutes | **Servings:** 6

Ingredients:

1 medium-sized cabbage head, chopped	1 medium-sized white onion, peeled and sliced
28-ounce of stewed tomatoes	3/4 teaspoon of salt
1/4 teaspoon of ground black pepper	10-ounce of tomato soup

Directions:
Using a 6 quarts slow cooker, place all the ingredients, and stir properly.

Cover it with the lid, plug in the slow cooker and let it cook at the high heat setting for 3 hours or until the vegetables get soft.

Serve right away.

Nutrition:
Calories:103 Cal, Carbohydrates:17g, Protein:4g, Fats:2g, Fiber:4g.

451. Awesome Spinach Artichoke Soup

Preparation Time: 15-30 minutes | **Cooking Time:** 4 hours and 45 minutes | **Servings:** 6

Ingredients:

15 ounce of cooked white beans	2 cups of frozen artichoke hearts, thawed
2 cups of spinach leaves	1 small red onion, peeled and chopped
1 teaspoon of minced garlic	1 teaspoon of salt
1/2 teaspoon of ground black pepper	2 teaspoons of dried basil
1 teaspoon of dried oregano	1/2 teaspoon of whole-grain mustard paste
2 1/2 tablespoons of nutritional yeast	1 1/2 teaspoons of white miso
4 tablespoons of lemon juice	16 fluid ounce of almond milk, unsweetened
3 cups of vegetable broth	1 cups of water

Directions:
Grease a 6-quarts slow cooker with a non-stick cooking spray, add the artichokes, spinach, onion, garlic, salt, black pepper, basil, and oregano.

Pour in the vegetable broth and water, stir properly and cover it with the lid.

Then plug in the slow cooker and let it cook at the high heat setting for 4 hours or until the vegetables get soft.

While waiting for that, place the white beans in a food processor, add the yeast, miso, mustard, lemon juice, and almond milk.

Mash until it gets smooth, and set it aside.

When the vegetables are cooked thoroughly, add the prepared bean mixture and continue cooking for 30 minutes at the high heat setting or until the soup gets slightly thick.

Garnish it with cheese and serve.

Nutrition:
Calories:200 Cal, Carbohydrates:13g, Protein:4g, Fats:12g, Fiber:2g.

452. Brazilian Black Bean Stew

Preparation Time: 15 minutes | **Cooking Time:** 30 minutes | **Servings:** 2

Ingredients:

½ tablespoon olive oil	1 medium onion, chopped
1 teaspoon garlic powder	½ cup sweet potatoes, peeled and diced
½ large red bell pepper, diced	1 cup diced tomatoes with juice
½ cup of corn	½ cup broccoli
1 small hot green chili pepper, diced	1 1/2 cups water
½ cup black beans	1 mango - peeled, seeded, and diced
¼ cup chopped fresh cilantro	¼ teaspoon salt

Directions:
Select the Sauté setting on the Instant Pot. Add olive oil and onions to the Instant Pot. Stir in garlic powder, and cook until tender, then mix in the sweet potatoes, bell pepper, tomatoes with juice, chili pepper, corn, broccoli, and water. Stir the beans into the Instant Pot. Select Pressure Cook or Manual, and adjust the pressure to High and the time to 12 minutes. After cooking, let the pressure release naturally for 10 minutes, then quickly release any remaining pressure.

Open the lid and mix in the mango and cilantro, and season with salt.

Nutrition:
Calories 434, Total Fat 5. 8g, Saturated Fat 1g, Cholesterol 0mg, Sodium 325mg, Total Carbohydrate 86. 6g, Dietary Fiber 16. 1g, Total Sugars 32. 4g, Protein 16. 3g

453. Split Pea and Carrot Stew

Preparation Time: 10 minutes | **Cooking Time:** 20 minutes | **Servings:** 2

Ingredients:

1 tablespoon avocado oil	1 small onion, diced
½ carrot, diced into small cubes	½ leek stick, diced into cubes
4–5 cloves garlic, diced finely	1 bay leaf
1 teaspoon paprika powder	1 1/2 teaspoons cumin powder
½ teaspoon salt	¼ teaspoon cinnamon powder
¼ teaspoon chili powder or cayenne pepper	2 cups green split peas (rinsed well
½ cup chopped tinned tomatoes	Juice of ½ lemon
2 cups vegetable stock	

Directions:
Press the Sauté key to the Instant Pot. Add the avocado oil, onions, carrots, and leeks and cook for 4 minutes, stirring a few times.

Add the rest of the ingredients and stir. Cancel the Sauté function by pressing the Keep Warm/Cancel button.

Place and lock the lid, make sure the steam releasing handle is pointing to Sealing. Press Manual and adjust to 10 minutes.

Once the timer goes off, allow the pressure to release for 4-5 minutes and then use the Quick-release method before opening the lid.

Serve.

Nutrition:
Calories 337, Total Fat 20. 5g, Saturated Fat 4. 2g, Cholesterol 0mg, Sodium 661mg, Total Carbohydrate 32. 6g, Dietary Fiber 16. 3g, Total Sugars 7. 9g, Protein 10g

Chapter 5: Snacks

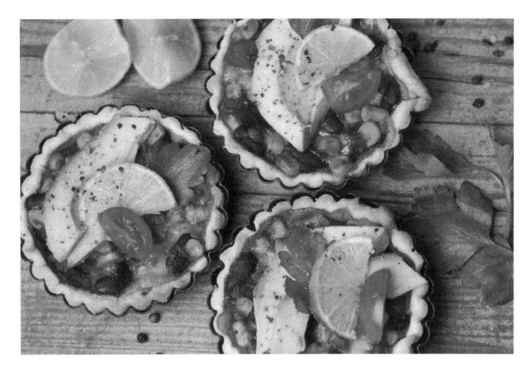

454. Beans, Tomato & Corn Quesadillas

Preparation Time: 15-30 minutes | **Cooking Time:** 35 minutes | **Servings:** 4

Ingredients:

1 tsp olive oil	1 small onion, chopped
½ medium red bell pepper, deseeded and chopped	1 (7 oz) can chopped tomatoes
1 (7 oz) can black beans, drained and rinsed	1 (7 oz) can sweet corn kernels, drained
4 whole-wheat tortillas	1 cup grated plant-based cheddar cheese

Directions:

Heat the olive oil in a medium skillet and sauté the onion and bell pepper until softened, 3 minutes.

Mix in the tomatoes, black beans, sweet corn, and cook until the tomatoes soften, 10 minutes. Season with salt and black pepper.

Heat another medium skillet over medium heat and lay in one tortilla. Spread a quarter of the tomato mixture on top, scatter a quarter of the plant cheese on the sauce, and cover with another tortilla. Cook until the cheese melts. Flip and cook further for 2 minutes.

Transfer to a plate and make one more piece using the remaining ingredients.

Cut each tortilla set into quarters and serve immediately.

Nutrition:

Calories 197 Fats 6. 4g Carbs 30. 2g Protein 6. 6g

455. Spinach and Mashed Tofu Salad

Preparation Time: 20 minutes | **Cooking Time:** 3-30 minutes | **Servings:** 4

Ingredients:

2 8-oz. blocks firm tofu, drained	4 cups baby spinach leaves
4 tbsp. cashew butter	1½ tbsp. soy sauce
1-inch piece ginger, finely chopped	1 tsp. red miso paste
2 tbsp. sesame seeds	1 tsp. organic orange zest
1 tsp. nori flakes	2 tbsp. water

Directions:

Use paper towels to absorb any excess water left in the tofu before crumbling both blocks into small pieces.

In a large bowl, combine the mashed tofu with the spinach leaves.

Mix the remaining ingredients in another small bowl and, if desired, add the optional water for a more smooth dressing.

Pour this dressing over the mashed tofu and spinach leaves.

Transfer the bowl to the fridge and allow the salad to chill for up to one hour. Doing so will guarantee a better flavor. Or, the salad can be served right away. Enjoy!

Nutrition:

Calories 166 Carbohydrates 5. 5 g Fats 10. 7 g Protein 11. 3 g

456. Cucumber Edamame Salad

Preparation Time: 5 minutes | **Cooking Time:** 8 minutes | **Servings:** 2

Ingredients:

3 tbsp. avocado oil	1 cup cucumber, sliced into thin rounds
½ cup fresh sugar snap peas, sliced or whole	½ cup fresh edamame
¼ cup radish, sliced	1 large Hass avocado, peeled, pitted, sliced
1 nori sheet, crumbled	2 tsp. roasted sesame seeds
1 tsp. salt	

Directions:

Bring a medium-sized pot filled halfway with water to a boil over medium-high heat.

Add the sugar snaps and cook them for about 2 minutes.

Take the pot off the heat, drain the excess water, transfer the sugar snaps to a medium-sized bowl, and set aside for now.

Fill the pot with water again, add the teaspoon of salt and bring to a boil over medium-high heat.

Add the edamame to the pot and let them cook for about 6 minutes.

Take the pot off the heat, drain the excess water, transfer the soybeans to the bowl with sugar snaps, and let them cool down for about 5 minutes.

Combine all ingredients, except the nori crumbs and roasted sesame seeds, in a medium-sized bowl.

Carefully stir, using a spoon, until all ingredients are evenly coated in oil.

Top the salad with the nori crumbs and roasted sesame seeds.

Transfer the bowl to the fridge and allow the salad to cool for at least 30 minutes. Serve chilled and enjoy!

Nutrition:

Calories 409 Carbohydrates 7. 1 g Fats 38. 25 g Protein 7. 6 g

457. Artichoke White Bean Sandwich Spread

Preparation Time: 10 minutes | **Cooking Time:** 3-30 minutes | **Servings:** 2

Ingredients:

½ cup raw cashews, chopped	Water
1 clove garlic, cut into half	1 tablespoon lemon zest
1 teaspoon fresh rosemary, chopped	¼ teaspoon salt
¼ teaspoon pepper	6 tablespoons almond, soy, or coconut milk
1 15. 5-ounce can cannellini beans, rinsed and drained well	3 to 4 canned artichoke hearts, chopped
¼ cup hulled sunflower seeds	Green onions, chopped, for garnish

Directions:

Soak the raw cashews for 15 minutes in enough water to cover them. Drain and dab with a paper towel to make them as dry as possible.

Transfer the cashews to a blender and add the garlic, lemon zest, rosemary, salt, and pepper. Pulse to break everything up and then add the milk, one tablespoon at a time, until the mixture is smooth and creamy.

Mash the beans in a bowl with a fork. Add the artichoke hearts and sunflower seeds. Toss to mix.

Pour the cashew mixture on top and season with more salt and pepper if desired. Mix the ingredients well and spread on whole-wheat bread, crackers, or a wrap.

Nutrition:
Calories 110 Carbohydrates 14 g Fats 4 g Protein 6 g

458. Buffalo Chickpea Wraps

Preparation Time: 20 minutes | **Cooking Time:** 5 minutes | **Servings:** 4

Ingredients:

¼ cup plus 2 tablespoons hummus	2 tablespoons lemon juice
1½ tablespoons maple syrup	1 to 2 tablespoons hot water
1 head Romaine lettuce, chopped	1 15-ounce can chickpeas, drained, rinsed, and patted dry
4 tablespoons hot sauce, divided	1 tablespoon olive or coconut oil
¼ teaspoon garlic powder	1 pinch sea salt
4 wheat tortillas	¼ cup cherry tomatoes, diced
¼ cup red onion, diced	¼ of a ripe avocado, thinly sliced

Directions:
Mix the hummus with lemon juice and maple syrup in a large bowl. Use a whisk and add the hot water, a little at a time until it is thick but spreadable.
Add the Romaine lettuce and toss to coat. Set aside.
Pour the prepared chickpeas into another bowl. Add three tablespoons of the hot sauce, olive oil, garlic powder, and salt; toss to coat.
Heat a metal skillet (cast iron works the best) over medium heat and add the chickpea mixture. Sauté for three to five minutes and mash gently with a spoon.
Once the chickpea mixture is slightly dried out, remove it from the heat and add the rest of the hot sauce. Stir it in well and set aside.
Lay the tortillas on a clean, flat surface and spread a quarter cup of the buffalo chickpeas on top. Top with tomatoes, onion, and avocado (optional) and wrap.

Nutrition:
Calories 254 Carbohydrates 39. 4 g Fats 6. 7 g Protein 9. 1 g

459. Coconut Veggie Wraps

Preparation Time: 5 minutes | **Cooking Time:** 3-30 minutes | **Servings:** 5

Ingredients:

1½ cups shredded carrots	1 red bell pepper, seeded, thinly sliced
2½ cups kale	1 ripe avocado, thinly sliced
1 cup fresh cilantro, chopped	5 coconut wraps
2/3 cups hummus	6½ cups green curry paste

Directions:
Slice, chop, and shred all the vegetables.
Lay a coconut wrap on a clean flat surface and spread two tablespoons of the hummus and one tablespoon of the green curry paste on top of the end closest to you.
Place some carrots, bell pepper, kale, and cilantro on the wrap and start rolling it up, starting from the edge closest to you. Roll tightly and fold in the ends.
Place the wrap, seam down, on a plate to serve.

Nutrition:
Calories 236 Carbohydrates 23. 6 g Fats 14. 3 g Protein 5. 5 g

460. Cucumber Avocado Sandwich

Preparation Time: 15 minutes | **Cooking Time:** 3-30 minutes | **Servings:** 2

Ingredients:

½ of a large cucumber, peeled, sliced	¼ teaspoon salt
4 slices whole-wheat bread	4 ounces goat cheese with or without herbs, at room temperature
2 Romaine lettuce leaves	1 large avocado, peeled, pitted, sliced
2 pinches lemon pepper	1 squeeze of lemon juice
½ cup alfalfa sprouts	

Directions:

Peel and slice the cucumber thinly. Lay the slices on a plate and sprinkle them with a quarter to a half teaspoon of salt. Let this sit for 10 minutes or until water appears on the plate.

Place the cucumber slices in a colander and rinse with cold water. Let these drain, then place them on a dry plate and pat dry with a paper towel.

Spread all slices with goat cheese and place lettuce leaves on the two bottom pieces of bread. Layer the cucumber slices and avocado atop the bread.

Sprinkle one pinch of lemon pepper over each sandwich and drizzle a little lemon juice over the top.

Top with the alfalfa sprouts and place another piece of bread, goat cheese down, on top.

Nutrition:

Calories 246 Carbohydrates 20 g Fats 12 g Protein 9 g

461. Fresh Puttanesca With Quinoa

Preparation Time: 15-30 minutes | **Cooking Time:** 30 minutes | **Servings:** 4

Ingredients:

1 cup brown quinoa	2 cups of water
1/8 tsp salt	4 cups plum tomatoes, chopped
4 pitted green olives, sliced	4 pitted Kalamata olives, sliced
1 ½ tbsp capers, rinsed and drained	2 garlic cloves, minced
1 tbsp olive oil	1 tbsp chopped fresh parsley
¼ cup chopped fresh basil	1/8 tsp red chili flakes

Directions:

Add the quinoa, water, and salt to a medium pot and cook covered over medium heat until tender and water is absorbed for about 10 to 15 minutes.

Meanwhile, in a medium bowl, mix the tomatoes, green olives, Kalamata olives, capers, garlic, olive oil, parsley, basil, and red chili flakes. Allow sitting for 5 minutes.

Serve the puttanesca with the quinoa.

Nutrition:

Calories 427 kcal Fats 7. 1g Carbs 88. 2g Protein 7. 2g

462. Quinoa Cherry Tortilla Wraps

Preparation Time: 15-30 minutes | **Cooking Time:** 25 minutes | **Servings:** 4

Ingredients:

½ cup brown quinoa	Salt and black pepper to taste
2 tsp olive oil	1 ½ cups shredded carrots
1 ¼ cups fresh cherries, pitted and halved	4 scallions, chopped
2 tbsp plain vinegar	2 tbsp low-sodium soy sauce
1 tbsp pure maple syrup	4 (8-inch) tortilla wraps

Directions:

Cook the quinoa in 1 cup of slightly salted water in a medium pot over medium heat until tender and the water absorbs, 10 minutes. Fluff and set aside to warm.

Heat the olive oil in a medium skillet and sauté the carrots, cherries, and scallions. While cooking, in a small bowl, mix the vinegar, soy sauce, and maple syrup. Stir the mixture into the vegetable mixture. Simmer for 5 minutes and turn the heat off.

Spread the tortillas on a flat surface, spoon the mixture at the center, fold the sides and ends to wrap in the filling.

Serve warm.

Nutrition:

Calories 282 kcal Fats 6. 5g Carbs 48g Protein 8. 3g

463. Quinoa With Mixed Herbs

Preparation Time: 15-30 minutes | **Cooking Time:** 20 minutes | **Servings:** 4

Ingredients:

1 cup quinoa, well-rinsed	2 cups vegetable broth
Salt to taste	2 garlic cloves, minced, divided

¼ cup chopped chives	2 tbsp finely chopped parsley
2 tbsp finely chopped basil	2 tbsp finely chopped mint
2 tbsp finely chopped soft sundried tomatoes	1 tbsp olive oil (optional)
½ tsp lemon zest	1 tbsp fresh lemon juice
2 tbsp minced walnuts	Salt and black pepper to taste

Directions:

In a medium pot, combine the quinoa, vegetable broth, ¼ tsp of salt, and half of the garlic in a medium saucepan. Boil until the quinoa is tender and the liquid absorbs, 10-15 minutes.

Open the lid, fluff with a fork, and stir in the chives, parsley, basil, mint, tomatoes, olive oil, zest, lemon juice, and walnuts. Warm for 5 minutes.

Dish the food and serve warm.

Nutrition:

Calories 393 kcal Fats 17. 1g Carbs 31. 9g Protein 27. 8g

464. Chickpea Avocado Pizza

Preparation Time: 15-30 minutes | **Cooking Time:** 40 minutes | **Servings:** 4

Ingredients:

For the pizza crust:

3 ½ cups whole-wheat flour	1 tsp yeast
1 tsp salt	1 pinch sugar
3 tbsp olive oil	1 cup of warm water

For the topping:

1 cup red pizza sauce	1 cup baby spinach
Salt and black pepper to taste	1 (15 oz) can chickpeas, drained and rinsed
1 medium avocado, pitted, peeled, and chopped	¼ cup grated plant-based Parmesan cheese

Directions:

Preheat the oven the 350 F and lightly grease a pizza pan with cooking spray.

In a medium bowl, mix the flour, nutritional yeast, salt, sugar, olive oil, and warm water until

smooth dough forms. Allow rising for an hour or until the dough doubles in size.

Spread the dough on the pizza pan and apply the pizza sauce on top.

Top with the spinach, chickpeas, avocado, and plant Parmesan cheese.

Bake the pizza for 20 minutes or until the cheese melts.

Remove from the oven, cool for 5 minutes, slice, and serve.

Nutrition:

Calories 678 kcal Fats 22. 7g Carbs 104. 1g Protein 23. 5g

465. White Bean Stuffed Squash

Preparation Time: 15-30 minutes | **Cooking Time:** 60 minutes | **Servings:** 4

Ingredients:

2 pounds large acorn squash	2 tbsp olive oil
3 garlic cloves, minced	1 (15 oz) can white beans, drained and rinsed
1 cup chopped spinach leaves	½ cup vegetable stock
Salt and black pepper to taste	½ tsp cumin powder
½ tsp chili powder	

Directions:

Preheat the oven to 350 F.

Cut the squash into half and scoop out the seeds. Season with salt and pepper and place face down on a sheet pan. Bake for 45 minutes.

While the squash cooks, heat the olive oil in a medium pot over medium heat.

Sauté the garlic until fragrant, 30 seconds, and mix in the beans. Cook for 1 minute.

Stir in the spinach, allow wilting for 2 minutes, and season with salt, black pepper, cumin powder, and chili powder. Cook for 2 minutes and turn the heat off.

When the squash is fork-tender, remove it from the oven and fill the holes with the bean and spinach mixture.

Serve warm.

Nutrition:

Calories 365 kcal Fats 34. 6g Carbs 16. 7g Protein 2. 3g

466. Grilled Zucchini And Spinach Pizza

Preparation Time: 15-30 minutes | **Cooking Time:** 30 minutes | **Servings:** 4

Ingredients:

For the pizza crust:

3 ½ cups whole-wheat flour	1 tsp yeast
1 tsp salt	1 pinch sugar
3 tbsp olive oil	1 cup of warm water

For the topping:

1 cup marinara sauce	2 large zucchinis, sliced
½ cup chopped spinach	¼ cup pitted and sliced black olives
½ cup grated plant Parmesan cheese	

Directions:

Preheat the oven the 350 F and lightly grease a pizza pan with cooking spray.

In a medium bowl, mix the flour, nutritional yeast, salt, sugar, olive oil, and warm water until smooth dough forms. Allow rising for an hour or until the dough doubles in size. Spread the dough on the pizza pan and apply the pizza sauce on top.

Meanwhile, heat a grill pan over medium heat, season the zucchinis with salt, black pepper, and cook in the pan until slightly charred on both sides.

Set the cucumbers on the pizza crust and top with the spinach, olives, and plant Parmesan cheese. Bake the pizza for 20 minutes or until the cheese melts. Remove from the oven, cool for 5 minutes, slice, and serve.

Nutrition:

Calories 519 kcal Fats 13. 4g Carbs 87. 5g Protein 19. 6g

467. Honey-Almond Popcorn

Preparation Time: 5 minutes | **Cooking Time:** 10 minutes | **Servings:** 4

Ingredients:

1/2 cup popcorn kernels	2 tablespoons honey
1/2 teaspoon sea salt	2 tablespoons coconut sugar
1 cup roasted almonds	1/4 cup walnut oil

Directions:

Take a pot, place it over medium-low heat, add oil and when it melts, add four kernels and wait until they sizzle.

Then add the remaining kernel, toss until coated, sprinkle with sugar, drizzle with honey, shut the pot with the lid, and shake the kernels until popped completely, adding almonds halfway.

Once all the kernels have popped, season them with salt and serve straight away.

Nutrition:

Calories: 120 Cal Fat: 4.5 g Carbs: 19 g Protein: 1 g Fiber: 1 g

468. Turmeric Snack Bites

Preparation Time: 35 minutes | **Cooking Time:** 0 minute | **Servings:** 10

Ingredients:

1 cup Medjool dates, pitted, chopped	1/2 cup walnuts
1 teaspoon ground turmeric	1 tablespoon cocoa powder, unsweetened
1/2 teaspoon ground cinnamon	1/2 cup shredded coconut, unsweetened

Directions:

Place all the ingredients in a food processor and pulse for 2 minutes until a smooth mixture comes together.

Tip the mixture in a bowl and then shape it into ten small balls, 1 tablespoon of the mixture per ball and then refrigerate for 30 minutes.

Serve straight away.

Nutrition:

Calories: 109 Cal Fat: 2 g Carbs: 13 g Protein: 1 g Fiber: 0 g

469. Watermelon Pizza

Preparation Time: 10 minutes | **Cooking Time:** 0 minute | **Servings:** 10

Ingredients:

1/2 cup strawberries, halved	1/2 cup blueberries
1 watermelon	1/2 cup raspberries
1 cup of coconut yogurt	1/2 cup pomegranate seeds

1/2 cup cherries   Maple syrup as needed

Directions:
Cut watermelon into 3-inch thick slices, then spread yogurt on one side, leaving some space in the edges, and then top evenly with fruits and drizzle with maple syrup.
Cut the watermelon into wedges and then serve.

Nutrition:
Calories: 150 Cal Fat: 4 g Carbs: 21 g Protein: 10 g Fiber: 2 g

470. Nooch Popcorn

Preparation Time: 10 minutes | **Cooking Time:** 10 minutes | **Servings:** 4

Ingredients:
1/3 cup nutritional yeast
1 teaspoon of sea salt
3 tablespoons coconut oil
½ cup popcorn kernels

Directions:
Place yeast in a large bowl, stir in salt and set aside until required.
Take a medium saucepan, place it over medium-high heat, add oil and when it melts, add four kernels and wait until they sizzle.
Then add the remaining kernel, toss until coated, shut the pan with the lid, and shake the kernels until popped completely.
When done, transfer popcorn to the yeast mixture, shut with lid, and shape well until coated.
Serve straight away

Nutrition:
Calories: 160 Cal Fat: 6 g Carbs: 28 g Protein: 3 g Fiber: 4 g

471. Masala Popcorn

Preparation Time: 5 minutes | **Cooking Time:** 15 minutes | **Servings:** 4

Ingredients:
3 cups popped popcorn
1 teaspoon ground cumin
1 teaspoon ground coriander

2 hot chili peppers, sliced
6 curry leaves

1/3 teaspoon salt

1/8 teaspoon chaat masala
¼ teaspoon red pepper flakes
1/3 cup olive oil

1/4 teaspoon turmeric powder
1/4 teaspoon garam masala

Directions:
Take a large pot, place it over medium heat, add half of the oil and when hot, add chili peppers and curry leaves and cook for 3 minutes until golden.
When done, transfer curry leaves and pepper to a plate lined with paper towels and set aside until required.
Add remaining oil into the pot, add remaining ingredients except for popcorns, stir until mixed and cook for 1 minute until fragrant.
Then tip in popcorns, remove the pan from heat, stir well until coated, and then sprinkle with bay leaves and red chili.
Toss until mixed and serve straight away.

Nutrition:
Calories: 150 Cal Fat: 9 g Carbs: 15 g Protein: 2 g Fiber: 4 g

472. Cauliflower Nuggets

Preparation Time: 35 minutes | **Cooking Time:** 0 minutes | **Servings:** 4

Ingredients:
3 tablespoon yeast flakes
½ cauliflower
½ cup breadcrumbs
Salt and pepper

60 ml of soy milk

2 tablespoons of oil
30 g flour

Directions:
Separate the cauliflower into florets and wash.
Mix the flour, yeast flakes, milk, salt, and pepper.
Roll the cauliflower in the mass and then roll in breadcrumbs.
Place on a baking sheet and drizzle with oil.
Bake for about 35 minutes at 200 degrees Celsius, until the cauliflower is cooked through.

Nutrition:
Calories: 279 Fat: 15.4g Carbs: 20.5g Protein: 12.1g Fiber: 3.2g

473. Cauliflower Potato Burgers

Preparation Time: 15 minutes | **Cooking Time:** 7 minutes | **Servings:** 2

Ingredients:

7 oz cauliflower rice	1/4 cup mashed potato
1 tablespoon almond flour	1 teaspoon salt
1 teaspoon white pepper	1 tablespoon coconut yogurt
1 tablespoon breadcrumbs	1/2 cup water, for cooking

Directions:

In the mixing bowl combine cauliflower rice and mashed potato.

Add almond flour, salt, white pepper, and coconut yogurt.

Then wear gloves and make medium size burgers from the mixture.

Sprinkle every burger with breadcrumbs and wrap it in the foil.

Pour water into the instant pot bowl and insert the steamer rack.

Place wrapped burgers on the steamer rack and close the lid.

Cook the meal on High (Manual mode) for 7 minutes. Then allow natural pressure release for 10 minutes.

Nutrition:

Calories: 163, Fat: 9, Fiber: 4.8, Carbs: 17, Protein: 6.6

474. Sweet Potato Burgers

Preparation Time: 10 minutes | **Cooking Time:** 20 minutes | **Servings:** 2

Ingredients:

1 sweet potato	1/2 onion, diced
1 teaspoon chives	1/2 teaspoon salt
1 teaspoon cayenne pepper	3 tablespoon flax meal
1/2 cup kale	1 teaspoon olive oil
1/2 cup water, for cooking	

Directions:

Pour water into the instant pot and insert the steamer rack.

Place sweet potato on the steamer rack and close the lid.

Cook the vegetables on Manual mode (High pressure) for 15 minutes (quick pressure release).

Meanwhile, place onion, chives, and kale in the blender. Blend until smooth.

Transfer the blended mixture to the mixing bowl. When the sweet potato is cooked – cut it into halves and scoop all the flesh into the kale mixture. Mix it up carefully with the help of the fork.

Add flax meal, salt, and cayenne pepper. Stir well. With the help of the fingertips make medium burgers.

Clean the instant pot bowl and put olive oil inside. Preheat for 2-3 minutes on Sauté mode.

Then add burgers and cook them for 2 minutes from each side on Sauté mode.

Nutrition:

Calories: 139, Fat: 6.4, Fiber: 6, Carbs: 19.7, Protein: 4.3

475. Potato Patties

Preparation Time: 10 minutes | **Cooking Time:** 15 minutes | **Servings:** 4

Ingredients:

3 russet potatoes, peeled	3 tablespoon aquafaba
1/2 teaspoon salt	1 teaspoon almond butter
1/2 teaspoon smoked paprika	1/4 teaspoon chili flakes
2 tablespoon wheat flour	

Directions:

With the help of the hand mixer, whisk aquafaba until you get soft peaks.

Then grate potatoes and combine them with aquafaba in the mixing bowl.

Add salt, smoked paprika, chili flakes, and wheat flour. Mix it up carefully.

Preheat the instant pot on Sauté mode for 4 minutes. Add almond butter and melt it.

Then with the help of the spoon make medium patties; press them a little with the help of hand palms and put in the hot almond butter.

Cook the patties for 3 minutes then flip into another side. Cook the patties for 4 minutes more.

Nutrition:
Calories: 150, Fat: 2.5, Fiber: 4.4, Carbs: 29, Protein: 4

476. Lentil Burgers

Preparation Time: 20 minutes | **Cooking Time:** 26 minutes | **Servings:** 7

Ingredients:

1 cup lentils, soaked overnight	1 cup of water
1/2 carrot, peeled	1 teaspoon cayenne pepper
4 tablespoon wheat flour	1 teaspoon salt
1 teaspoon olive oil	1 tablespoon dried dill

Directions:
Put lentils in the Instant pot together with water, carrot, salt, and cayenne pepper.
Close the lid and set Manual mode (High pressure).
Cook the ingredients for 25 minutes and allow natural pressure release for 10 minutes.
Transfer the cooked ingredients in the blender and blend until smooth.
Add wheat flour and dried dill. Mix it up until smooth. If the mixture is liquid – add more flour.
Make the burgers and place them together with the olive oil in the instant pot.
Set Manual mode (High pressure) for 1 minute (quick pressure release).
It is recommended to serve burgers warm.

Nutrition:
Calories 122, Fat 1.1, Fiber 8.7, Carbs 20.7, Protein 7.7

477. Scrumptious Baked Potatoes

Preparation Time: 15-30 minutes | **Cooking Time:** 8 hours and 10 minutes | **Servings:** 8

Ingredients:

8 potatoes	Salt to taste for serving
Ground black pepper to taste for serving	

Directions:
Rinse potatoes until clean, wipe dry and then prick with a fork.
Wrap each potato in an aluminum foil and place in a 6 to 8 quarts slow cooker.
Cover with a lid, and then plug in the slow cooker and let cook on a low heat setting for 8 hours or until tender.
When the cooking time is over, unwrap potatoes and prick with a fork to check if potatoes are tender or not.
Sprinkle potatoes with salt, black pepper, and your favorite seasoning and serve.

Nutrition:
Calories:93 Cal, Carbohydrates:3g, Protein:3g, Fats:1g, Fiber:2g.

478. Fantastic Butternut Squash & Vegetables

Preparation Time: 15-30 minutes | **Cooking Time:** 4 hours and 15 minutes | **Servings:** 6

Ingredients:

1 1/2 cups of corn kernels	2 pounds of butternut squash
1 medium-sized green bell pepper	14 1/2 ounce of diced tomatoes
1/2 cup of chopped white onion	1/2 teaspoon of minced garlic
1/2 teaspoon of salt	1/4 teaspoon of ground black pepper
1 tablespoon and 2 teaspoons of tomato paste	1/2 cup of vegetable broth

Directions:
Peel, centralize the butternut squash and dice and place it into a 6-quarts slow cooker.
Create a hole on the green bell pepper, then cut it into 1/2 inch pieces and add it to the slow cooker.
Add the remaining ingredients into the slow cooker except for tomato paste, stir properly and cover it with the lid.
Then plug in the slow cooker and let it cook on the low heat setting for 6 hours or until the vegetables get soft.
When 6 hours of the cooking time is done, remove 1/2 cup of the cooking liquid from the slow cooker.

Then pour the tomato mixture into this cooking liquid, stir properly and place it in the slow cooker.

Stir properly and continue cooking for 30 minutes or until the mixture becomes slightly thick.

Serve right away.

Nutrition:
Calories:134 Cal, Carbohydrates:23g, Protein:6g, Fats:2g, Fiber:4g.

479. Balls from Beetroot

Preparation Time: 35 minutes | **Cooking Time:** 0 minutes | **Servings:** 4

Ingredients:

4 sprigs of parsley	2 tablespoon walnuts
260 g beetroot	½ onion
1 clove of garlic	Salt and pepper

Directions:
Boil the beetroot, peel, and grate coarsely with a kitchen grater.

Roast the walnuts and process them into flour in a food processor.

Cut the onion into small cubes, peel the garlic clove and mash it with a fork.

Wash, shake, and chop the parsley.

Mix all **Ingredients:** in a bowl and season with salt and a little pepper.

Shape into balls of the same size and let stand for a few minutes.

Nutrition:
Calories: 239 Fat: 11.4g Carbs: 10.5g Protein: 12.1g Fiber: 3.2g

480. Polenta Skewers

Preparation Time: 35 minutes | **Cooking Time:** 0 minutes | **Servings:** 4

Ingredients:

½ avocado	10 cherry tomatoes
1 mini zucchini	150 g corn grits
2 tablespoon olive oil	1 teaspoon sesame seeds, black
10 basil leaves	10 toothpicks
450 ml of vegetable stock	Salt and pepper

Directions:
The day before, bring the corn grits to the boil in the broth and cook for a few minutes, stirring constantly. Pour into a square form and chill until the next day.

Cut the polenta into small cubes and fry in a pan in a little olive oil.

Wash the zucchini, cut into thin slices, and fry in the pan once the polenta is ready.

Wash the tomatoes and cut them in half, pluck the basil leaves from the branches.

Stone the avocado and cut it into thin slices.

Skewer a polenta cube, a zucchini, a tomato, a slice of avocado, and a basil leaf onto a toothpick.

Serve with sesame seeds.

Nutrition:
Calories: 259 Fat: 15.4g Carbs: 20.5g Protein: 12.1g Fiber: 3.2g

481. Börek with Spinach Filling

Preparation Time: 25 minutes | **Cooking Time:** 0 minutes | **Servings:** 10

Ingredients:

10 yufka sheets	2 cloves of garlic
1 small onion	3 tablespoon soy yogurt
4 tablespoon soy milk	400 g spin nat
3 tablespoons of oil	1 pinch of nutmeg
Salt and pepper	

Directions:
Wash the spinach, peel the garlic and onion and cut into small cubes.

Steam the spinach, onion, and garlic in oil in a deep pan.

After a few minutes, season with nutmeg, salt, and pepper and stir in the yogurt.

Lay the Yufka leaves and brush with the spinach filling.

Roll up and brush with a little milk.

Then place on a baking sheet and bake in the oven at 180 degrees Celsius for about 15 minutes.

Nutrition:
Calories: 219 Fat: 9.4g Carbs: 10.5g Protein: 11.1g Fiber: 3.2g

482. Taler With Avocado Cream

Preparation Time: 25 minutes | **Cooking Time:** 0 minutes | **Servings:** 5

Ingredients:

20 pumpernickels, round	1 chili pepper
1 lime	2 avocados
6 beetroot chips	50 g vegan cream cheese
Salt and pepper	

Directions:

Cut the chili pepper lengthways and scrape out the stones.

Halve the avocados, core them and scrape the pulp into a blender jar.

Add the cream cheese and a little lime juice.

Mix a homogeneous cream from the chili pepper, avocado, lime, cream cheese, and a little salt and pepper.

Put the little Pumpernickel Taler ready and put a serving of avocado cream on each with a piping bag.

Crumble the chips and sprinkle them over the talers.

Nutrition:

Calories: 243 Fat: 10.4g Carbs: 12.5g Protein: 9.1g Fiber: 3.2g

483. Pumpernickel with Avocado

Preparation Time: 10 minutes | **Cooking Time:** 0 minutes | **Servings:** 2

Ingredients:

6 small slices of pumpernickel	1 avocado
1 roll of vegan cheese spread	1 tablespoon chives
Salt and pepper	

Directions:

Halve the avocado, remove the seeds, and carefully remove them from the skin. Cut into slices and place on a plate.

Spread cheese on the bread, then top with avocado, and then sprinkle with a little pepper and chopped chives.

Nutrition:

Calories: 159 Fat: 9.4g Carbs: 10.5g Protein: 9.1g Fiber: 3.2g

484. Savory Mushroom Cakes

Preparation Time: 30 minutes | **Cooking Time:** 0 minutes | **Servings:** 4

Ingredients:

1 bun	1 small onion
1 clove of garlic	500 g mushrooms
1 pinch of marjoram	2 tablespoons of oil
1 tablespoon flaxseed, crushed	3 tablespoon soy milk
Salt and pepper	

Directions:

Clean the mushrooms and cut them into small cubes. Peel the onion and garlic, then also dice.

Crumble the bun and mix in a bowl with the mushrooms, garlic, and onion.

Add marjoram, salt, and pepper, and fold in the flax seeds as well.

Add soy milk so that the mixture sticks well.

Heat the oil in a non-stick pan, form small meatballs and fry them until golden brown on both sides.

Nutrition:

Calories: 129 Fat: 12.4g Carbs: 11.5g Protein: 9.1g Fiber: 3.2g

485. Churros With Chocolate

Preparation Time: 35 minutes | **Cooking Time:** 0 minutes | **Servings:** 6

Ingredients:

2 teaspoons of baking powder	1 ¼ cup of flour
2 cups of oil	1 pinch of salt
50 g sugar	1 cup of soy milk
100 g vegan chocolate	cinnamon and sugar

Directions:

Mix the sugar, baking powder, flour, and salt. Then stir in ¾ of the soy milk until a velvety batter is formed.

Heat the oil in a saucepan and roll the churro batter into a long line.

When the oil is hot, cut the thin roll into pieces with scissors and bake them in the oil until they are evenly golden yellow on all sides.

In Zimt and roll sugar and heat the chocolate with the remaining soy milk.

Nutrition:
Calories: 209 Fat: 15.4g Carbs: 20.5g Protein: 12.1g Fiber: 3.2g

486. Zucchini Rolls with Cream Cheese

Preparation Time: 35 minutes | **Cooking Time:** 0 minutes | **Servings:** 4

Ingredients:

1 tablespoon oil	60 g apricots, dried
350 g zucchini	Salt and pepper
1 sprig of thyme	½ lime

Directions:
Turn after a minute and fry the same way on the other side.

Let cool on a plate and in the meantime prepare the filling.

Let the apricots soak a little and then chop them.

Mix with cream cheese, chopped thyme, and a little pepper. Season to taste with salt and prepare.

Brush the zucchini slices with some filling and roll-up.

Add a few squirts of lime juice to serve.

Nutrition:
Calories: 235 Fat: 15.4g Carbs: 20.5g Protein: 12.1g Fiber: 3.2g

487. Spinach Burgers

Preparation Time: 10 minutes | **Cooking Time:** 10 minutes | **Servings:** 7

Ingredients:

3 cups spinach, chopped	2 tablespoon coconut shreds
4 tablespoon panko breadcrumbs	1 teaspoon salt
1/2 teaspoon chili flakes	2 tablespoon flax meal
6 tablespoon hot water	1 teaspoon olive oil

1 tablespoon coconut yogurt

Directions:
In the mixing bowl mix up together flax meal and hot water. Whisk the mixture.

Then add coconut shred, panko breadcrumbs, spinach, chili flakes, coconut yogurt, and salt.

Mix up the mixture until homogenous.

Set the Saute mode in Instant pot and preheat it until it shows "Hot".

Then brush the instant bowl with olive oil from inside.

Make patties from the spinach mixture with the help of 2 spoons and place them in the instant pot.

Saute them for 10 minutes. You can flip the patties during cooking if desired.

Nutrition:
Calories: 47, Fat: 2.9, Fiber: 1.3, Carbs: 4.5, Protein: 1.5

488. Tempeh Patties

Preparation Time: 15 minutes | **Cooking Time:** 11 minutes | **Servings:** 5

Ingredients:

10 oz tempeh	1 carrot, peeled
4 tablespoon oatmeal	1/4 teaspoon minced garlic
1 teaspoon onion powder	1/2 teaspoon salt
2 oz black beans, canned	1 tablespoon tomato sauce
1 teaspoon golden syrup	1/2 cup water, for cooking

Directions:
Cut tempeh into chunks and place it on the steamer rack.

Pour water into the instant pot and insert the steamer rack with tempeh.

Close the lid and cook on Manual mode (High pressure) for 7 minutes. Then use quick pressure release.

Meanwhile, chop the carrot and place it in the food processor.

Add minced garlic, oatmeal onion powder, salt, canned beans, tomato sauce, and golden syrup.

Blend the mixture for 2-3 minutes.

Then add cooked tempeh and keep blending for 1 minute more. The final mixture texture shouldn't be too smooth.

Use the burger mold and make burgers. Freeze them until solid.

Then wrap every burger in foil or use non-stick paper and place in the cleaned instant pot bowl. Cook the burgers on High (Manual mode) for 4 minutes. Then allow natural pressure release for 10 minutes.

Nutrition:
Calories: 175, Fat: 6.6, Fiber: 2.5, Carbs: 18, Protein: 13.7

489. Pumpkin Burgers

Preparation Time: 10 minutes | **Cooking Time:** 3 minutes | **Servings:** 2

Ingredients:

2 hamburger buns	1 tablespoon pumpkin seeds
1 tablespoon pumpkin powder	3 tablespoon pumpkin puree
2 tablespoons breadcrumbs	1/2 teaspoon chili flakes
1 teaspoon turmeric	1 tablespoon flax meal
3 tablespoons hot water	

Directions:
In the mixing bowl combine flax meal and hot water. Whisk the mixture and add pumpkin powder, pumpkin puree, breadcrumbs, chili flakes, and turmeric.

Mix up the mixture. Add pumpkin seeds.

With the help of the burger mold, make 2 burgers.

Place them in the instant pot bowl and close the lid.

Set Manual mode (High pressure) and cook for 3 minutes.

Then use quick pressure release and open the lid. Fill the burger buns with pumpkin burgers.

Nutrition:
Calories: 197, Fat: 5.6, Fiber: 3.3, Carbs: 30.5, Protein: 7.2

490. Fabulous Glazed Carrots

Preparation Time: 15-30 minutes | **Cooking Time:** 2 hours and 20 minutes | **Servings:** 5

Ingredients:

1 pound of carrots	2 teaspoons of chopped cilantro
1/4 teaspoon of salt	1/4 cup of brown sugar
1/4 teaspoon of ground cinnamon	1/8 teaspoon of ground nutmeg
1 tablespoon of cornstarch	1 tablespoon of olive oil
2 tablespoons of water	1 large orange, juiced and zested

Directions:
Peel the carrots, rinse, cut them into 1/4 inch thick rounds and place them in a 6 quarts slow cooker.

Add the salt, sugar, cinnamon, nutmeg, olive oil, orange zest, juice, and stir properly.

Cover it with the lid, then plug in the slow cooker and let it cook on the high heat setting for 2 hours or until the carrots become soft.

Stir properly the cornstarch and water until it blends well. Thereafter, add this mixture to the slow cooker.

Continue cooking for 10 minutes or until the sauce in the slow cooker gets slightly thick.

Sprinkle the cilantro over carrots and serve.

Nutrition:
Calories:160 Cal, Carbohydrates:40g, Protein:1g, Fats:0. 3g, Fiber:2. 3g.

491. Flavorful Sweet Potatoes with Apples

Preparation Time: 15-30 minutes | **Cooking Time:** 5 hours | **Servings:** 6

Ingredients:

3 medium-sized apples, peeled and cored	6 medium-sized sweet potatoes, peeled and cored
1/4 cup of pecans	1/4 teaspoon of ground cinnamon
1/4 teaspoon of ground nutmeg	2 tablespoons of vegan butter, melted
1/4 cup of maple syrup	

Directions:

Cut the sweet potatoes and the apples into 1/2 inch slices.

Grease a 6-quarts slow cooker with a non-stick cooking spray and arrange the sweet potato slices in the bottom of the cooker.

Top it with the apple slices; sprinkle it with the cinnamon and nutmeg, before garnishing it with butter.

Cover it with the lid, plug in the slow cooker and let it cook on the low heat setting for 4 hours or until the sweet potatoes get soft.

When done, sprinkle it with pecans and continue cooking for another 30 minutes.

Serve right away.

Nutrition:

Calories:120 Cal, Carbohydrates:24g, Protein:1g, Fats:3g, Fiber:2g.

492. Buttery Baby Potatoes

Preparation Time: 15-30 minutes | **Cooking Time:** 40 minutes | **Servings:** 4

Ingredients:

4 tbsp unsalted plant butter, melted	4 garlic cloves, minced
3 tbsp chopped chives	Salt and black pepper to taste
2 tbsp grated plant-based Parmesan cheese	1 ½ lb baby potatoes, rinsed and drained

Directions:

Preheat the oven to 400 F.

In a large bowl, mix the butter, garlic, chives, salt, black pepper, and plant Parmesan cheese. Toss the potatoes in the butter mixture until well coated.

Spread the mixture into a baking sheet, cover with foil, and roast in the oven for 30 minutes or until tender.

Remove the potatoes from the oven and toss in the remaining butter mixture. Serve.

Nutrition:

Calories 192 kcal Fats 8. 8g Carbs 25. 7g Protein 4. 1g

493. Sweetened Carrots With Parsley Drizzle

Preparation Time: 15-30 minutes | **Cooking Time:** 14 minutes | **Servings:** 4

Ingredients:

1 lb baby carrots	2 tbsp plant butter
2 tbsp pure maple syrup	1 tbsp freshly squeezed lemon juice
½ tsp black pepper	¼ cup chopped fresh parsley

Directions:

Boil some water in a medium pot. Add some salt and cook the carrots until tender, 5 to 6 minutes. Drain the carrots.

Melt the butter in a large skillet and mix in the maple syrup and lemon juice.

Toss in the carrots, season with black pepper, and toss in the parsley.

Serve the carrots.

Nutrition:

Calories 120 kcal Fats 6g Carbs 16. 8g Protein 1. 1g

494. Chipotle and Lime Tortilla Chips

Preparation Time: 10 minutes | **Cooking Time:** 15 minutes | **Servings:** 4

Ingredients:

12 ounces whole-wheat tortillas	4 tablespoons chipotle seasoning 1 tablespoon olive oil
4 limes, juiced	

Directions:

Whisk together oil and lime juice, brush it well on tortillas, then sprinkle with chipotle seasoning and bake for 15 minutes at 350 degrees F until crispy, turning halfway.

When done, let the tortilla cool for 10 minutes, then break it into chips and serve.

Nutrition:

Calories: 150 Cal Fat: 7 g Carbs: 18 g Protein: 2 g Fiber: 2 g

495. Carrot and Sweet Potato Fritters

Preparation Time: 10 minutes | **Cooking Time:** 8 minutes | **Servings:** 10

Ingredients:

1/3 cup quinoa flour	1½ cups shredded sweet potato
1 cup grated carrot	1/3 teaspoon ground black pepper
2/3 teaspoon salt	2 teaspoons curry powder
2 flax eggs	2 tablespoons coconut oil

Directions:

Place all the ingredients in a bowl, except for oil, stir well until combined, and then shape the mixture into ten small patties

Take a large pan, place it over medium-high heat, add oil and when it melts, add patties in it and cook for 3 minutes per side until browned.

Serve straight away

Nutrition:
Calories: 70 Cal Fat: 3 g Carbs: 8 g Protein: 1 g Fiber: 1 g

496. Wonderful Glazed Root Vegetables

Preparation Time: 15-30 minutes | **Cooking Time:** 4 hours and 20 minutes | **Servings:** 6

Ingredients:

6 medium-sized carrots	4 medium-sized parsnips
1 pound of sweet potatoes	2 medium-sized red onions
1 teaspoon of salt	1/2 teaspoon of ground black pepper
5 teaspoons of chopped thyme	3 tablespoons of honey
1 tablespoon of apple cider vinegar	1 tablespoon of olive oil

Directions:

Peel the carrots, parsnip, sweet potatoes, onions, and cut them into 1-inch pieces.

Grease a 6 quarts slow cooker with a non-stick cooking spray, place the carrots, parsnip, onion in the bottom and then top it with the sweet potatoes.

Using a bowl whisk the salt, black pepper, 2 teaspoons of thyme, honey, and oil properly.

Pour this mixture over on the vegetables and toss it to coat.

Cover it with the lid, then plug in the slow cooker and let it cook at the low heat setting for 4 hours or until the vegetables get tender.

When cooked, pour in the vinegar, stir, sprinkle it with the remaining thyme and serve.

Nutrition:
Calories:137 Cal, Carbohydrates:26g, Protein:2g, Fats:4g, Fiber:3g.

497. Super Aubergines

Preparation Time: 15-30 minutes | **Cooking Time:** 8 hours and 15 minutes | **Servings:** 6

Ingredients:

1 pound of eggplant	10-ounce of tomatoes, quartered
2-ounce of sun-dried tomatoes	1 small fennel bulb, sliced
1 medium-sized red onion, peeled and sliced	1/2 cup of chopped parsley
1/4 cup of chopped basil	1/4 cup of chopped chives
2 teaspoons of capers	1 teaspoon of minced garlic
1 1/2 teaspoon of salt	1 teaspoon of ground black pepper
1 teaspoon of coriander seeds	1 lemon, juiced
6 tablespoons of olive oil, divided	

Directions:

Using a 6 quarts slow cooker, add 2 tablespoons of olive oil, top it with onions and garlic.

Remove the stem of the eggplant, cut it into 1/2-inch thick slices and brush 2 tablespoons of oil on both sides of the eggplant slices.

Garnish the onion with the eggplant slices and cover it with tomato pieces, sun-dried tomatoes, and fennel slices.

Sprinkle it with salt, black pepper, and coriander seeds.

Cover it with the lid, then plug in the slow cooker and let it cook at the low heat setting for 6 to 8 hours or until vegetables get tender.

While doing that, place the parsley, basil, and chives in a food processor.

Add the remaining 2 tablespoons of olive oil along with the lemon juice, caper, and pulse it until it gets smooth.

When the vegetables are cooked, transfer them to a serving platter and drizzle them with the prepared herbs mixture.

Serve right away with crusty bread.

Nutrition:
Calories:62 Cal, Carbohydrates:12g, Protein:2g, Fats:2g, Fiber:4g.

498. Sweet and Spicy Red Thai Vegetable Curry

Preparation Time: 15-30 minutes | **Cooking Time:** 4 hours and 45 minutes | **Servings:** 6

Ingredients:

1/2 head cauliflower, chopped into florets	2 medium-sized sweet potatoes, peeled and cubed
1 cup of cooked green peas	8 ounce of chopped white mushrooms
1/4 cup of chopped cilantro, chopped	1 small white onion, sliced
1/2 teaspoon of salt	1 tablespoon of brown sugar
1/2 cup of toasted cashews	3 tablespoon of red curry paste
3 tablespoons of soy sauce	2 teaspoons of Sriracha sauce
14-ounce of coconut milk	

Directions:
Grease a 6-quarts slow cooker with a non-stick cooking spray and add the cauliflower florets, sweet potatoes, and onion.

Using a bowl, stir properly the salt, sugar, red curry paste, soy sauce, Sriracha sauce, and coconut milk.

Pour this mixture on top of the vegetables in the slow cooker and toss it to coat properly.

Cover it with the lid, then plug in the slow cooker and let it cook at the low heat setting for 4 hours or until the vegetables get soft.

Then add the mushrooms, peas, to the slow cooker and continue cooking for 30 minutes. Garnish it with cilantro and serve.

Nutrition:
Calories:141 Cal, Carbohydrates:13g, Protein:0g, Fats:9g, Fiber:3g.

499. Vibrant Minestrone

Preparation Time: 15-30 minutes | **Cooking Time:** 6 hours and 25 minutes | **Servings:** 6

Ingredients:

30 ounce of cooked cannellini beans	8 ounces of uncooked small pasta
12 thin asparagus spears	3 carrots, peeled and sliced
6 ounce of chopped spinach	28 ounce of diced tomatoes
1 cup of cooked peas	1 medium-sized white onion, peeled and diced
1 1/2 teaspoon of minced garlic	1 teaspoon of salt
1/2 teaspoon of ground black pepper	3 cups of vegetable stock
3 cups of water	1/3 cup of grated parmesan cheese

Directions:
Grease a 6-quarts slow cooker with a non-stick cooking spray, add the beans, carrots, tomatoes, onion, garlic, vegetable stock, and water.

Stir properly and cover it with the lid.

Then plug in the slow cooker and let it cook at the low heat setting for 4 hours or until the vegetables get soft.

While doing that cut the asparagus into three and when the vegetables are cooked add the asparagus to the slow cooker along with the peas, salt, black pepper, spinach, and pasta.

Continue cooking for 15 minutes.

Garnish it with cheese and serve.

Nutrition:
Calories:110 Cal, Carbohydrates:18g, Protein:5g, Fats:2g, Fiber:4g.

500. Broccoli Tots

Preparation Time: 15-30 minutes | **Cooking Time:** 30 minutes | **Servings:** 4

Ingredients:

1 tbsp flax seed powder + 3 tbsp water	1 large head broccoli, cut into florets
2/3 cup toasted almond flour	2 garlic cloves, minced
2 cups grated plant-based Parmesan cheese	Salt to taste

Directions:

Preheat the oven to 350 F and line a baking sheet with parchment paper.

In a small bowl, mix the flax seed powder with the water and allow thickening for 5 minutes to make the flax egg.

Place the broccoli in a safe microwave bowl, sprinkle with 2 tbsp of water, and steam in the microwave for 1 minute or until softened.

Transfer the broccoli to a food processor and add the flax egg, almond flour, garlic, plant cheese, and salt. Blend until coarsely smooth and well combined.

Pour the mixture into a bowl and form 2-inch oblong balls from the mixture.

Place the tots on the baking sheet and bake in the oven for 15 to 20 minutes or until firm and compacted.

Remove the tots from the oven and serve warm with tomato dipping sauce.

Nutrition:

Calories 216 Fats 14. 08g Carbs 7. 78g Protein 14. 66g

501. Summer Vegetable Mix

Preparation Time: 15-30 minutes | **Cooking Time:** 40 minutes | **Servings:** 4

Ingredients:

2 medium zucchinis, chopped	2 medium yellow squash, chopped
1 medium red onion, cut into 1-inch wedges	1 medium red bell pepper, deseeded and cut into 1-inch dices
1 cup cherry tomatoes, halved	4 tbsp olive oil
Salt and black pepper to taste	3 garlic cloves, minced
2/3 cup whole-wheat breadcrumbs	1 lemon, zested
1/4 cup chopped fresh basil	

Directions:

Preheat the oven to 450 F and lightly grease a large baking sheet with cooking spray.

In a medium bowl, add the zucchini, yellow squash, red onion, bell pepper, tomatoes, olive oil, salt, black pepper, and garlic. Toss well and spread the mixture on the baking sheet.

Roast in the oven for 25 to 30 minutes or until the vegetables are tender while stirring every 5 minutes.

Meanwhile, heat the olive oil in a medium skillet and sauté the garlic until fragrant. Mix in the breadcrumbs, lemon zest, and basil. Cook for 2 to 3 minutes.

Remove the vegetables from the oven and toss in the breadcrumb's mixture.

Serve warm.

Nutrition:

Calories 258 kcal Fats 14. 5g Carbs 30. 4g Protein 5. 5g

502. Mixed Seed Crackers

Preparation Time: 15-30 minutes | **Cooking Time:** 50 minutes | **Servings:** 4

Ingredients:

1/3 cup coconut flour	1/3 cup sesame seeds
1/3 cup sunflower seeds	1/3 cup chia seeds
1/3 cup pumpkin seeds	1 tsp salt
1/4 cup plant butter, melted	1 cup boiling water

Directions:

Preheat an oven to 300 F and line a baking sheet with parchment paper.

In a medium bowl, mix the coconut flour, sesame seeds, sunflower seeds, chia seeds, pumpkin seeds, and salt.

Add the plant butter, boiling water, and mix until well combined.

Spread the mixture on the baking sheet and bake in the oven for 45 minutes until the crackers are firm.

Remove the crackers and allow cooling for 10 minutes.
Break the crackers into pieces and enjoy!

Nutrition:
Calories 725 Fats 67. 2g Carbs 18. 1g Protein 24. 3g

503. Seitan Bell Pepper Balls

Preparation Time: 15-30 minutes | **Cooking Time:** 25 minutes | **Servings:** 4

Ingredients:

1 tbsp flax seed powder + 3 tbsp water	1 lb seitan, crumbled
¼ cup chopped mixed bell peppers	Salt and black pepper to taste
1 tbsp almond flour	1 tsp garlic powder
1 tsp onion powder	1 tsp tofu mayonnaise
Olive oil for brushing	

Directions:
Preheat the oven to 400 F and line a baking sheet with parchment paper.
In a medium bowl, mix the flax seed powder with water and allow thickening for 5 minutes.
Add the seitan, bell peppers, salt, black pepper, almond flour, garlic powder, onion powder, and tofu mayonnaise. Mix well and form 1-inch balls from the mixture.
Arrange on the baking sheet, brush with cooking spray, and bake in the oven for 15 to 20 minutes or until brown and compacted.
Remove from the oven and serve.

Nutrition:
Calories 492 Fats 41. 3g Carbs 4. 1g Protein 26. 5g

504. Quinoa Stuffed Tomatoes

Preparation Time: 15-30 minutes | **Cooking Time:** 50 minutes | **Servings:** 4

Ingredients:

8 medium-sized tomatoes	¾ cup quinoa, rinsed and drained
1 ½ cups water	1 tbsp olive oil
1 small onion, diced	3 garlic cloves, minced
Salt and black pepper to taste	1 cup chopped spinach

1 (7 oz) can chickpeas, drained and rinsed	½ cup chopped fresh basil

Directions:
Preheat the oven to 400 F.
Cut off the heads of tomatoes and use a paring knife to scoop the inner pulp of the tomatoes. Season with some olive oil, salt, and black pepper.
Add the quinoa and water to a medium pot, season with salt, and cook for 10 to 15 minutes until the quinoa is tender and the water is absorbed. Fluff and set aside.
Heat the remaining olive oil in a medium skillet and sauté the onion and garlic until softened and fragrant, 30 seconds.
Mix in the spinach and cook until wilted, 2 minutes. Stir in the basil, chickpeas, and quinoa; allow warming from 2 minutes.
Spoon the mixture into the tomatoes, place the tomatoes into the baking dish and bake in the oven for 20 minutes or until the tomatoes soften. Remove the tomatoes from the oven and dish the food. Serve warm.

Nutrition:
Calories 296 kcal Fats 7. 5g Carbs 48. 3g Protein 12g

505. Cajun Sweet Potato Chips

Preparation Time: 15-30 minutes | **Cooking Time:** 55 minutes | **Servings:** 4

Ingredients:

2 sweet potatoes, peeled and thinly sliced	Salt to season
2 tbsp melted plant butter	1 tbsp Cajun seasoning

Directions:
Preheat the oven to 400 F and line a baking sheet with parchment paper.
In a medium bowl, add the sweet potatoes, salt, plant butter, and Cajun seasoning. Toss well. Spread the chips on the baking sheet making sure not to overlap and bake in the oven for 50 minutes to 1 hour or until crispy.
Remove the sheet and pour the chips into a large bowl.
Allow cooling and enjoy.

Nutrition:
Calories 65 Fats 5. 9g Carbs 2. 8g Protein 1g

506. Maple Cinnamon Popcorn

Preparation Time: 15-30 minutes | **Cooking Time:** 15 minutes | **Servings:** 4

Ingredients:

½ cup popcorn kernels	¼ tsp cinnamon powder
½ tsp pure maple syrup	1 tsp plant butter, melted
Salt to taste	

Directions:
Pour the popcorn kernels into a large pot and set over medium heat. Cover the lid and allow the kernels to pop completely. Shake the pot a few times to ensure even popping, 10 minutes.
Meanwhile, in a small bowl, mix the cinnamon powder, maple syrup, butter, and salt. When the popcorn is ready, turn the heat off, and toss in the cinnamon mixture until well distributed. Pour the popcorn into serving bowls, allow cooling, and enjoy.

Nutrition:
Calories 15 Fats 1g Carbs 1. 5g Protein 0. 2g

507. Skewers of Mozzarella And Tomato

Preparation Time: 15 minutes | **Cooking Time:** 0 minutes | **Servings:** 8

Ingredients:

1 teaspoon pesto	250 g cherry tomatoes
250 g vegan mozzarella	1 bunch of basil
3 tablespoon olive oil	

Directions:
Wash and prepare the tomatoes.
Pluck the basil leaves, cut the mozzarella into small cubes.
Mix the pesto with the olive oil in a small bowl.
Prepare wooden skewers and place two tomatoes, two basil leaves, and two cubes of mozzarella alternately on the skewers.
Brush with a little pesto to serve.

Nutrition:
Calories: 259 Fat: 15.4g Carbs: 20.5g Protein: 12.1g Fiber: 3.2g

508. Filled Mushrooms

Preparation Time: 55 minutes | **Cooking Time:** 0 minutes | **Servings:** 2

Ingredients:

30 g pine nuts	½ lime
½ bunch of basil	8 large mushrooms
50 ml of water	115 g cashew nuts
2 tablespoon coconut milk	Salt and pepper

Directions:
Soak the cashew nuts in water the evening before.
The drain water and fill the cores together with the basil, the coconut milk, the water, and the lime juice in a food processor.
Process into a creamy puree.
Clean the mushrooms and brush with the filling.
Then bake in the oven at 180 degrees Celsius for about 15 minutes.
In the meantime, toast the pine nuts in a small non-stick pan.
Sprinkle the pine nuts over the mushrooms to serve.

Nutrition:
Calories: 239 Fat: 11.4g Carbs: 10.5g Protein: 11.1g Fiber: 3.2g

509. Pizza Bites

Preparation Time: 95 minutes | **Cooking Time:** 0 minutes | **Servings:** 8

Ingredients:

200 g flour	1 teaspoon salt
180 ml of water	½ cubes of yeast
1 teaspoon of sugar	250 g vegan salami
250 g vegan Gouda	

Directions:
Mix sugar, flour, and salt in a bowl.
Make a well and crumble the yeast into it. Warm the water slightly and gradually pour it into the hollow.
Mix the yeast and let it rise briefly, then work all the Ingredients in the bowl into a smooth dough.

Let rise for 50 minutes, then roll out.

Cut the cheese and salami into thin slices.

Cut rectangles from the dough and cover the lower edge with cheese and salami. Roll up a little, cover again, and close the dough.

Bake at 240 degrees Celsius for 10 to 12 minutes.

Nutrition:
Calories: 289 Fat: 15.4g Carbs: 20.5g Protein: 12.1g Fiber: 3.2g

510. Filled Dough Pieces In Carrot Shape

Preparation Time: 30 minutes | **Cooking Time:** 0 minutes | **Servings:** 8

Ingredients:

400 ml vegetable stock	200 g red lentils
1 tablespoon almond butter	1 pack. Pizza dough
salt and pepper	1 bunch of parsley

Directions:
Do not make funnels out of aluminum paper to hold the pizza dough in the shape of a carrot.

Roll out the dough, cut into strips and wrap around the funnels.

Then bake at 200 degrees Celsius for about 10 minutes until they are golden brown.

In the meantime, bring the broth to a boil and cook the lentils in it.

Season with almond butter, salt, and pepper and let cool slightly.

Fill the funnels with lentils and finally put a bunch of parsley on top.

These bites go perfectly with an Easter brunch.

Nutrition:
Calories: 229 Fat: 9.4g Carbs: 11.5g Protein: 12.1g Fiber: 3.2g

511. Banana Cream Stuffed Strawberries

Preparation Time: 15-30 minutes | **Cooking Time:** 10 minutes | **Servings:** 4

Ingredients:

12 fresh strawberries, heads removed	¼ cup cashew cream
¼ tsp banana extract	1 tbsp unsweetened coconut flakes

Directions:
Use a teaspoon to scoop out some of the strawberries pulp to create a hole within.

In a small bowl, mix the cashew cream, banana extract, and maple syrup.

Spoon the mixture into the strawberries and garnish with the coconut flakes. Serve.

Nutrition:
Calories 47 Fats 3. 38g Carbs 4. 11g Protein 0. 69g

512. Tahini String Beans

Preparation Time: 15-30 minutes | **Cooking Time:** 10 minutes | **Servings:** 4

Ingredients:

1 tbsp sesame oil	1 cup string beans, trimmed
Salt to taste	2 tbsp pure tahini
2 tbsp coarsely chopped mint leaves	¼ tsp red chili flakes for topping

Directions:
Pour the string beans into a medium safe microwave dish, sprinkle with 1 tbsp of water, and steam in the microwave until softened, 1 minute.

Heat the sesame oil in a large skillet and toss in the string beans until well coated in the butter.

Season with salt and mix in the tahini and mint leaves. Cook for 1 to 2 minutes and turn the heat off.

Plate the string beans and serve.

Nutrition:
Calories 79 kcal Fats 4. 3g Carbs 9. 5g Protein 1. 27g

513. Black Beans Burger

Preparation Time: 15 minutes | **Cooking Time:** 5 minutes | **Servings:** 5

Ingredients:

1 cup black beans, cooked	2 tablespoons bread crumbs
1 teaspoon salt	1/4 cup sweet corn, cooked

1 teaspoon turmeric

1 tablespoon fresh parsley, chopped

1/2 yellow sweet pepper, chopped

1/2 cup of water

Directions:

Mash the black beans until you get puree and combine them with salt, sweet corn, turmeric, parsley, and sweet pepper.

Mix it up carefully with the help of a spoon.

Add breadcrumbs and stir again.

Pour water into the instant pot bowl and insert the steamer rack.

Make the burgers from the black bean mixture and freeze them for 30 minutes.

Then wrap every burger in the foil and place it on the steamer rack.

Close the lid and cook on Manual mode (High pressure) for 5 minutes.

Then allow natural pressure release for 5 minutes.

Remove the foil from the burgers and transfer it to the plate. Garnish burgers with lettuce leaves if desired.

Nutrition:

Calories: 155, Fat: 0.9, Fiber: 6.5, Carbs: 28.8, Protein: 9.2

514. Mushroom Burger

Preparation Time: 10 minutes | **Cooking Time:** 14 minutes | **Servings:** 4

Ingredients:

2 cups mushrooms, chopped

1 onion, diced

1/2 cup silken tofu

1/2 teaspoon salt

1/2 teaspoon chili flakes

1 tablespoon dried parsley

1 teaspoon dried dill

3 tablespoon flax meal

1/2 teaspoon olive oil

Directions:

Put mushrooms in the blender and grind.

Then transfer the vegetables to the instant pot together with onion, and olive oil.

Stir gently and close the lid. Cook **Ingredients:** on Sauté mode for 10 minutes.

Meanwhile, mash silken tofu until you get a puree. Mix it up with salt, chili flakes, dried

parsley, and dried dill. Add flax meal and pulse for 10 seconds.

When the mushroom mixture is cooked transfer it to a bowl and combine it with the silken tofu. Stir well.

Make the burgers.

Line the instant pot pan with baking paper and place burgers on it.

Close the lid and meal for 4 minutes on High. Then use quick pressure release.

Chill the burgers to room temperature before serving.

Nutrition:

Calories: 47, Fat: 2.6, Fiber: 2.5, Carbs: 5.4, Protein: 2.6

515. Seitan Burgers

Preparation Time: 10 minutes | **Cooking Time:** 2 minutes | **Servings:** 1

Ingredients:

1 burger bun

1 teaspoon mustard

1 teaspoon soy sauce

1 seitan steak

1 teaspoon onion powder

1 teaspoon olive oil

1 tablespoon apple cider vinegar

Directions:

Make the sauce for seitan steak: mix up together soy sauce, onion powder, olive oil, and apple cider vinegar.

Brush seitan steak with sauce from each side and place in the instant pot.

Close the lid and cook on Manual mode (High pressure) for 2 minutes (quick pressure release).

Meanwhile, cut the burger bun into halves and spread with mustard.

Place seitan steak on the one half of the burger bun and cover with the second one.

Nutrition:

Calories: 303, Fat: 8.8, Fiber: 2.8, Carbs: 24.9, Protein: 26.8

516. Maple Roasted Squash

Preparation Time: 15-30 minutes | **Cooking Time:** 40 minutes | **Servings:** 4

Ingredients:

1 large butternut squash, deseeded and cubed	2 tbsp olive oil
4 garlic cloves, minced	¼ cup pure maple syrup
Salt and black pepper to taste	1 tsp red chili flakes
1 tsp coriander seeds	

Directions:

Preheat the oven to 375 F.

In a medium bowl, toss the squash with the olive oil, garlic, maple syrup, salt, black pepper, red chili flakes, and coriander seeds.

Spread the mixture on a baking sheet and roast in the oven for 25 to 30 minutes or until the potatoes soften and golden brown.

Remove from the oven, plate, and serve warm.

Nutrition:

Calories 126 kcal Fats 7. 1g Carbs 15. 6g Protein 1. 1g

517. Carrot And Red Onion Sauté

Preparation Time: 15-30 minutes | **Cooking Time:** 20 minutes | **Servings:** 4

Ingredients:

2 beets, peeled and cut into wedges	3 small carrots, cut crosswise
2 tbsp plant butter	1 medium red onion, cut into wedges
½ tsp dried oregano	1/8 tsp salt

Directions:

Steam the beets and carrots in a medium safe microwave bowl until softened, 6 minutes. Meanwhile, melt the butter in a large skillet and sauté the onion until softened, 3 minutes. Stir in the carrots, beets, oregano, and salt. Mix well and cook for 5 minutes. Dish the food into serving bowls and serve warm.

Nutrition:

Calories 95 kcal Fats 6g Carbs 10. 2g Protein 1. 4g

518. Avocado Tomato Bruschetta

Preparation Time: 10 minutes | **Cooking Time:** 0 minute | **Servings:** 4

Ingredients:

3 slices of whole-grain bread	6 chopped cherry tomatoes
½ of sliced avocado	½ teaspoon minced garlic
½ teaspoon ground black pepper	2 tablespoons chopped basil
½ teaspoon of sea salt	1 teaspoon balsamic vinegar

Directions:

Place tomatoes in a bowl, and then stir in vinegar until mixed. Top bread slices with avocado slices, then top evenly with tomato mixture, garlic, and basil, and season with salt and black pepper.

Serve straight away

Nutrition:

Calories: 131 Cal
Fat: 7.3 g
Carbs: 15 g
Protein: 2.8 g
Fiber: 3.2 g

519. Thai Snack Mix

Preparation Time: 15 minutes | **Cooking Time:** 90 minutes | **Servings:** 4

Ingredients:

5 cups mixed nuts	1 cup chopped dried pineapple
1 cup pumpkin seed	1 teaspoon garlic powder
1 teaspoon onion powder	2 teaspoons paprika
1 teaspoon of sea salt	1/4 cup coconut sugar
1/2 teaspoon red chili powder	1/2 teaspoon ground black pepper
1 tablespoon red pepper flakes	1/2 tablespoon red curry powder
2 tablespoons soy sauce	2 tablespoons coconut oil

Directions:

Switch on the slow cooker, add all the ingredients in it except for dried pineapple and red pepper flakes, stir until combined, and cook for 90 minutes at a high heat setting, stirring every 30 minutes.

When done, spread the nut mixture on a baking sheet lined with parchment paper and let it cool. Then spread dried pineapple on top, sprinkle with red pepper flakes and serve.

Nutrition:
Calories: 230 Cal Fat: 17.5 g Carbs: 11.5 g Protein: 6.5 g Fiber: 2 g

520. Zucchini Fritters

Preparation Time: 10 minutes | **Cooking Time:** 6 minutes | **Servings:** 12

Ingredients:

1/2 cup quinoa flour	3 1/2 cups shredded zucchini
1/2 cup chopped scallions	1/3 teaspoon ground black pepper
1 teaspoon salt	2 tablespoons coconut oil
2 flax eggs	

Directions:
Squeeze moisture from the zucchini by wrapping it in a cheesecloth and then transfer it to a bowl.

Add remaining ingredients, except for oil, stir until combined, and then shape the mixture into twelve patties.

Take a skillet pan, place it over medium-high heat, add oil and when hot, add patties and cook for 3 minutes per side until brown.

Serve the patties with your favorite vegan sauce.

Nutrition:
Calories: 37 Cal Fat: 1 g Carbs: 4 g Protein: 2 g Fiber: 1 g

521. Zucchini Chips

Preparation Time: 10 minutes | **Cooking Time:** 120 minutes | **Servings:** 4

Ingredients:

1 large zucchini, thinly sliced	1 teaspoon salt
2 tablespoons olive oil	

Directions:
Pat dry zucchini slices and then spread them in an even layer on a baking sheet lined with parchment sheet.

Whisk together salt and oil, brush this mixture over zucchini slices on both sides and then bake for 2 hours or more until brown and crispy.

When done, let the chips cool for 10 minutes and then serve straight away.

Nutrition:
Calories: 54 Cal Fat: 5 g Carbs: 1 g Protein: 0 g

522. Rosemary Beet Chips

Preparation Time: 10 minutes | **Cooking Time:** 20 minutes | **Servings:** 3

Ingredients:

3 large beets, scrubbed, thinly sliced	1/8 teaspoon ground black pepper
¼ teaspoon of sea salt	3 sprigs of rosemary, leaves chopped
4 tablespoons olive oil	

Directions:
Spread beet slices in a single layer between two large baking sheets, brush the slices with oil, then season with spices and rosemary, toss until well coated, and bake for 20 minutes at 375 degrees F until crispy, turning halfway.

When done, let the chips cool for 10 minutes and then serve.

Nutrition:
Calories: 79 Cal Fat: 4.7 g Carbs: 8.6 g Protein: 1.5 g Fiber: 2.5 g

523. Quinoa Broccoli Tots

Preparation Time: 10 minutes | **Cooking Time:** 20 minutes | **Servings:** 16

Ingredients:

2 tablespoons quinoa flour	2 cups steamed and chopped broccoli florets
1/2 cup nutritional yeast	1 teaspoon garlic powder
1 teaspoon miso paste	2 flax eggs
2 tablespoons hummus	

Directions:

Place all the ingredients in a bowl, stir until well combined, and then shape the mixture into sixteen small balls.

Arrange the balls on a baking sheet lined with parchment paper, spray with oil and bake at 400 degrees F for 20 minutes until brown, turning halfway.

When done, let the tots cool for 10 minutes and then serve straight away.

Nutrition:

Calories: 19 Cal Fat: 0 g Carbs: 2 g Protein: 1 g Fiber: 0.5 g

524. Spicy Roasted Chickpeas

Preparation Time: 10 minutes | **Cooking Time:** 20 minutes | **Servings:** 6

Ingredients:

30 ounces cooked chickpeas	½ teaspoon salt
2 teaspoons mustard powder	½ teaspoon cayenne pepper
2 tablespoons olive oil	

Directions:

Place all the ingredients in a bowl and stir until well coated and then spread the chickpeas in an even layer on a baking sheet greased with oil.

Bake the chickpeas for 20 minutes at 400 degrees F until golden brown and crispy and then serve straight away.

Nutrition:

Calories: 187.1 Cal Fat: 7.4 g Carbs: 24.2 g Protein: 7.3 g Fiber: 6.3 g

525. Nacho Kale Chips

Preparation Time: 10 minutes | **Cooking Time:** 14 hours | **Servings:** 10

Ingredients:

2 bunches of curly kale	2 cups cashews, soaked, drained
1/2 cup chopped red bell pepper	1 teaspoon garlic powder
1 teaspoon salt	2 tablespoons red chili powder
1/2 teaspoon smoked paprika	1/2 cup nutritional yeast
1 teaspoon cayenne	3 tablespoons lemon juice
3/4 cup water	

Directions:

Place all the ingredients except for kale in a food processor and pulse for 2 minutes until smooth. Place kale in a large bowl, pour in the blended mixture, mix until coated, and dehydrate for 14 hours at 120 degrees F until crispy.

If a dehydrator is not available, spread kale between two baking sheets and bake for 90 minutes at 225 degrees F until crispy, flipping halfway.

When done, let chips cool for 15 minutes and then serve.

Nutrition:

Calories: 191 Cal Fat: 12 g Carbs: 16 g Protein: 9 g Fiber: 2 g

526. Roasted Brussels Sprouts With Cranberries

Preparation Time: 15-30 minutes | **Cooking Time:** 50 minutes | **Servings:** 4

Ingredients:

1 pound Brussels sprouts, halved	3 tbsp olive oil
Salt and black pepper to taste	1 medium white onion, chopped
½ cup dried cranberries	1 lemon, juiced
1 tbsp chopped fresh basil	

Directions:

Preheat the oven to 425 F.

Spread the Brussels sprouts on a roasting sheet, drizzle with olive oil, and season with salt and black pepper.

Mix the seasoning onto the vegetables and roast in the oven until light brown and tender, 20 to 25 minutes.

Transfer the Brussels sprouts to a large salad bowl and mix in the onion, cranberries, lemon juice, and basil. Serve immediately.

Nutrition:

Calories 144 kcal Fats 10. 4g Carbs 12. 7g Protein 2. 1g

527. Roasted Garlic Asparagus With Dijon Mustard

Preparation Time: 15-30 minutes | **Cooking Time:** 35 minutes | **Servings:** 4

Ingredients:

2 tbsp plant butter

2 garlic cloves, minced

1 tbsp freshly squeezed lemon juice

1 lb asparagus, hard part trimmed

1 tsp Dijon mustard

Directions:

Melt the butter in a large skillet and sauté the asparagus until softened with some crunch, 7 minutes. Mix in the garlic and cook until fragrant, 30 seconds.

Meanwhile, in a small bowl, quickly whisk the mustard, lemon juice and pour the mixture over the asparagus. Cook for 2 minutes and plate the asparagus. Serve warm.

Nutrition:

Calories 77 Fats 6g Carbs 5. 2g Protein 2. 7g

528. Tofu Zucchini Kabobs

Preparation Time: 15-30 minutes | **Cooking Time:** 10 minutes | **Servings:** 4

Ingredients:

1 (14 oz) block extra-firm tofu, pressed and cut into 1-inch cubes

1 tbsp olive oil

1 tsp smoked paprika

1 tsp garlic powder

1 medium zucchini, cut into 2-inch rounds

2 tbsp freshly squeezed lemon juice

1 tsp cumin powder

Directions:

Preheat a grill to medium heat.

Meanwhile, thread the tofu and zucchini alternately on the wooden skewers.

In a small bowl, whisk the olive oil, lemon juice, paprika, cumin powder, and garlic powder. Brush the skewers all around with the mixture and place them on the grill grate.

Cook on both sides until golden brown, 5 minutes. Serve afterward.

Nutrition:

Calories 147 Fats 10. 3g Carbs 5g Protein 11. 9g

529. Chili Toasted Nuts

Preparation Time: 15-30 minutes | **Cooking Time:** 35 minutes | **Servings:** 4

Ingredients:

1 cup mixed nuts

¼ tsp hot sauce

¼ tsp onion powder

1 tbsp plant butter, melted

¼ tsp garlic powder

Directions:

Preheat the oven to 350 F and line a baking sheet with baking paper.

In a medium bowl, mix the nuts, butter, hot sauce, garlic powder, and onion powder. Spread the mixture on the baking sheet and toast in the oven for 10 minutes.

Remove the sheet, allow complete cooling, and serve.

Nutrition:

Calories 267 Fats 28. 3g Carbs 4. 9g Protein 2. 7g

530. Tangy Cabbage Stir-Fry

Preparation Time: 15-30 minutes | **Cooking Time:** 15 minutes | **Servings:** 4

Ingredients:

2 tbsp soy sauce

1 tbsp hot sauce

½ tbsp olive oil

2 carrots, julienned

2 garlic cloves, minced

Salt and black pepper to taste

1 tbsp toasted sesame oil

½ tbsp pure date sugar

1 head green cabbage, shredded

3 green onions, thinly sliced

1 tbsp fresh grated ginger

1 tbsp sesame seeds

Directions:

In a small bowl, mix the soy sauce, sesame oil, hot sauce, and date sugar.

Heat the olive oil in a large skillet and sauté the cabbage, carrots, green onion, garlic, and ginger until softened, 5 minutes.

Mix in the prepared sauce and toss well. Cook for 1 to 2 minutes. Dish the food and garnish with the sesame seeds.

Nutrition:
Calories 126 kcal Fats 8. 2g Carbs 12. 6g Protein
2. 4g

531. Marinated Mushrooms

Preparation Time: 10 minutes | **Cooking Time:**
7 minutes | **Servings:** 6

Ingredients:

12 ounces small button mushrooms	1 teaspoon minced garlic
1/4 teaspoon dried thyme	1/2 teaspoon sea salt
1/2 teaspoon dried basil	1/2 teaspoon red pepper flakes
1/4 teaspoon dried oregano	1/2 teaspoon maple syrup
1/4 cup apple cider vinegar	1/4 cup and 1 teaspoon olive oil
2 tablespoons chopped parsley	

Directions:

Take a skillet pan, place it over medium-high heat, add 1 teaspoon oil and when hot, add mushrooms and cook for 5 minutes until golden brown.

Meanwhile, prepare the marinade and for this, place the remaining ingredients in a bowl and whisk until combined.

When mushrooms have cooked, transfer them into the bowl of marinade and toss until well coated.

Serve straight away

Nutrition:

Calories: 103 Cal Fat: 9 g Carbs: 2 g Protein: 1 g

532. Hummus Quesadillas

Preparation Time: 5 minutes | **Cooking Time:**
15 minutes | **Servings:** 1

Ingredients:

1 tortilla, whole wheat	1/4 cup diced roasted red peppers
1 cup baby spinach	1/3 teaspoon minced garlic
1/4 teaspoon salt	1/4 teaspoon ground black pepper
1/4 teaspoon olive oil Oil as needed	1/4 cup hummus

Directions:

Place a large pan over medium heat, add oil and when hot, add red peppers and garlic, season with salt and black pepper, and cook for 3 minutes until sauté.

Then stir in spinach, cook for 1 minute, remove the pan from heat and transfer the mixture to a bowl.

Prepare quesadilla and for this, spread hummus on one-half of the tortilla, then spread spinach mixture on it, cover the filling with the other half of the tortilla and cook in a pan for 3 minutes per side until browned.

When done, cut the quesadilla into wedges and serve.

Nutrition:

Calories: 187 Cal Fat: 9 g Carbs: 16.3 g Protein: 10.4 g Fiber: 0 g

533. Peanut Butter Blossom Biscuits

Preparation Time: 15-30 minutes | **Cooking Time:** 15 minutes + 1-hour chilling | **Servings:** 4

Ingredients:

1 tbsp flax seed powder + 3 tbsp water	1 cup pure date sugar + more for dusting
½ cup unsalted butter softened	½ cup creamy peanut butter
1 large egg, at room temperature	1 tsp vanilla extract
1 ¾ cup whole-wheat flour	1 tsp baking soda
¼ tsp salt	¼ cup unsweetened chocolate chips

Directions:

In a small bowl, mix the flax seed powder with water and allow thickening for 5 minutes to make the flax egg.

In a medium bowl using an electric mixer, whisk the date sugar, plant butter, and peanut butter until light and fluffy.

Mix in the flax egg and vanilla until well combined. Add the flour, baking soda, salt, and whisk well again.

Fold in the chocolate chips, cover the bowl with a plastic wrap, and refrigerate for 1 hour. After, preheat the oven to 375 F and line a baking sheet with parchment paper.

Use a cookie sheet to scoop mounds of the batter onto the sheet with 1-inch intervals. Bake in the oven for 9 to 10 minutes or until golden brown and slightly cracked on top.

Remove the cookies from the oven, cool for 3 minutes, roll in some date sugar, and serve.

Nutrition:
Calories 839 Fats 52. 5g Carbs 77. 9g Protein 21. 1g

534. Black Bean and Corn Quesadillas

Preparation Time: 15 minutes | **Cooking Time:** 30 minutes | **Servings:** 4

Ingredients:
For the Black Beans and Corn:

1/2 of a medium white onion, peeled, chopped	1/2 cup cooked black beans
1/2 cup cooked corn kernels	1 teaspoon minced garlic
½ of jalapeno, deseeded, diced	1/2 teaspoon salt
1 teaspoon red chili powder	1 teaspoon cumin
1 tablespoon olive oil	

For the Quesadillas:

4 large corn tortillas	4 green onions, chopped
½ cup vegan nacho cheese sauce	½ cup chopped cilantro
1 large tomato, diced	Salsa as needed for dipping

Directions:
Prepare beans and for this, take a frying pan, place it over medium-high heat, add oil, and when hot, add onion, jalapeno, and garlic and cook for 3 minutes.

Then add remaining ingredients, stir until mixed and cook for 2 minutes until hot.

Take a large skillet pan, place over medium heat, place the tortilla in it and cook for 1 minute until toasted, and then flip it.

Spread some of the cheese sauce on one half of the top, spread with bean mixture, top with cilantro, onion, and tomato, and then fold the filling with the other side of the tortilla.

Pat down the tortilla, cook it for 2 minutes, then carefully flip it, continue cooking for 2 minutes until hot, and then slide to a plate.

Cook remaining quesadilla in the same manner, then cut them into wedges and serve.

Nutrition:
Calories: 251 Cal Fat: 9.5 g Carbs: 30.6 g Protein: 15.6 g Fiber: 12.1 g

535. Oven-Dried Grapes

Preparation Time: 5 minutes | **Cooking Time:** 4 hours | **Servings:** 4

Ingredients:
3 large bunches of grapes, seedless
Olive oil as needed for greasing

Directions:
Spread grapes into two greased baking sheets and bake for 4 hours at 225 degrees F until semi-dried.

When done, let the grape cool completely and then serve.

Nutrition:
Calories: 299 Cal Fat: 1 g Carbs: 79 g Protein: 3.1 g Fiber: 3.7 g

536. Stuffed Peppers

Preparation Time: 25 minutes | **Cooking Time:** 30-120 minutes | **Servings:** 5

Ingredients:

5 bell peppers, seeds removed	1 medium-sized onion, peeled and finely chopped
7 oz button mushrooms, sliced	4 garlic cloves, peeled and crushed
4 tbsp of extra-virgin olive oil	1 tsp of salt
¼ tsp of freshly ground black pepper	¼ cup of rice
½ tbsp. of cayenne pepper	

Directions:
Use package instructions to pre-cook the rice, or simply place ¼ cup of rice in 1 cup of water and bring it to a boil. Cook for 10 minutes.

With the cooker's lid off, heat two tablespoons of olive oil and place the onion and crushed garlic in the stainless steel insert. Press "Saute" and stir-fry until translucent and add mushrooms, salt, pepper, and cayenne pepper.

Mix well and continue to cook until the water evaporates. Remove from the heat and combine with rice.

Using a wooden spoon, combine the ingredients, and add the remaining olive oil.

Use the mixture to stuff the pepper and gently transfer them to your instant pot.

Securely lock the lid and press the "Manual" button. Set the timer for 10 minutes and adjust the steam release handle. Cook on high pressure. When done, press the "Cancel" button and release the steam naturally.

Enjoy!

Nutrition:
Calories:680, Total Fat:71.8g, Saturated Fat:20.9g, Total Carbs:10g, Dietary Fiber:7g, Sugar:2g, Protein:3g, Sodium:525mg

537. Quorn Sausage Frittata

Preparation Time: 10 minutes | **Cooking Time:** 33 minutes | **Servings:** 4

Ingredients:

12 whole eggs	1 cup plain unsweetened yogurt
Salt and ground black pepper to taste	1 tbsp butter
1 celery stalk, chopped	12 oz Quorn sausages
¼ cup shredded cheddar cheese	

Directions:
Preheat the oven to 350 F.

In a medium bowl, whisk the eggs, plain yogurt, salt, and black pepper.

Melt the butter in a large (safe oven skillet over medium heat. Sauté the celery until soft, 5 minutes. Transfer the celery into a plate and set aside.

Add the Quorn sausages to the skillet and cook until brown with frequent stirring to break the lumps that form for about 8 minutes.

Flatten the Quorn sausage in the bottom of the skillet using the spoon, scatter the celery on top,

pour the egg mixture all over, and sprinkle with the cheddar cheese.

Put the skillet in the oven and bake until the eggs are set and cheese melts for about 20 minutes. Remove the skillet, slice the frittata, and serve warm with kale salad.

Nutrition:
Calories:293, Total Fat:27.9g, Saturated Fat:2.9g, Total Carbs:11g, Dietary Fiber:4g, Sugar:2g, Protein:5g, Sodium:20mg

Chapter 6: Desserts

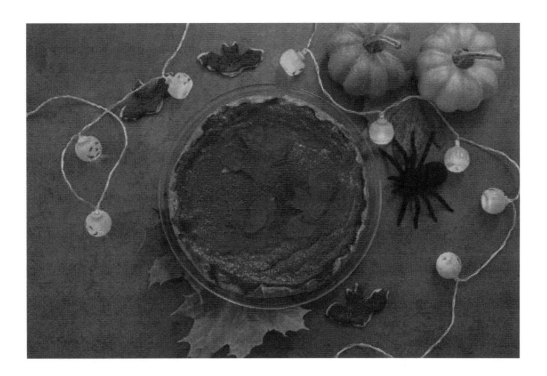

538. Brownie Energy Bites

Preparation Time: 1 hour and 10 minutes | **Cooking Time:** 0 minute | **Servings:** 2

Ingredients:

1/2 cup walnuts	1 cup Medjool dates, chopped
1/2 cup almonds	1/8 teaspoon salt
1/2 cup shredded coconut flakes	1/3 cup and 2 teaspoons cocoa powder, unsweetened

Directions:

Place almonds and walnuts in a food processor and pulse for 3 minutes until the dough starts to come together.

Add remaining ingredients, reserving ¼ cup of coconut, and pulse for 2 minutes until incorporated.

Shape the mixture into balls, roll them in remaining coconut until coated, and refrigerate for 1 hour.

Serve straight away

Nutrition:
Calories: 174.6 Cal Fat: 8.1 g Carbs: 25.5 g Protein: 4.1 g Fiber: 4.4 g

539. Strawberry Coconut Ice Cream

Preparation Time: 5 minutes | **Cooking Time:** 0 minute | **Servings:** 4

Ingredients:

4 cups frozen strawberries	1 vanilla bean, seeded
28 ounces coconut cream	1/2 cup maple syrup

Directions:

Place cream in a food processor and pulse for 1 minute until soft peaks come together.

Then tip the cream in a bowl, add remaining ingredients in the blender and blend until a thick mixture comes together.

Add the mixture into the cream, fold until combined, and then transfer ice cream into a freezer-safe bowl and freeze for 4 hours until firm, whisking every 20 minutes after 1 hour.

Serve straight away.

Nutrition:
Calories: 100 Cal
Fat: 100 g
Carbs: 100 g
Protein: 100 g
Fiber: 100 g

540. Salted Caramel Chocolate Cups

Preparation Time: 5 minutes | **Cooking Time:** 2 minutes | **Servings:** 12

Ingredients:

¼ teaspoon sea salt granules	1 cup dark chocolate chips, unsweetened
2 teaspoons coconut oil	6 tablespoons caramel sauce

Directions:
Take a heatproof bowl, add chocolate chips and oil, stir until mixed, then microwave for 1 minute until melted, stir chocolate and continue heating in the microwave for 30 seconds.

Take twelve mini muffin tins, line them with muffin liners, spoon a little bit of chocolate mixture into the tins, spread the chocolate in the bottom and along the sides, and freeze for 10 minutes until set.

Then fill each cup with ½ tablespoon of caramel sauce, cover with remaining chocolate and freeze for another 2salt0 minutes until set.

When ready to eat, peel off liner from the cup, sprinkle with sauce, and serve.

Nutrition:
Calories: 80 Cal Fat: 5 g Carbs: 10 g Protein: 1 g Fiber: 0.5 g

541. Chocolate Peanut Butter Energy Bites

Preparation Time: 1 hour and 5 minutes | **Cooking Time:** 0 minute | **Servings:** 4

Ingredients:

1/2 cup oats, old-fashioned	1/3 cup cocoa powder, unsweetened
1 cup dates, chopped	1/2 cup shredded coconut flakes, unsweetened

1/2 cup peanut butter

Directions:
Place oats in a food processor along with dates and pulse for 1 minute until the paste starts to come together.

Then add remaining ingredients, and blend until incorporated and a very thick mixture comes together.

Shape the mixture into balls, refrigerate for 1 hour until set and then serve.

Nutrition:
Calories: 88.6 Cal Fat: 5 g Carbs: 10 g Protein: 2.3 g Fiber: 1.6 g

542. Mango Coconut Cheesecake

Preparation Time: 4 hours and 10 minutes | **Cooking Time:** 0 minute | **Servings:** 4

Ingredients:

For the Crust:

1 cup macadamia nuts	1 cup dates, pitted, soaked in hot water for 10 minutes

For the Filling:

2 cups cashews, soaked in warm water for 10 minutes	1/2 cup and 1 tablespoon maple syrup
1/3 cup and 2 tablespoons coconut oil	1/4 cup lemon juice
1/2 cup and 2 tablespoons coconut milk, unsweetened, chilled	

For the Topping:
1 cup fresh mango slices

Directions:
Prepare the crust, and for this, place nuts in a food processor and process until mixture resembles crumbs.

Drain the dates, add them to the food processor and blend for 2 minutes until a thick mixture comes together.

Take a 4-inch cheesecake pan, place date mixture in it, spread and press evenly, and set aside.

Prepare the filling and for this, place all its ingredients in a food processor and blend for 3 minutes until smooth.

Pour the filling into the crust, spread evenly, and then freeze for 4 hours until set.

Top the cake with mango slices and then serve.

Nutrition:
Calories: 200 Cal Fat: 11 g Carbs: 22.5 g Protein: 2 g Fiber: 1 g

543. Rainbow Fruit Salad

Preparation Time: 10 minutes | **Cooking Time:** 0 minute | **Servings:** 4

Ingredients:
For the Fruit Salad:

1 pound strawberries, hulled, sliced	1 cup kiwis, halved, cubed
1 1/4 cups blueberries	1 1/3 cups blackberries
1 cup pineapple chunks	

For the Maple Lime Dressing:

2 teaspoons lime zest	1/4 cup maple syrup
1 tablespoon lime juice	

Directions:
Prepare the salad, and for this, take a bowl, place all its ingredients and toss until mixed.

Prepare the dressing, and for this, take a small bowl, place all its ingredients and whisk well.

Drizzle the dressing over salad, toss until coated, and serve.

Nutrition:
Calories: 88.1 Cal Fat: 0.4 g Carbs: 22.6 g Protein: 1.1 g Fiber: 2.8 g

544. Cookie Dough Bites

Preparation Time: 4 hours and 10 minutes | **Cooking Time:** 0 minute | **Servings:** 18

Ingredients:

15 ounces cooked chickpeas	1/3 cup vegan chocolate chips
1/3 cup and 2 tablespoons peanut butter	8 Medjool dates pitted
1 teaspoon vanilla extract, unsweetened	2 tablespoons maple syrup

1 1/2 tablespoons almond milk, unsweetened

Directions:
Place chickpeas in a food processor along with dates, butter, and vanilla and then process for 2 minutes until smooth.

Add remaining ingredients, except for chocolate chips, and then pulse for 1 minute until blended and dough comes together.

Add chocolate chips, stir until just mixed, then shape the mixture into 18 balls and refrigerate for 4 hours until firm.

Serve straight away

Nutrition:
Calories: 200 Cal Fat: 9 g Carbs: 26 g Protein: 1 g Fiber: 0 g

545. Chocolate & Almond Butter Barks

Preparation Time: 15-30 minutes | **Cooking Time:** 35 minutes | **Servings:** 4

Ingredients:

1/3 cup coconut oil, melted	¼ cup almond butter, melted
2 tbsp unsweetened coconut flakes.	1 tsp pure maple syrup
A pinch of ground rock salt	¼ cup unsweetened cocoa nibs

Directions:
Line a baking tray with baking paper and set aside.

In a medium bowl, mix the coconut oil, almond butter, coconut flakes, maple syrup, and then fold in the rock salt and cocoa nibs.

Pour and spread the mixture on the baking sheet, chill in the refrigerator for 20 minutes or until firm.

Remove the dessert, break it into shards, and enjoy it immediately.

Preserve extras in the refrigerator.

Nutrition:
Calories 279 Fats 28. 1g Carbs 8. 6g Protein 4. 4g

546. Mini Berry Tarts

Preparation Time: 15-30 minutes | **Cooking Time:** 35 minutes + 1-hour chilling | **Servings:** 4

Ingredients:

For the pie crust:

4 tbsp flax seed powder + 12 tbsp water	1/3 cup whole-wheat flour + more for dusting
½ tsp salt	¼ cup plant butter, cold and crumbled
3 tbsp pure malt syrup	1 ½ tsp vanilla extract

For the filling:

6 oz cashew cream	6 tbsp pure date sugar
¾ tsp vanilla extract	1 cup mixed frozen berries

Directions:

Preheat the oven to 350 F and grease a mini pie pan with cooking spray.

In a medium bowl, mix the flax seed powder with water and allow soaking for 5 minutes.

In a large bowl, combine the flour and salt. Add the butter and using an electric hand mixer, whisk until crumbly. Pour in the flax egg, malt syrup, vanilla, and mix until smooth dough forms.

Flatten the dough on a flat surface, cover with plastic wrap, and refrigerate for 1 hour.

After, lightly dust a working surface with some flour, remove the dough onto the surface, and using a rolling pin, flatten the dough into a 1-inch diameter circle,

Use a large cookie cutter, cut out rounds of the dough and fit into the pie pans. Use a knife to trim the edges of the pan. Lay a parchment paper on the dough cups, pour on some baking beans, and bake in the oven until golden brown, 15 to 20 minutes.

Remove the pans from the oven, pour out the baking beans, and allow cooling.

In a medium bowl, mix the cashew cream, date sugar, and vanilla extract.

Divide the mixture into the tart cups and top with berries. Serve immediately.

Nutrition:

Calories 545 Fats 33. 5g Carbs 53. 6g Protein 10. 6g

547. Mixed Nut Chocolate Fudge

Preparation Time: 15-30 minutes | **Cooking Time:** 2 hours 10 minutes | **Servings:** 4

Ingredients:

3 cups unsweetened chocolate chips	¼ cup thick coconut milk
1 ½ tsp vanilla extract	A pinch salt
1 cup chopped mixed nuts	

Directions:

Line a 9-inch square pan with baking paper and set aside.

Melt the chocolate chips, coconut milk, and vanilla in a medium pot over low heat.

Mix in the salt and nuts until well distributed and pour the mixture into the square pan.

Refrigerate for at least 2 hours.

Remove from the fridge, cut into squares, and serve.

Nutrition:

Calories 907 Fats 31. 5g Carbs 152. 1g Protein 7. 7g

548. Date Cake Slices

Preparation Time: 15-30 minutes | **Cooking Time:** 1 hour 20 minutes | **Servings:** 4

Ingredients:

½ cup cold plant butter, cut in pieces, plus extra for greasing	1 tbsp flax seed powder + 3 tbsp water
½ cup whole-wheat flour, plus extra for dusting	¼ cup chopped pecans and walnuts
1 tsp baking powder	1 tsp baking soda
1 tsp cinnamon powder	1 tsp salt
1/3 cup water	1/3 cup pitted dates, chopped
½ cup pure date sugar	1 tsp vanilla extract
¼ cup pure date syrup for drizzling.	

Directions:

Preheat the oven to 350 F and lightly grease a round baking dish with some plant butter.

In a small bowl, mix the flax seed powder with water and allow thickening for 5 minutes to make the flax egg.

In a food processor, add the flour, nuts, baking powder, baking soda, cinnamon powder, and salt. Blend until well combined.

Add the water, dates, date sugar, and vanilla. Process until smooth with tiny pieces of dates evident.

Pour the batter into the baking dish and bake in the oven for 1 hour and 10 minutes or until a toothpick inserted comes out clean. Remove the dish from the oven, invert the cake onto a serving platter to cool, drizzle with the date syrup, slice, and serve.

Nutrition:
Calories 850 Fats 61. 2g Carbs 65. 7g Protein 12. 8g

549. Chocolate Mousse Cake

Preparation Time: 15-30 minutes | **Cooking Time:**40 minutes + 6 hours 30 minutes chilling | **Servings:** 4

Ingredients:

2/3 cup toasted almond flour	¼ cup unsalted plant butter, melted
2 cups unsweetened chocolate bars, broken into pieces	2 ½ cups coconut cream
Fresh raspberries or strawberries for topping	

Directions:
Lightly grease a 9-inch springform pan with some plant butter and set aside.

Mix the almond flour and plant butter in a medium bowl and pour the mixture into the springform pan. Use the spoon to spread and press the mixture into the bottom of the pan. Place in the refrigerator to firm for 30 minutes.

Meanwhile, pour the chocolate into a safe microwave bowl and melt for 1 minute stirring every 30 seconds.

Remove from the microwave and mix in the coconut cream and maple syrup.

Remove the cake pan from the oven, pour the chocolate mixture on top making sure to shake

the pan and even the layer. Chill further for 4 to 6 hours.

Take out the pan from the fridge, release the cake and garnish with the raspberries or strawberries.

Slice and serve.

Nutrition:
Calories 608 Fats 60. 5g Carbs 19. 8g Protein 6. 3g

550. Apple Raspberry Cobbler

Preparation Time: 15-30 minutes | **Cooking Time:**50 minutes | **Servings:** 4

Ingredients:

3 apples, peeled, cored, and chopped	2 tbsp pure date sugar
1 cup fresh raspberries	2 tbsp unsalted plant butter
½ cup whole-wheat flour	1 cup toasted rolled oats
2 tbsp pure date sugar	1 tsp cinnamon powder

Directions:
Preheat the oven to 350 F and grease a baking dish with some plant butter.

Add the apples, date sugar, and 3 tbsp of water to a medium pot. Cook over low heat until the date sugar melts and then, mix in the raspberries. Cook until the fruits soften, 10 minutes.

Pour and spread the fruit mixture into the baking dish and set aside.

In a blender, add the plant butter, flour, oats, date sugar, and cinnamon powder. Pulse a few times until crumbly.

Spoon and spread the mixture on the fruit mix until evenly layered.

Bake in the oven for 25 to 30 minutes or until golden brown on top.

Remove the dessert, allow cooling for 2 minutes, and serve.

Nutrition:
Calories 539 Fats 12g Carbs 105. 7g Protein 8. 2g

551. White Chocolate Pudding

Preparation Time: 15-30 minutes | **Cooking Time:** 4 hours 20 minutes | **Servings:** 4

Ingredients:

3 tbsp flaxseed + 9 tbsp water	3 tbsp cornstarch
¼ tbsp salt	1 cup cashew cream
2 ½ cups almond milk	½ pure date sugar
1 tbsp vanilla caviar	6 oz unsweetened white chocolate chips
Whipped coconut cream for topping	Sliced bananas and raspberries for topping

Directions:

In a small bowl, mix the flax seed powder with water and allow thickening for 5 minutes to make the flax egg.

In a large bowl, whisk the cornstarch and salt, and then slowly mix in the cashew cream until smooth. Whisk in the flax egg until well combined.

Pour the almond milk into a pot and whisk in the date sugar. Cook over medium heat while frequently stirring until the sugar dissolves. Reduce the heat to low and simmer until steamy and bubbly around the edges.

Pour half of the almond milk mixture into the flax egg mix, whisk well and pour this mixture into the remaining milk content in the pot. Whisk continuously until well combined.

Bring the new mixture to a boil over medium heat while still frequently stirring and scraping all the corners of the pot, 2 minutes.

Turn the heat off, stir in the vanilla caviar, then the white chocolate chips until melted. Spoon the mixture into a bowl, allow cooling for 2 minutes, cover with plastic wraps making sure to press the plastic onto the surface of the pudding, and refrigerate for 4 hours.

Remove the pudding from the fridge, take off the plastic wrap, and whip for about a minute. Spoon the dessert into serving cups, swirl some coconut whipping cream on top, and top with the bananas and raspberries. Enjoy immediately.

Nutrition:

Calories 654 Fats 47. 9g Carbs 52. 1g Protein 7. 3g

552. Cardamom Coconut Fat Bombs

Preparation Time: 5minutes | **Cooking Time:** 2minutes | **Servings:** 6

Ingredients:

½ cup unsweetened grated coconut	3 oz. unsalted butter, room temperature
¼ tsp green cardamom powder	½ tsp vanilla extract
¼ tsp cinnamon powder	

Directions:

Pour the grated coconut into a skillet and roast until lightly brown. Set aside to cool.

In a bowl, combine the butter, half of the coconut, cardamom, vanilla, and cinnamon.

Use your hands to form bite-size balls from the mixture and roll each in the remaining coconut. Refrigerate the balls until ready to serve.

Nutrition:

Calories: 687, Total Fat: 54.5g, Saturated Fat: 27.4 g, Total Carbs: 9g, Dietary Fiber: 2g, Sugar: 4g, Protein: 38g, Sodium: 883 mg

553. Berries, Nuts, and Cream Bowl

Preparation Time: 10minutes | **Cooking Time:** 20minutes | **Servings:** 6

Ingredients:

For the dark chocolate cake:

5 tbsp flax seed powder + 2/3 cup water	1 cup dairy-free dark chocolate
1 cup butter	1 pinch salt
1 tsp vanilla extract	

For the topping:

2 cups fresh blueberries	4 tbsp lemon juice
1 tsp vanilla extract	2 cups coconut cream
4 oz. walnuts, chopped	½ cup roasted unsweetened coconut chips

Directions:

Preheat the oven to 320 F; grease a 9-inch springform pan with cooking spray and line with parchment paper.

In a bowl, mix the flax seed powder with water and allow thickening for 5 minutes.

Then, break the chocolate and butter into a bowl and melt in the microwave for 1 to 2 minutes.

Share the flax egg into two bowls; whisk the salt into one portion and then, 1 teaspoon of vanilla into the other.

Pour the chocolate mixture into the vanilla mixture and combine well. Then, fold into the other flax egg mixture.

Pour the batter into the springform pan and bake for 15 to 20 minutes or until a knife inserted into the cake comes out clean.

When ready, slice the cake into squares and share it into serving bowls. Set aside.

Pour the blueberries, lemon juice, and the remaining vanilla into a small bowl. Use a fork to break the blueberries and allow sitting for a few minutes.

Whip the coconut cream with a whisk until a soft peak forms.

To serve, spoon the cream on the cakes, top with the blueberry mixture, and sprinkle with the walnuts and coconut flakes.

Serve immediately.

Nutrition:
Calories: 49, Total Fat: 45g, Saturated Fat: 29.9g, Total Carbs: 12 g, Dietary Fiber: 3g, Sugar: 6g, Protein: 3g, Sodium: 48mg

554. Chocolate Peppermint Mousse

Preparation Time: 10minutes, 30minutes refrigeration | **Cooking Time:** 30-120 minutes | **Servings:** 4

Ingredients:

¼ cup swerve sugar, divided	4 oz. dairy-free cashew cream softened
3 tbsp unsweetened cocoa powder	¾ tsp peppermint extract
¼ cup of warm water	½ tsp vanilla extract
1/3 cup coconut cream	

Directions:
Put 2 tablespoons of swerve sugar, the cashew cream, and cocoa powder in a blender. Add the peppermint extract, warm water, and process until smooth.

In a large bowl, whip the vanilla extract, coconut cream, and the remaining swerve sugar using a whisk. Fetch out 5 to 6 tablespoons for garnishing.

Next, fold in the cocoa mixture until thoroughly combined.

Spoon the mousse into serving cups and chill in the fridge for 30 minutes.

Garnish with the reserved whipped cream and serve immediately.

Nutrition:
Calories: 70, Total Fat7.4: g, Saturated Fat: 4.6g, Total Carbs: 1g, Dietary Fiber: 0g, Sugar: 0 g, Protein: 0g, Sodium: 8 mg

555. Keto Brownies

Preparation Time: 10minutes | **Cooking Time:** 20minutes, 2hour refrigeration | **Servings:** 4

Ingredients:

2 tbsp flax seed powder + 6 tbsp water	1/4 cup unsweetened cocoa powder
1/2 cup almond flour	1/2 tsp baking powder
½ cup erythritol	10 tablespoons butter
	1/2 cup + 2 tbsp
2 oz dairy-free dark chocolate	½ teaspoon vanilla extract optional

Directions:
Preheat the oven to 375 F and line a baking sheet with parchment paper. Set aside.

Mix the flaxseed powder with water in a bowl and allow thickening for 5 minutes.

In a separate bowl, mix the cocoa powder, almond flour, baking powder, and erythritol until no lumps from the erythritol remain.

In another bowl, add the butter and dark chocolate and melt both in the microwave for 30 seconds to 1 minute.

Whisk the flax egg and vanilla into the chocolate mixture, then pour the mixture into the dry ingredients. Combine evenly.

Pour the batter onto the paper-lined baking sheet and bake in the oven for 20 minutes or until a toothpick inserted into the cake comes out clean.

Remove from the oven to cool completely and refrigerate for 30 minutes to 2 hours.

When ready, slice into squares, and serve.

Nutrition:
Calories: 321, Total Fat: 40.3g, Saturated Fat: 18 g, Total Carbs: 19 g, Dietary Fiber: 5g, Sugar: 4 g, Protein: 2 g, Sodium: 265 mg

556. Ambrosia Salad With Pecans

Preparation Time: 15-30 minutes | **Cooking Time:** 15 minutes + 1-hour chilling | **Servings:** 4

Ingredients:

1 cup pure coconut cream	½ tsp vanilla extract
2 medium bananas, peeled and cut into chunks	1 ½ cups unsweetened coconut flakes
4 tbsp toasted pecans, chopped	1 cup pineapple tidbits, drained
1 (11 oz) can mandarin oranges, drained	¾ cup maraschino cherries stems removed

Directions:
In a medium bowl, mix the coconut cream and vanilla extract until well combined.

In a larger bowl, combine the bananas, coconut flakes, pecans, pineapple, oranges, and cherries until evenly distributed.

Pour on the coconut cream mixture and fold well into the salad.

Chill in the refrigerator for 1 hour and serve afterward.

Nutrition:
Calories 648 Fats 36g Carbs 85. 7g Protein 6. 6g

557. Chocolate and Avocado Pudding

Preparation Time: 3 hours and 10 minutes | **Cooking Time:** 0 minute | **Servings:** 1

Ingredients:

1 small avocado, pitted, peeled	1 small banana, mashed
1/3 cup cocoa powder, unsweetened	1 tablespoon cacao nibs, unsweetened
1/4 cup maple syrup	1/3 cup coconut cream

Directions:
Add avocado in a food processor along with cream and then pulse for 2 minutes until smooth.

Add remaining ingredients, blend until mixed, and then tip the pudding in a container.

Cover the container with a plastic wrap; it should touch the pudding and refrigerate for 3 hours.

Serve straight away.

Nutrition:
Calories: 87 Cal Fat: 7 g Carbs: 9 g Protein: 1.5 g Fiber: 3.2 g

558. Chocolate Avocado Ice Cream

Preparation Time: 1 hour and 10 minutes | **Cooking Time:** 0 minute | **Servings:** 2

Ingredients:

4.5 ounces avocado, peeled, pitted	1/2 cup cocoa powder, unsweetened
1 tablespoon vanilla extract, unsweetened	1/2 cup and 2 tablespoons maple syrup
13.5 ounces coconut milk, unsweetened	1/2 cup water

Directions:
Add avocado in a food processor along with milk and then pulse for 2 minutes until smooth.

Add remaining ingredients, blend until mixed, and then tip the pudding in a freezer-proof container.

Place the container in a freezer and chill for freeze for 4 hours until firm, whisking every 20 minutes after 1 hour.

Serve straight away.

Nutrition:
Calories: 80.7 Cal Fat: 7.1 g Carbs: 6 g Protein: 0.6 g Fiber: 2 g

559. Watermelon Mint Popsicles

Preparation Time: 8 hours and 5 minutes | **Cooking Time:** 0 minute | **Servings:** 8

Ingredients:

20 mint leaves, diced	6 cups watermelon chunks

3 tablespoons lime juice

Directions:
Add watermelon in a food processor along with lime juice and then pulse for 15 seconds until smooth.

Pass the watermelon mixture through a strainer placed over a bowl, remove the seeds and then stir mint into the collected watermelon mixture. Take eight Popsicle molds, pour in prepared watermelon mixture, and freeze for 2 hours until slightly firm.

Then insert popsicle sticks and continue freezing for 6 hours until solid.

Serve straight away

Nutrition:
Calories: 90 Cal Fat: 0 g Carbs: 23 g Protein: 0 g Fiber: 0 g

560.   Mango Coconut Chia Pudding

Preparation Time: 2 hours and 5 minutes | **Cooking Time:** 0 minute | **Servings:** 1

Ingredients:
1 medium mango, peeled, cubed	1/4 cup chia seeds
2 tablespoons coconut flakes	1 cup coconut milk, unsweetened
1 1/2 teaspoons maple syrup	

Directions:
Take a bowl, place chia seeds in it, whisk in milk until combined, and then stir in maple syrup.

Cover the bowl with a plastic wrap; it should touch the pudding mixture and refrigerate for 2 hours until the pudding has set.

Then puree mango until smooth, top it evenly over pudding, sprinkle with coconut flakes, and serve.

Nutrition:
Calories: 159 Cal Fat: 9 g Carbs: 17 g Protein: 3 g Fiber: 6 g

561.   Apricot Tarte Tatin

Preparation Time: 15-30 minutes | **Cooking Time:** 30 minutes + 1-hour chilling | **Servings:** 4

Ingredients:
For the pie crust:
4 tbsp flax seed powder + 12 tbsp water	¼ cup almond flour + extra for dusting
3 tbsp whole-wheat flour	½ tsp salt
¼ cup plant butter, cold and crumbled	3 tbsp pure maple syrup
1 ½ tsp vanilla extract	

For the filling:
4 tbsp melted plant butter + more for brushing	3 tsp pure maple syrup
1 tsp vanilla extract	1 lemon, juiced
12 apricots, halved and pitted	½ cup coconut cream
3 to 4 fresh basil leaves to garnish	

Directions:
Preheat the oven to 350 F and grease a large pie pan with cooking spray.

In a medium bowl, mix the flax seed powder with water and allow thickening for 5 minutes.

In a large bowl, combine the flour and salt. Add the plant butter and using an electric hand mixer, whisk until crumbly. Pour in the flax egg, maple syrup, vanilla, and mix until smooth dough forms. Flatten the dough on a flat surface, cover with plastic wrap, and refrigerate for 1 hour.

Lightly dust a working surface with almond flour, remove the dough onto the surface, and using a rolling pin, flatten the dough into a 1-inch diameter circle. Set aside.

In a large bowl, mix the plant butter, maple syrup, vanilla, and lemon juice. Add the apricots to the mixture and coat well.

Arrange the apricots (open side down) in the pie pan and lay the dough on top. Press to fit and cut off the dough hanging on the edges. Brush the top with more plant butter and bake in the oven for 35 to 40 minutes or until golden brown, and puffed up.

Remove the pie pan from the oven, allow cooling for 5 minutes, and run a butter knife around the edges of the pastry. Invert the dessert onto a large plate, spread the coconut cream on top, and garnish with the basil leaves. Slice and serve.

Nutrition:
Calories 484 Fats 33. 8g Carbs 46. 4g Protein 2. 8g

562. Chocolate & Pistachio Popsicles

Preparation Time: 15-30 minutes | **Cooking Time:** 5 minutes + 3 hours chilling | **Servings:** 4

Ingredients:

½ cup unsweetened chocolate chips, melted	1 ½ cups oat milk
1 tbsp unsweetened cocoa powder	3 tbsp pure date syrup
1 tsp vanilla extract	A handful of pistachios, chopped

Directions:
In a blender, add chocolate, oat milk, cocoa powder, date syrup, vanilla, pistachios, and process until smooth. Divide the mixture into popsicle molds and freeze for 3 hours.
Dip the popsicle molds in warm water to loosen the popsicles and pull out the popsicles.

Nutrition:
Calories 315 Fats 17. 8g Carbs 34. 9g Protein 11. 9g

563. Strawberry Cupcakes With Cashew Cheese Frosting

Preparation Time: 15-30 minutes | **Cooking Time:** 35 minutes + 30 minutes chilling | **Servings:** 4

Ingredients:
For the cupcakes:

2 cups whole-wheat flour	¼ cup cornstarch
2 ½ tsp baking powder	1 ½ cups pure date sugar
½ tsp salt	¾ cup unsalted plant butter, room temperature
3 tsp vanilla extract	1 cup strawberries, pureed

1 cup oat milk, room temperature	

For the frosting:

¾ cup cashew cream	2 tbsp coconut oil, melted
3 tbsp pure maple syrup	1 tsp vanilla extract
1 tsp freshly squeezed lemon juice	¼ tsp salt
2-4 tbsp water as needed for blending	

Directions:
Preheat the oven to 350 F and line a 12-holed muffin tray with cupcake liners. Set aside.
In a large bowl, mix the flour, cornstarch, baking powder, date sugar, and salt.
Using an electric mixer, whisk in the plant butter, vanilla extract, strawberries, and oat milk until well combined.
Divide the mixture into the muffin cups two-thirds way up and bake in the oven for 20 to 25 minutes or until golden brown on top and a toothpick inserted comes out clean. Remove the cupcakes and allow cooling while you make the frosting.
In a blender, add the cashew cream, coconut oil, maple syrup, vanilla, lemon juice, and salt. Process until smooth. If the mixture is too thick, add some water to lighten the consistency a little. Pour the frosting into medium and chill for 30 minutes.
Transfer the mixture into a piping bag and swirl mounds of the frosting onto the cupcakes. Serve immediately.

Nutrition:
Calories 853 Fats 42g Carbs 112. 8g Protein 14. 3g

564. Nut Stuffed Sweet Apples

Preparation Time: 15-30 minutes | **Cooking Time:** 35 minutes | **Servings:** 4

Ingredients:

4 gala apples	3 tbsp pure maple syrup
4 tbsp almond flour	6 tbsp pure date sugar
6 tbsp plant butter, cold and cubed	1 cup chopped mixed nuts

Directions:

Preheat the oven to 400 F.

Slice off the top of the apples and use a melon baller or spoon to scoop out the cores of the apples. In a bowl, mix the maple syrup, almond flour, date sugar, butter, and nuts.

Spoon the mixture into the apples and then bake in the oven for 25 minutes or until the nuts are golden brown on top and the apples soft. Remove the apples from the oven, allow cooling, and serve.

Nutrition:

Calories 581 Fats 43. 6g Carbs 52. 1g Protein 3. 6g

565. Classic Pecan Pie

Preparation Time: 15-30 minutes | **Cooking Time:** 50 minutes + 1-hour chilling | **Servings:** 4

Ingredients:

For the pie crust:

4 tbsp flax seed powder + 12 tbsp water	1/3 cup whole-wheat flour + more for dusting
½ tsp salt	¼ cup plant butter, cold and crumbled
3 tbsp pure malt syrup	1 ½ tsp vanilla extract.

For the filling:

3 tbsp flax seed powder + 9 tbsp water	2 cups toasted pecans, coarsely chopped
1 cup light corn syrup	½ cup pure date sugar
1 tbsp pure pomegranate molasses	4 tbsp plant butter, melted
½ tsp salt	2 tsp vanilla extract

Directions:

Preheat the oven to 350 F and grease a large pie pan with cooking spray.

In a medium bowl, mix the flax seed powder with water and allow thickening for 5 minutes. Do this for the filling's flax egg too in a separate bowl.

In a large bowl, combine the flour and salt. Add the plant butter and using an electric hand mixer, whisk until crumbly. Pour in the crust's flax egg, maple syrup, vanilla, and mix until smooth dough forms.

Flatten the dough on a flat surface, cover with plastic wrap, and refrigerate for 1 hour.

Lightly dust a working surface with flour, remove the dough onto the surface, and using a rolling pin, flatten the dough into a 1-inch diameter circle.

Lay the dough on the pie pan and press to fit the shape of the pan. Use a knife to trim the edges of the pan. Lay a parchment paper on the dough, pour on some baking beans, and bake in the oven until golden brown, 15 to 20 minutes. Remove the pan from the oven, pour out the baking beans, and allow cooling.

In a large bowl, mix the filling's flax egg, pecans, corn syrup, date sugar, pomegranate molasses, plant butter, salt, and vanilla. Pour and spread the mixture on the pie crust. Bake further for 20 minutes or until the filling sets. Remove from the oven, decorate with more pecans, slice, and cool. Slice and serve.

Nutrition:

Calories 992 Fats 59. 8g Carbs 117. 6 g Protein 8g

566. Asian Fruit Salad

Preparation Time: 30 minutes | **Cooking Time:** 0 minutes | **Servings:** 8

Ingredients:

Passion fruit, one-half cup (about six of the fruit)	Papaya, one chopped
Pineapple, one cup chunked	Oranges, two separated into segments
Star fruit, three sliced thin	Mangoes, two large, peeled and chunked
Mint, fresh, one-third cup chopped coarsely	Lime juice, one third cup
Lime zest, one tablespoon	Ginger, ground, one tablespoon
Vanilla extract, one tablespoon	Brown sugar, one half cup
Water, four cups	

Directions:

Mix the water and the sugar in a medium-sized saucepan and put it over medium to high heat until the sugar is dissolved.

Let this simmer for five minutes over very low heat, so the sugar does not burn. Add in the vanilla extract and the ginger and stir well.

Let this cook for ten more minutes. Let the mix cool off the heat until it is room temperature, and then add in the mint, juice, and zest.

During the time the sauce is cooling, mix the remainder of the Ingredients in a large-sized bowl.

Pour the syrup mixture over the fruit in the bowl and mix gently to coat all pieces with the sauce.

Put the bowl in the refrigerator until the fruit is cold then serve.

Nutrition:
Calories: 220 Protein: 3g Fat: 1g Carbs: 56g

567. Mimosa Salad

Preparation Time: 10 minutes | **Cooking Time:** 0 minutes | **Servings:** 8

Ingredients:

Mint, fresh, one half cup	Orange juice, one half cup
Pineapple, one cup cut into small pieces	Strawberries, one cup cut into quarters
Blueberries, one cup	Blackberries, one cup
Kiwi, three peeled and sliced	

Directions:
In a large-sized bowl, mix all of the fruits and then top with the orange juice and the fresh mint.

Toss gently together all of the fruit until they are well mixed.

Nutrition:
Calories: 215 Protein: 3g Fat: 1g Carbs: 49g

568. Summer Banana Pudding

Preparation Time: 15-30 minutes | **Cooking Time:** 25 minutes + 1 hour | **Servings:** 4

Ingredients:

1 cup unsweetened almond milk	2 cups cashew cream
¾ cup + 1 tbsp pure date sugar	¼ tsp salt
3 tbsp cornstarch	2 tbsp cold plant butter, cut into 4 pieces
1 tsp vanilla extract	2 medium banana, peeled and sliced

Directions:
In a medium pot, mix the almond milk, cashew cream, date sugar, and salt. Cook over medium heat until slightly thickened, 10 to 15 minutes. Stir in the cornstarch, plant butter, vanilla extract, and banana extract. Cook further for 1 to 2 minutes or until the pudding thickens. Dish the pudding into 4 serving bowls and chill in the refrigerator for at least 1 hour. To serve, top with the bananas and enjoy!

Nutrition:
Calories 466 Fats 29. 9g Carbs 47. 8g Protein 4. 3g

569. Cranberry Truffles

Preparation Time: 15-30 minutes | **Cooking Time:** 15 minutes | **Servings:** 4

Ingredients:

2 cups fresh cranberries	2 tbsp pure date syrup
1 tsp vanilla extract	16 oz cashew cream
4 tbsp plant butter	3 tbsp unsweetened cocoa powder
2 tbsp pure date sugar	

Directions:
Set a silicone egg tray aside.

Puree the cranberries, date syrup, and vanilla in a blender until smooth.

Add the cashew cream and plant butter to a medium pot. Heat over medium heat until the mixture is well combined. Turn the heat off.

Mix in the cranberry mixture and divide the mixture into the muffin holes. Refrigerate for 40 minutes or until firm.

Remove the tray and pop out the truffles.

Meanwhile, mix the cocoa powder and date sugar on a plate. Roll the truffles in the mixture until well dusted and serve.

Nutrition:
Calories 882 Fats 66. 35g Carbs 64. 5g Protein 19. 95g

570. Mango & Lemon Cheesecake

Preparation Time: 15-30 minutes | **Cooking Time:**20 minutes + 3 hours 30 minutes chilling | **Servings:** 4

Ingredients:

2/3 cup toasted rolled oats

¼ cup plant butter, melted

3 tbsp pure date sugar

6 oz cashew cream cheese

¼ cup of coconut milk

1 lemon, zested and juiced

¼ cup just-boiled water

3 tsp agar agar powder

1 large ripe mangoes, peeled and chopped

Directions:

Process the oats, butter, and date sugar in a blender until smooth.

Pour the mixture into a greased 9-inch springform pan and press the mixture onto the bottom of the pan. Refrigerate for 30 minutes until firm while you make the filling.

In a large bowl, using an electric mixer, whisk the cashew cream cheese until smooth. Beat in the coconut milk, lemon zest, and lemon juice.

Mix the boiled water and agar-agar powder until dissolved and whisk this mixture into the creamy mix. Fold in the mangoes.

Remove the cake pan from the fridge and pour in the mango mixture. Shake the pan to ensure a smooth layering on top. Refrigerate further for at least 3 hours.

Remove the cheesecake from the fridge, release the cake pan, slice, and serve.

Nutrition:
Calories 337 Fats 28g Carbs 21. 3g Protein 5. 4g

571. Plum Cashew Cheesecake

Preparation Time: 15-30 minutes | **Cooking Time:**20 minutes + 3 hours 30 minutes chilling | **Servings:** 4

Ingredients:

2/3 cup toasted rolled oats

¼ cup plant butter, melted

3 tbsp pure date sugar

6 oz cashew cream cheese

¼ cup oats milk

¼ cup just-boiled water

3 tsp agar agar powder

4 plums, cored and finely diced

2 tbsp toasted cashew nuts, chopped

Directions:

Process the oats, butter, and date sugar in a blender until smooth.

Pour the mixture into a greased 9-inch springform pan and press the mixture onto the bottom of the pan. Refrigerate for 30 minutes until firm while you make the filling.

In a large bowl, using an electric mixer, whisk the cashew cream cheese until smooth. Beat in the oats milk.

Mix the boiled water and agar-agar powder until dissolved and whisk this mixture into the creamy mix. Fold in the plums.

Remove the cake pan from the fridge and pour in the plum mixture. Shake the pan to ensure a smooth layering on top. Refrigerate further for at least 3 hours.

Take out the cake pan, release the cake, and garnish with the cashew nuts.

Slice and serve.

Nutrition:
Calories 354 Fats 26. 7g Carbs 27. 7g Protein 6. 4g

572. Matcha Cheesecake

Preparation Time: 15-30 minutes | **Cooking Time:**20 minutes + 3 hours 30 minutes chilling | **Servings:** 4

Ingredients:

2/3 cup toasted rolled oats

¼ cup plant butter, melted

3 tbsp pure date sugar

6 oz cashew cream cheese

¼ cup almond milk

1 tbsp matcha powder

¼ cup just-boiled water

3 tsp agar agar powder

2 tbsp toasted hazelnuts, chopped

Directions:

Process the oats, butter, and date sugar in a blender until smooth.

Pour the mixture into a greased 9-inch springform pan and press the mixture onto the bottom of the pan. Refrigerate for 30 minutes until firm while you make the filling.

In a large bowl, using an electric mixer, whisk the cashew cream cheese until smooth. Beat in the almond milk and mix in the matcha powder until smooth.

Mix the boiled water and agar-agar until dissolved and whisk this mixture into the creamy mix. Fold in the hazelnuts until well distributed.

Remove the cake pan from the fridge and pour in the cream mixture. Shake the pan to ensure a smooth layering on top. Refrigerate further for at least 3 hours.

Take out the cake pan, release the cake, slice, and serve.

Nutrition:
Calories 650 Fats 59. 33g Carbs 25. 84g Protein 13. 54g

573. Brown Butter Pumpkin Pie

Preparation Time: 15-30 minutes | **Cooking Time:** 1 hour 10 minutes + 1-hour chilling | **Servings:** 4

Ingredients:
For the pie crust:

4 tbsp flax seed powder + 12 tbsp water	1/3 cup whole-wheat flour
½ tsp salt	¼ cup plant butter, cold and crumbled
3 tbsp pure malt syrup	1 ½ tsp vanilla extract

For the filling:

2 tbsp flax seed powder + 6 tbsp water	4 tbsp plant butter
¼ cup pure maple syrup	¼ cup pure date sugar
1 tsp cinnamon powder	½ tsp ginger powder
1/8 tsp cloves powder	¼ tsp salt
1 (15 oz) can pumpkin purée	1 cup almond milk

Directions:
Preheat the oven to 350 F. In a bowl, mix flax seed powder with water and allow thickening for 5 minutes. Do this for the filling's flax seed too in a separate bowl. In a bowl, combine the and salt. Add in plant butter and whisk until crumbly. Pour in the crust's flax egg, maple syrup, vanilla, and mix until smooth dough forms. Flatten the dough on a flat surface, cover with plastic wrap, and refrigerate for 1 hour.

Lightly dust a working surface with flour, remove the dough onto the surface, and using a rolling pin, flatten the dough into a 1-inch diameter circle. Lay the dough on a greased pie pan and press to fit the shape of the pan. Use a knife to trim the edges of the pan. Lay a parchment paper on the dough, pour on some baking beans and bake for 15-20 minutes. Remove, pour out the baking beans, and allow cooling.

In a bowl, whisk the filling's flaxseed, butter, maple syrup, date sugar, cinnamon powder, ginger powder, cloves powder, salt, pumpkin puree, and almond milk. Pour the mixture onto the pie crust and bake further for 35-40 minutes. Slice and serve afterward.

Nutrition:
Calories 544 Fats 31g Carbs 58. 4g Protein 9. 8g

574. Key Lime Pie

Preparation Time: 3 hours and 15 minutes | **Cooking Time:** 0 minute | **Servings:** 12

Ingredients:
For the Crust:

¾ cup coconut flakes, unsweetened	1 cup dates, soaked in warm water for 10 minutes in water, drained

For the Filling:

¾ cup of coconut meat	1 ½ avocado, peeled, pitted
2 tablespoons key lime juice	¼ cup agave

Directions:
Prepare the crust, and for this, place all its ingredients in a food processor and pulse for 3 to 5 minutes until the thick paste comes together.

Take an 8-inch pie pan, grease it with oil, pour crust mixture in it and spread and press the mixture evenly in the bottom and along the sides, and freeze until required.

Prepare the filling and for this, place all its ingredients in a food processor, and pulse for 2 minutes until smooth.

Pour the filling into the prepared pan, smooth the top, and freeze for 3 hours until set.

Cut pie into slices and then serve.

Nutrition:
Calories: 213 Cal Fat: 10 g Carbs: 29 g Protein: 1200 g Fiber: 6 g

575. Chocolate Mint Grasshopper Pie

Preparation Time: 4 hours and 15 minutes | **Cooking Time:** 0 minute | **Servings:** 4

Ingredients:
For the Crust:

1 cup dates, soaked in warm water for 10 minutes in water, drained	1/8 teaspoons salt
1/2 cup pecans	1 teaspoons cinnamon
1/2 cup walnuts	

For the Filling:

½ cup mint leaves	2 cups of cashews, soaked in warm water for 10 minutes in water, drained
2 tablespoons coconut oil	1/4 cup and 2 tablespoons of agave
1/4 teaspoons spirulina	1/4 cup water

Directions:
Prepare the crust, and for this, place all its ingredients in a food processor and pulse for 3 to 5 minutes until the thick paste comes together.

Take a 6-inch springform pan, grease it with oil, place crust mixture in it and spread and press the mixture evenly in the bottom and along the sides, and freeze until required.

Prepare the filling and for this, place all its ingredients in a food processor, and pulse for 2 minutes until smooth.

Pour the filling into the prepared pan, smooth the top, and freeze for 4 hours until set.

Cut pie into slices and then serve.

Nutrition:
Calories: 223.7 Cal Fat: 7.5 g Carbs: 36 g Protein: 2.5 g Fiber: 1 g

576. Peanut Butter Energy Bars

Preparation Time: 5 hours and 15 minutes | **Cooking Time:** 5 minutes | **Servings:** 16

Ingredients:

1/2 cup cranberries	12 Medjool dates, pitted
1 cup roasted almond	1 tablespoon chia seeds
1 1/2 cups oats	1/8 teaspoon salt
1/4 cup and 1 tablespoon agave nectar	1/2 teaspoon vanilla extract, unsweetened
1/3 cup and 1 tablespoon peanut butter, unsalted	2 tablespoons water

Directions:
Place an almond in a food processor, pulse until chopped, and then transfer into a large bowl.

Add dates into the food processor along with oats, pour in water, and pulse for dates are chopped.

Add dates mixture into the almond mixture, add chia seeds and berries and stir until mixed.

Take a saucepan, place it over medium heat, add remaining butter and remaining ingredients, stir and cook for 5 minutes until mixture reaches a liquid consistency.

Pour the butter mixture over the date mixture, and then stir until well combined.

Take an 8 x 8 inches baking tray, line it with a parchment sheet, add date mixture in it, spread and press it evenly and refrigerate for 5 hours.

Cut it into sixteen bars and serve.

Nutrition:
Calories: 187 Cal Fat: 7.5 g Carbs: 27.2 g Protein: 4.7 g Fiber: 2 g

577. Black Bean Brownie Pops

Preparation Time: 45 minutes | **Cooking Time:** 2 minutes | **Servings:** 12

Ingredients:

3/4 cup chocolate chips	15 ounce cooked black beans
1 tablespoon maple syrup	5 tablespoons cacao powder
1/8 teaspoon sea salt	2 tablespoons sunflower seed butter

Directions:

Place black beans in a food processor, add remaining ingredients, except for chocolate, and pulse for 2 minutes until combined and the dough starts to come together.

Shape the dough into twelve balls, arrange them on a baking sheet lined with parchment paper, then insert a toothpick into each ball and refrigerate for 20 minutes.

Then meat chocolate in the microwave for 2 minutes, and dip brownie pops in it until covered.

Return the pops into the refrigerator for 10 minutes until set and then serve.

Nutrition:
Calories: 130 Cal Fat: 6 g Carbs: 17 g Protein: 4 g Fiber: 1 g

578. Lemon Cashew Tart

Preparation Time: 3 hours and 15 minutes | **Cooking Time:** 0 minute | **Servings:** 12

Ingredients:
For the Crust:

1 cup almonds	4 dates, pitted, soaked in warm water for 10 minutes in water, drained
1/8 teaspoon crystal salt	1 teaspoon vanilla extract, unsweetened

For the Cream:

1 cup cashews, soaked in warm water for 10 minutes in water, drained	1/4 cup water
1/4 cup coconut nectar	1 teaspoon coconut oil
1 teaspoon vanilla extract, unsweetened	1 lemon, Juiced
1/8 teaspoon crystal salt	

For the Topping:
Shredded coconut as needed

Directions:

Prepare the cream and for this, place all its ingredients in a food processor, pulse for 2 minutes until smooth, and then refrigerate for 1 hour.

Then prepare the crust, and for this, place all its ingredients in a food processor and pulse for 3 to 5 minutes until the thick paste comes together.

Take a tart pan, grease it with oil, place crust mixture in it and spread and press the mixture evenly in the bottom and along the sides, and freeze until required.

Pour the filling into the prepared tart, smooth the top, and refrigerate for 2 hours until set.

Cut tart into slices and then serve.

Nutrition:
Calories: 166 Cal Fat: 10 g Carbs: 15 g Protein: 5 g Fiber: 1 g

579. Peppermint Oreos

Preparation Time: 2 hours | **Cooking Time:** 0 minute | **Servings:** 12

Ingredients:
For the Cookies:

1 cup dates	2/3 cup brazil nuts
3 tablespoons carob powder	2/3 cup almonds
1/8 teaspoon sea salt	3 tablespoons water

For the Crème:

2 tablespoons almond butter	1 cup coconut chips
2 tablespoons melted coconut oil	1 cup coconut shreds
3 drops of peppermint oil	1/2 teaspoon vanilla powder

For the Dark Chocolate:

3/4 cup cacao powder	1/2 cup date paste
1/3 cup coconut oil, melted	

Directions:

Prepare the cookies, and for this, place all its ingredients in a food processor and pulse for 3 to 5 minutes until the dough comes together.

Then place the dough between two parchment sheets, roll the dough, then cut out twenty-four cookies of the desired shape and freeze until solid.

Prepare the crème, and for this, place all its ingredients in a food processor and pulse for 2 minutes until smooth.

When cookies have hardened, sandwich crème in between the cookies by placing dollops on top of a cookie and then pressing it with another cookie.

Freeze the cookies for 30 minutes and in the meantime, prepare chocolate and for this, place all its ingredients in a bowl and whisk until combined.

Dip frozen cookie sandwich into chocolate, at least two times, and then freeze for another 30 minutes until chocolate has hardened.

Serve straight away.

Nutrition:
Calories: 470 Cal Fat: 32 g Carbs: 51 g Protein: 7 g Fiber: 12 g

580. Caramel Brownie Slice

Preparation Time: 4 hours | **Cooking Time:** 0 minute | **Servings:** 16

Ingredients:
For the Base:

¼ cup dried figs	1 cup dried dates
½ cup cacao powder	½ cup pecans
½ cup walnuts	

For the Caramel Layer:

¼ teaspoons sea salt	2 cups dried dates, soaked in water for 1 hour
3 Tablespoons coconut oil	5 Tablespoons water

For the Chocolate Topping:

1/3 cup agave nectar	½ cup cacao powder
¼ cup of coconut oil	

Directions:
Prepare the base, and for this, place all its ingredients in a food processor and pulse for 3 to 5 minutes until the thick paste comes together.

Take an 8 x 8 inches baking dish, grease it with oil, place the base mixture in it and spread and press the mixture evenly in the bottom, and freeze until required.

Prepare the caramel layer, and for this, place all its ingredients in a food processor and pulse for 2 minutes until smooth.

Pour the caramel into the prepared baking dish, smooth the top, and freeze for 20 minutes.

Then prepare the topping and for this, place all its ingredients in a food processor, and pulse for 1 minute until combined.

Gently spread the chocolate mixture over the caramel layer and then freeze for 3 hours until set.

Serve straight away.

Nutrition:
Calories: 128 Cal Fat: 12 g Carbs: 16 g Protein: 2 g Fiber: 3 g

581. Snickers Pie

Preparation Time: 4 hours | **Cooking Time:** 0 minute | **Servings:** 16

Ingredients:
For the Crust:

12 Medjool dates, pitted	1 cup dried coconut, unsweetened
5 tablespoons cocoa powder	1/2 teaspoon sea salt
1 teaspoon vanilla extract, unsweetened	1 cup almonds

For the Caramel Layer:

10 Medjool dates, pitted, soaked for 10 minutes in warm water, drained	2 teaspoons vanilla extract, unsweetened
3 teaspoons coconut oil	3 tablespoons almond butter, unsalted

For the Peanut Butter Mousse:

3/4 cup peanut butter	2 tablespoons maple syrup
1/2 teaspoon vanilla extract, unsweetened	1/8 teaspoon sea salt
28 ounces coconut milk, chilled	

Directions:
Prepare the crust, and for this, place all its ingredients in a food processor and pulse for 3 to 5 minutes until the thick paste comes together.

Take a baking pan, line it with parchment paper, place crust mixture in it and spread and press the mixture evenly in the bottom, and freeze until required.

Prepare the caramel layer, and for this, place all its ingredients in a food processor and pulse for 2 minutes until smooth.

Pour the caramel on top of the prepared crust, smooth the top and freeze for 30 minutes until set.

Prepare the mousse and for this, separate coconut milk and its solid, then add solid from coconut milk into a food processor, add remaining ingredients and then pulse for 1 minute until smooth.

Top prepared mousse over caramel layer, and then freeze for 3 hours until set.

Serve straight away.

Nutrition:
Calories: 456 Cal Fat: 33 g Carbs: 37 g Protein: 8.3 g Fiber: 5 g

582. Double Chocolate Orange Cheesecake

Preparation Time: 4 hours | **Cooking Time:** 0 minute | **Servings:** 12

Ingredients:
For the Base:

9 Medjool dates, pitted	1/3 cup Brazil nuts
2 tablespoons maple syrup	1/3 cup walnuts
2 tablespoons water	3 tablespoons cacao powder

For the Chocolate Cheesecake:

1/2 cup cacao powder	1 1/2 cups cashews, soaked for 10 minutes in warm water, drained
1/3 cup liquid coconut oil	1 teaspoon vanilla extract, unsweetened
1/3 cup maple syrup	1/3 cup water

For the Orange Cheesecake:

2 oranges, juiced	1/4 cup maple syrup
1 cup cashews, soaked for 10 minutes in warm water, drained	1 teaspoon vanilla extract, unsweetened
2 tablespoons coconut butter	1/2 cup liquid coconut oil
2 oranges, zested	4 drops of orange essential oil

For the Chocolate Topping:

3 tablespoons cacao powder	3 drops of orange essential oil
2 tablespoons liquid coconut oil	3 tablespoons maple syrup

Directions:
Prepare the base, and for this, place all its ingredients in a food processor and pulse for 3 to 5 minutes until the thick paste comes together.

Take a cake tin, place crust mixture in it and spread and press the mixture evenly in the bottom, and freeze until required.

Prepare the chocolate cheesecake, and for this, place all its ingredients in a food processor and pulse for 2 minutes until smooth.

Pour the chocolate cheesecake mixture on top of the prepared base, smooth the top and freeze for 20 minutes until set.

Then prepare the orange cheesecake and for this, place all its ingredients in a food processor, and pulse for 2 minutes until smooth

Top orange cheesecake mixture over chocolate cheesecake, and then freeze for 3 hours until hardened.

Then prepare the chocolate topping and for this, take a bowl, add all the ingredients in it and stir until well combined.

Spread chocolate topping over the top, freeze the cake for 10 minutes until the topping has hardened, and then slice to serve.

Nutrition:
Calories: 508 Cal Fat: 34.4 g Carbs: 44 g Protein: 8 g Fiber: 3 g

583. Cinnamon Bananas

Preparation Time: 5 minutes | **Cooking Time:** 8 minutes | **Servings:** 2

Ingredients:

2 bananas, peeled, sliced	1 teaspoon cinnamon
2 tablespoons granulated Splenda	1/4 teaspoon nutmeg

Directions:
Prepare the cinnamon mixture and for this, place all the ingredients in a bowl, except for banana, and stir until mixed.

Take a large skillet pan, place it over medium heat, spray with oil, add banana slices and sprinkle with half of the prepared cinnamon mixture.

Cook for 3 minutes, then sprinkle with the remaining prepared cinnamon mixture and

continue cooking for 3 minutes until tender and hot.
Serve straight away.

Nutrition:
Calories: 155 Cal Fat: 2 g Carbs: 39 g Protein: 1 g Fiber: 3 g

584. Salted Almonds

Preparation Time: 5 minutes | **Cooking Time:** 20 minutes | **Servings:** 4

Ingredients:
2 cups almonds   4 tablespoons salt
1 cup boiling water

Directions:
Stir the salt into the boiling water in a pan, then add almonds to it and let them soak for 20 minutes.
Then drain the almonds, spread them in an even layer on a baking sheet lined with baking paper and sprinkle with salt.
Roast the almonds for 20 minutes at 300 degrees F, then cool them for 10 minutes and serve.

Nutrition:
Calories: 170 Cal Fat: 16 g Carbs: 5 g Protein: 6 g Fiber: 3 g

585. Pumpkin Cake Pops

Preparation Time: 10 minutes | **Cooking Time:** 10 minutes | **Servings:** 4

Ingredients:
1 cup coconut flour   ¼ teaspoon cinnamon
1/4 cup coconut sugar   1/4 cup chocolate
                        chips, unsweetened
3/4 cup pumpkin
puree

Directions:
Place all the ingredients in a bowl, except for chocolate chips, stir until incorporated, and then fold in chocolate chips until combined.
Shape the mixture into small balls, then place them on a cookie sheet greased with oil and bake for 10 minutes at 350 degrees F until done.
Let the balls cool completely and then serve.

Nutrition:
Calories: 82.5 Cal Fat: 3.4 g Carbs: 12.3 g Protein: 0.7 g Fiber: 0.05 g

586. Zucchini Cake Slices

Preparation Time: 10munites | **Cooking Time:** 20minutes | **Servings:** 4

Ingredients:
1 cup butter, softened 1 cup erythritol
+ extra for greasing
4 eggs   2/3 cup coconut flour
2 tsp baking powder   2/3 cup ground
                        almonds
1 lemon, zested and   1 cup finely grated
juiced   zucchini
1 cup crème fraiche,   1 tbsp chopped
for serving   walnuts

Directions:
Preheat the oven to 375 F, grease a springform pan with cooking spray, and line with parchment paper.
In a bowl, beat the butter and erythritol until creamy and pale. Add the eggs one after another while whisking. Sift the coconut flour and baking powder into the mixture and stir along with the ground almonds, lemon zest, juice, and zucchini.
Spoon the mixture into the springform pan and bake in the oven for 40 minutes or until risen and a toothpick inserted into the cake comes out clean.
Remove the cake from the oven when ready; allow cooling in the pan for 10 minutes, and transfer to a wire rack.
Spread the crème fraiche on top of the cake and sprinkle with the walnuts. Slice and serve.

Nutrition:
Calories: 262, Total Fat: 27.7g, Saturated Fat: 13.3g, Total Carbs: 4g, Dietary Fiber: 0g, Sugar: 6g, Protein: 2g, Sodium: 215 mg

587. Mixed Berry Pie

Preparation Time: 10minutes | **Cooking Time:** 20minutes, 2hour refrigeration | **Servings:** 4

Ingredients:
For the pie crust:

¼ cup almond flour + extra for dusting

3 tbsp coconut flour

½ tsp salt

¼ cup butter, cold and crumbled

3 tbsp erythritol
4 whole eggs

1 ½ tsp vanilla extract

For the filling:

2 ¼ cup strawberries and blackberries

1 cup erythritol + extra for sprinkling

1 vanilla pod, bean paste extracted

1 egg, beaten

Directions:

Preheat the oven to 350 F and grease a pie pan with cooking spray

In a large bowl, mix the almond flour, coconut flour, and salt.

Add the butter and mix with an electric hand mixer until crumbly. Add the erythritol and vanilla extract until mixed in. Then, pour in the 4 eggs one after another while mixing until formed into a ball.

Flatten the dough on a clean flat surface, cover in plastic wrap, and refrigerate for 1 hour.

After, lightly dust a clean flat surface with almond flour, unwrap the dough, and roll out the dough into a large rectangle, ½ - inch thickness and fit into a pie pan.

Pour some baking beans onto the pastry and bake in the oven until golden. Remove after, pour out the baking beans, and allow cooling.

In a bowl, mix the berries, erythritol, and vanilla bean paste. Spoon the mixture into the pie, level with a spoon, and use the pastry strips to create a lattice top over the berries. Brush with the beaten egg, sprinkle with more erythritol, and bake for 30 minutes or until the fruit is bubbling and the pie golden brown.

Remove from the oven, allow cooling, slice, and serve with whipped cream

Nutrition:

Calories: 238, Total Fat: 26.3g, Saturated Fat: 14.9g, Total Carbs: 1g, Dietary Fiber: 0g, Sugar: 0 g, Protein: 1 g, Sodium: 183 mg

588. Blackberry Lemon Tarte Tatin

Preparation Time: 10minutes | **Cooking Time:** 40minutes | **Servings:** 4

Ingredients:

For the pie crust:

¼ cup almond flour + extra for dusting

3 tbsp coconut flour

½ tsp salt

¼ cup butter, cold and crumbled

3 tbsp erythritol
4 whole eggs

1 ½ tsp vanilla extract

For the filling:

4 tbsp melted butter

3 tsp swerve brown sugar

1 cup fresh blackberries

1 tsp vanilla extract

1 lemon, juiced

1 cup ricotta cheese

3 to 4 fresh basil leaves to garnish

1 egg, lightly beaten

Directions:

For the pie crust:

Preheat the oven to 350 F and grease a pie pan with cooking spray

In a large bowl, mix the almond flour, coconut flour, and salt.

Add the butter and mix with an electric hand mixer until crumbly. Add the erythritol and vanilla extract until mixed in. Then, pour in the 4 eggs one after another while mixing until formed into a ball.

Flatten the dough on a clean flat surface, cover in plastic wrap, and refrigerate for 1 hour.

After, lightly dust a clean flat surface with almond flour, unwrap the dough, and roll out the dough into a 1-inch diameter circle.

For the filling:

In a 10-inch shallow baking pan, mix the butter, swerve brown sugar, blackberries, vanilla extract, and lemon juice. Arrange the blackberries uniformly across the pan.

Lay the pastry over the fruit filling and tuck the sides into the pan. Brush with the beaten egg and bake in the oven for 35 to 40 minutes or until golden and puffed up.

Remove, allow cooling for 5 minutes, and then run a knife around the pan to lose the pastry. Turn the pie over onto a plate, crumble the ricotta cheese on top, and garnish with the basil leaves.

Nutrition:
Calories: 15, Total Fat: 1.3g, Saturated Fat: 0.1g, Total Carbs: 1g, Dietary Fiber: 0g, Sugar: 1 g, Protein: 1g, Sodium: 8 mg

589. Lemon Sponge Cake with Cream

Preparation Time: 10minutes | **Cooking Time:** 30minutes | **Servings:** 4

Ingredients:
For the lemon puree:
4 large lemons   ¼ cup sugar-free
                           maple syrup

¼ tsp salt
For the cake:
½ cup unsalted butter   ½ cup erythritol
softened
1 tsp vanilla extract   ½ cup almond flour
                           sifted
3 large eggs, lightly   ½ cup heavy cream
beaten
1 tbsp Swerve
confectioner's sugar,
for dusting

Directions:
For the lemon puree:
Peel and juice the lemon. Strain or remove any white strains from the peel and transfer both peels and juice to a small saucepan. Add the erythritol and salt and simmer over low heat for 30 minutes.
Pour the mixture into a blender and process until smooth. Pour into a jar and set aside.
For the cake:
Preheat the oven to 350 F, grease two (2 x 8 inch) springform pans with cooking spray and line with parchment paper.
In a large mixing bowl, cream the butter, erythritol, and vanilla extract with an electric whisk until light and fluffy. Pour in the eggs gradually while beating until fully mixed. Carefully fold in the almond flour and share the mixture into the cake pans.
Bake in the oven for 25 to 30 minutes or until springy when touched and a toothpick inserted comes out clean.

Remove and allow cooling in the pans for 5 minutes before turning out onto a wire rack.
In a bowl, whip the double cream until a soft peak forms. Spoon onto the bottom sides of the cake and spread the lemon puree on top. Sandwich both cakes and sift the confectioner's sugar on top.
Slice and serve.

Nutrition:
Calories: 304, Total Fat: 29g, Saturated Fat: 23.5g, Total Carbs: 8g, Dietary Fiber: 3g, Sugar: 1 g, Protein: 8 g, Sodium: 8mg

590. Dark Chocolate Fudge

Preparation Time: 10minutes | **Cooking Time:** 20minutes | **Servings:** 4

Ingredients:
4 large eggs   1 cup swerve sugar
1 cup unsweetened   ½ cup melted butter
dark chocolate, melted
1/3 cup coconut flour

Directions:
Preheat the oven to 350 F and line a rectangular baking tray with parchment paper.
In a large mixing bowl, cream the eggs with swerve sugar until smooth. Add the melted chocolate, butter, and whisk until evenly combined. Carefully fold in the coconut flour to incorporate and pour the mixture into the baking tray.
Bake in the oven for 20 minutes or until a toothpick inserted comes out clean.
Remove from the oven and allow cooling in the tray. After, cut into squares and serve.

Nutrition:
Calories: 412, Total Fat: 43g, Saturated Fat: 37g, Total Carbs: 9g, Dietary Fiber: 3g, Sugar: 0 g, Protein: 5g, Sodium: 12 mg

591. Walnut Chocolate Squares

Preparation Time: 5minutes | **Cooking Time:** 3minutes | **Servings:** 6

Ingredients:
3½ oz. dairy-free dark   4 tbsp butter
chocolate,
unsweetened

1 pinch salt
½ tsp vanilla extract
¼ cup walnut butter
¼ cup chopped walnuts to garnish

Directions:

Pour the chocolate and butter into a safe microwave bowl and melt in the microwave for about 1 to 2 minutes.

Remove the bowl from the microwave and mix in the salt, walnut butter, and vanilla extract.

Grease a small baking sheet with cooking spray and line with parchment paper. Pour in the batter and use a spatula to spread out into a 4 x 6-inch rectangle.

Top with the chopped walnuts and chill in the refrigerator.

Once set, cut into 1 x 1-inch squares.

Serve while firming.

Nutrition:

Calories: 132, Total Fat: 11.5g, Saturated Fat: 4.3g, Total Carbs: 7g, Dietary Fiber: 4g, Sugar: 2 g, Protein: 1g, Sodium: 10 mg

592. Cacao Nut Bites

Preparation Time: 2 minutes | **Cooking Time:** 2 minutes | **Servings:** 4

Ingredients:

3½ oz. dairy-free dark chocolate

2 tbsp roasted unsweetened coconut chips

Sea salt

½ cup mixed nuts (hazelnuts, walnuts, pecans

1 tbsp sunflower seeds

Directions:

Pour the chocolate into a safe microwave bowl and melt in the microwave for 1 to 2 minutes.

Into 10 small cupcake liners (2-inches in diameters), share the chocolate.

Drop in the nuts, coconut chips, sunflower seeds and sprinkle with some salt.

Chill in the refrigerator until firm.

Serve immediately.

Nutrition:

Calories: 130, Total Fat: 12.4g, Saturated Fat: 4.3g, Total Carbs: 6g, Dietary Fiber: 4g, Sugar: 0 g, Protein: 1g, Sodium: 5mg

593. Cinnamon Tofu Pudding

Preparation Time: 17minutes | **Cooking Time:** 30-120 minutes | **Servings:** 6

Ingredients:

1¼ cups coconut cream

1 tsp cinnamon powder

2 oz. fresh strawberries

1 tsp vanilla extract

1 cup tofu cheese

Directions:

Pour the coconut cream into a bowl and whisk until a soft peak forms. Mix in the vanilla and cinnamon.

Lightly fold in the tofu cheese and refrigerate for 10 to 15 minutes to set.

Spoon into serving glasses, top with the strawberries and serve immediately.

Nutrition:

Calories: 114, Total Fat: 11.8g, Saturated Fat: 7.4g, Total Carbs: 1g, Dietary Fiber: 1g, Sugar: 1g, Protein: 1 g, Sodium: 39mg

594. Raspberries Turmeric Panna Cotta

Preparation Time: 3minutes, 2hours refrigeration | **Cooking Time:** 4minutes | **Servings:** 6

Ingredients:

½ tbsp unflavored powdered vegan + ½ tsp water

¼ tsp vanilla extract

1 tbsp erythritol

12 fresh raspberries

2 cups coconut cream

1 pinch turmeric powder

1 tbsp chopped toasted pecans

Directions:

Mix the vegan and water and allow sitting to dissolve.

Pour the coconut cream, vanilla extract, turmeric, and erythritol into a saucepan and bring to a boil over medium heat, then, simmer for 2 minutes. Turn the heat off.

Pour the mixture into 6 glasses, cover with a plastic wrap, and refrigerate for 2 hours or more.

Remove, top with the pecans and raspberries, and serve immediately.

Nutrition:
Calories: 830, Total Fat: 86.9g, Saturated Fat: 44.7g, Total Carbs: 12g, Dietary Fiber: 3g, Sugar: 7g, Protein: 6g, Sodium: 395mg

595. White Chocolate Fudge

Preparation Time: 5minutes | **Cooking Time:** 15 minutes, 4 hours refrigeration | **Servings:** 6

Ingredients:

2 cups coconut cream	1 tsp vanilla extract
3 oz. butter	3 oz. unsweetened white chocolate
Swerve sugar for sprinkling	

Directions:
Pour the coconut cream and vanilla into a saucepan and bring to a boil over medium heat, then simmer until reduced by half, about 15 minutes.
Stir in the butter until the batter is smooth; turn the heat off.
Chop the white chocolate into small bits and stir into the cream until melted.
Pour the mixture into a 7 x 7 baking sheet and chill in the fridge for 3 to 4 hours.
After, cut into squares, sprinkle with a little swerve sugar, and serve.

Nutrition:
Calories: 297, Total Fat: 31.3g, Saturated Fat: 25g, Total Carbs: 5g, Dietary Fiber: 1g, Sugar: 1 g, Protein: 3g, Sodium: 14 mg

596. Mint Chocolate Cheesecake

Preparation Time: 10minutes | **Cooking Time:** 5minutes, 3.5 hours refrigeration | **Servings:** 4

Ingredients:
For the crust:

1 cup of raw almonds	½ cup salted butter, melted
2 tbsp swerve sugar	

For the cake:

4 tbsp unsalted butter, melted	2 vegan sheets
2 tbsp lime juice	2/3 cup unsweetened dark chocolate, chopped + extra for garnishing
1 ½ cups cashew cream	½ cup swerve sugar
1 cup Greek sugar-free coconut yogurt	1 tbsp mint extract

Directions:
For the crust:
Preheat the oven to 350 F.
In a blender, process the almonds until finely ground. Add the butter and sweetener, and mix until combined.
Press the crust mixture into the bottom of the cake pan until firm.
Bake for 5 minutes. Place in the fridge to chill afterward.
For the cake:
In a small pot, combine the vegan with the lime juice, and a tablespoon of water. Allow sitting for 5 minutes and then, place the pot over medium heat to dissolve the vegan. Set aside.
Pour the dark chocolate into a bowl and melt in the microwave for 1 minute, stirring at every 10 seconds interval. Set aside.
In another, beat the cashew cream and swerve sugar using an electric mixer until smooth. Stir in the sugar-free coconut yogurt and vegan until evenly combined. After, fold in the melted dark chocolate and then the mint extract.
Remove the pan from the fridge and pour the cream mixture on top. Tap the side gently to release any trapped air bubbles and transfer to the fridge to chip for 3 hours or more.
When ready, remove and release the pan's locker, garnish the top of the cake with more dark chocolate, and slice.
Serve immediately.

Nutrition:
Calories: 687, Total Fat: 54.4g, Saturated Fat: 27.4g, Total Carbs: 9g, Dietary Fiber: 2g, Sugar: 4 g, Protein: 38 g, Sodium: 883mg

597. Cheesecake with Blueberries

Preparation Time: 4minutes | **Cooking Time:** 1hour, 28minutes, overnight refrigeration | **Servings:** 6

Ingredients:
For the pie crust:
  2 oz. butter
  2 tbsp Swerve sugar
  1¼ cups almond flour
  ½ tsp vanilla extract
For the filling:
  3 tbsp flax seed powder + 9 tbsp water
  2 cups dairy-free cashew cream
  ½ cup coconut cream
  1 tbsp Swerve sugar
  1 tsp lemon zest
  ½ tsp vanilla extract
  2 oz. fresh blueberries

Directions:
Preheat the oven to 350 F and grease a 9-inch springform pan with cooking spray. Line with parchment paper.

To make the crust, melt the butter in a skillet over low heat until nutty in flavor. Turn the heat off and stir in the almond flour, swerve sugar, and vanilla until a dough forms.

Press the mixture into the springform pan and bake in the oven until the crust is lightly golden about 8 minutes.

For the filling, mix the flax seed powder with water and allow sitting for 5 minutes to thicken. In a bowl, evenly combine the cashew cream, coconut cream, swerve sugar, lemon zest, vanilla extract, and flax egg.

Remove the crust from the oven and pour the mixture on top. Use a spatula to layer evenly. Bake the cake for 15 minutes at 400 F.

Then, reduce the heat to 230 F and bake further for 45 to 60 minutes.

Remove to cool completely. Refrigerate overnight and scatter the blueberries on top.

Unlock, lift the pan, and slice the cake into wedges. Serve immediately.

Nutrition:
Calories: 598, Total Fat: 56g, Saturated Fat: 18.8g, Total Carbs: 12g, Dietary Fiber: 3g, Sugar: 5 g, Protein: 15 g, Sodium: 762 mg

598. Lime Ice Cream

Preparation Time: 10minutes | **Cooking Time:** 30-120 minutes | **Servings:** 4

Ingredients:
  2 large avocados, pitted
  Juice and zest of 3 limes
  1/3 cup erythritol
  1¾ cups coconut cream
  ¼ tsp vanilla extract

Directions:
In a blender, combine the avocado pulp, lime juice and zest, erythritol, coconut cream, and vanilla extract. Process until the mixture is smooth.

Pour the mixture into your ice cream maker and freeze based on the manufacturer's instructions. When ready, remove and scoop the ice cream into bowls. Serve immediately.

Nutrition:
Calories: 129, Total Fat: 8.2g, Saturated Fat: 5.2g, Total Carbs: 7g, Dietary Fiber: 1g, Sugar: 4g, Protein: 7 g, Sodium: 52mg

599. Berry Coconut Yogurt Ice Pops

Preparation Time: 2 minutes, 8 hours refrigeration | **Cooking Time:** 30-120 minutes | **Servings:** 6

Ingredients:
  2/3 cup avocado, halved and pitted
  2/3 cup frozen strawberries & blueberries, thawed
  1 cup dairy-free sugar-free coconut yogurt
  ½ cup coconut cream
  1 tsp vanilla extract

Directions:
Pour the avocado pulp, berries, dairy-free sugar-free coconut yogurt, coconut cream, and vanilla extract. Process until smooth.

Pour into ice pop sleeves and freeze for 8 or more hours.

Enjoy the ice pops when ready.

Nutrition:
Calories: 240, Total Fat: 22.5g, Saturated Fat: 13.8g, Total Carbs: 9g, Dietary Fiber: 2g, Sugar: 6g, Protein: 3 g, Sodium: 37mg

600. Fruits Stew

Preparation Time: 10 minutes | **Cooking Time:** 10 minutes | **Servings:** 4

Ingredients:

1 avocado, peeled, pitted, and sliced	1 cup plums, stoned and halved
2 cups of water	2 teaspoons vanilla extract
1 tablespoon lemon juice	2 tablespoons stevia

Directions:
In a pan, combine the avocado with the plums, water, and the other ingredients, bring to a simmer and cook over medium heat for 10 minutes.
Divide the mix into bowls and serve cold.

Nutrition:
Calories 178, Fat 4.4, Fiber 2, Carbs 3, Protein 5

601. Plums and Nuts Bowls

Preparation Time: 5 minutes | **Cooking Time:** 0 minutes | **Servings:** 2

Ingredients:

2 tablespoons stevia	1 cup walnuts, chopped
1 cup plums, pitted and halved	1 teaspoon vanilla extract

Directions:
In a bowl, mix the plums with the walnuts and the other ingredients, toss, divide into 2 bowls and serve cold.

Nutrition:
Calories 400, Fat 23, Fiber 4, Carbs 6, Protein 7

602. Avocado and Strawberries Salad

Preparation Time: 5 minutes | **Cooking Time:** 0 minutes | **Servings:** 4

Ingredients:

2 avocados, pitted, peeled, and cubed	1 cup strawberries, halved
Juice of 1 lime	1 teaspoon almond extract
2 tablespoons almonds, chopped	1 tablespoon stevia

Directions:
In a bowl, combine the avocados with the strawberries, and the other ingredients, toss, and serve.

Nutrition:
Calories 150, Fat 3, Fiber 3, Carbs 5, Protein 6

603. Chocolate Watermelon Cups

Preparation Time: 2 hours | **Cooking Time:** 0 minutes | **Servings:** 4

Ingredients:

2 cups watermelon, peeled and cubed	1 tablespoon stevia
1 cup coconut cream	1 tablespoon cocoa powder
1 tablespoon mint, chopped	

Directions:
In a blender, combine the watermelon with the stevia and the other ingredients, pulse well, divide into cups and keep in the fridge for 2 hours before serving.

Nutrition:
Calories 164, Fat 14.6, Fiber 2.1, Carbs 9.9, Protein 2.1

604. Vanilla Raspberries Mix

Preparation Time: 10 minutes | **Cooking Time:** 10 minutes | **Servings:** 4

Ingredients:

1 cup of water	1 cup raspberries
3 tablespoons stevia	1 teaspoon nutmeg, ground

½ teaspoon vanilla extract

Directions:
In a pan, combine the raspberries with the water and the other ingredients, toss, cook over medium heat for 10 minutes, divide into bowls and serve.

Nutrition:
Calories 20, Fat 0.4, Fiber 2.1, Carbs 4, Protein 0.4

605. Ginger Cream

Preparation Time: 10 minutes | **Cooking Time:** 10 minutes | **Servings:** 4

Ingredients:

2 tablespoons stevia	2 cups coconut cream
1 teaspoon vanilla extract	1 tablespoon cinnamon powder
¼ tablespoon ginger, grated	

Directions:
In a pan, combine the cream with the stevia and other ingredients, stir, cook over medium heat for 10 minutes, divide into bowls and serve cold.

Nutrition:
Calories 280, Fat 28.6, Fiber 2.7, Carbs 7, Protein 2.8

606. Chocolate Ginger Cookies

Preparation Time: 10 minutes | **Cooking Time:** 20 minutes | **Servings:** 6

Ingredients:

2 cups almonds, chopped	2 tablespoons flaxseed mixed with 3 tablespoons water
¼ cup avocado oil	2 tablespoons stevia
¼ cup of cocoa powder	1 teaspoon baking soda

Directions:
In your food processor, combine the almonds with the flaxseed mix and the other ingredients, pulse well, scoop tablespoons out of this mix, arrange them on a lined baking sheet, flatten them a bit and cook at 360 degrees F for 20 minutes.

Serve the cookies cold.

Nutrition:
Calories 252, Fat 41.6, Fiber 6.5, Carbs 11.7, Protein 3

607. Mint Cookies

Preparation Time: 10 minutes | **Cooking Time:** 20 minutes | **Servings:** 6

Ingredients:

2 cups coconut flour	3 tablespoons flaxseed mixed with 4 tablespoons water
½ cup coconut cream	½ cup coconut oil, melted
3 tablespoons stevia	2 teaspoons mint, dried
2 teaspoons baking soda	

Directions:
In a bowl, mix the coconut flour with the flaxseed, coconut cream, and the other ingredients, and whisk well.
Shape balls out of this mix, place them on a lined baking sheet, flatten them, introduce them in the oven at 370 degrees F and bake for 20 minutes.
Serve the cookies cold.

Nutrition:
Calories 190, Fat 7.32, Fiber 2.2, Carbs 4, Protein 3

608. Berry Hazelnut Trifle

Preparation Time: 5minutes | **Cooking Time:** 30-120 minutes | **Servings:** 4

Ingredients:

1 ½ ripe avocado	¾ cup coconut cream
Zest and juice of ½ a lemon	1 tbsp vanilla extract
3 oz. fresh strawberries	2 oz. toasted hazelnuts

Directions:
In a bowl, add the avocado pulp, coconut cream, lemon zest and juice, and half of the vanilla extract. Mix the ingredients with an immersion blender.

Put the strawberries and remaining vanilla in another bowl and use a fork to mash the fruits.

In a tall glass, alternate layering the cream and strawberry mixtures.

Drop a few hazelnuts on each and serve the dessert immediately.

Nutrition:
Calories: 321, Total Fat: 31.4g, Saturated Fat: 19.2g, Total Carbs: 10g, Dietary Fiber: 5g, Sugar: 4 g, Protein: 2g, Sodium: 298mg

609. Avocado Truffles

Preparation Time: 4minutes | **Cooking Time:** 1minutes | **Servings:** 6

Ingredients:

1 ripe avocado, pitted	½ tsp vanilla extract
½ tsp lemon zest	1 pinch salt
5 oz. dairy-free dark chocolate, unsweetened	1 tbsp coconut oil
1 tbsp unsweetened cocoa powder	

Directions:
Scoop the pulp of the avocado into a bowl and mix with the vanilla using an immersion blender. Stir in the lemon zest and a pinch of salt.

Pour the chocolate and coconut oil into a safe microwave bowl and melt in the microwave for 1 minute.

Add to the avocado mixture and stir. Allow cooling to firm up a bit.

Oil your hands with a little oil and form balls out of the mix.

Roll each ball in the cocoa powder and serve immediately.

Nutrition:
Calories: 503, Total Fat: 50g, Saturated Fat: 30.9g, Total Carbs: 13g, Dietary Fiber: 4g, Sugar: 7g, Protein: 4 g, Sodium: 49mg

610. Mint Ice Cream

Preparation Time: 10minutes, refrigeration time | **Cooking Time:** 30-120 minutes | **Servings:** 4

Ingredients:

2 avocados, pitted	1¼ cups coconut cream
½ tsp vanilla extract	2 tbsp erythritol
2 tsp chopped mint leaves	

Directions:
Into a blender, spoon the avocado pulps, pour in the coconut cream, vanilla extract, erythritol, and mint leaves.

Process until smooth.

Pour the mixture into your ice cream maker and freeze according to the manufacturer's instructions.

When ready, remove and scoop the ice cream into bowls. Serve immediately.

Nutrition:
Calories: 373, Total Fat: 39.8 g, Saturated Fat: 24.7g, Total Carbs: 2 g, Dietary Fiber: 0g, Sugar: 2 g, Protein: 2g, Sodium: 147 mg

611. Chia Bars

Preparation Time: 10 minutes | **Cooking Time:** 20 minutes | **Servings:** 6

Ingredients:

1 cup coconut oil, melted	½ teaspoon baking soda
3 tablespoons chia seeds	2 tablespoons stevia
1 cup coconut cream	3 tablespoons flaxseed mixed with 4 tablespoons water

Directions:
In a bowl, combine the coconut oil with the cream, the chia seeds, and the other ingredients, whisk well, pour everything into a square baking dish, introduce in the oven at 370 degrees F and bake for 20 minutes.

Cool down, slice into squares and serve.

Nutrition:
Calories 220, Fat 2, Fiber 0.5, Carbs 2, Protein 4

612. Mint Avocado Bars

Preparation Time: 10 minutes | **Cooking Time:** 25 minutes | **Servings:** 6

Ingredients:

1 teaspoon almond extract	½ cup coconut oil, melted
2 tablespoons stevia	1 avocado, peeled, pitted, and mashed
2 cups coconut flour	1 tablespoon cocoa powder

Directions:

In a bowl, combine the coconut oil with the almond extract, stevia, and the other ingredients and whisk well.

Transfer this to a baking pan, spread evenly, introduce in the oven and cook at 370 degrees F and bake for 25 minutes.

Cool down, cut into bars, and serve.

Nutrition:

Calories 230, Fat 12.2, Fiber 4.2, Carbs 15.4, Protein 5.8

613. Coconut Chocolate Cake

Preparation Time: 10 minutes | **Cooking Time:** 30 minutes | **Servings:** 12

Ingredients:

4 tablespoons flaxseed mixed with 5 tablespoons water	1 cup coconut flesh, unsweetened and shredded
1 teaspoon vanilla extract	2 tablespoons cocoa powder
1 teaspoon baking soda	2 cups almond flour
4 tablespoons stevia	2 tablespoons lime zest
2 cups coconut cream	

Directions:

In a bowl, combine the flax meal with the coconut, the vanilla, and the other ingredients, whisk well and transfer to a cake pan.

Cook the cake at 360 degrees F for 30 minutes, cool down, and serve.

Nutrition:

Calories 268, Fat 23.9, Fiber 5.1, Carbs 9.4, Protein 6.1

614. Mint Chocolate Cream

Preparation Time: 10 minutes | **Cooking Time:** 0 minutes | **Servings:** 6

Ingredients:

1 cup coconut oil, melted	4 tablespoons cocoa powder
1 teaspoon vanilla extract	1 cup mint, chopped
2 cups coconut cream	4 tablespoons stevia

Directions:

In your food processor, combine the coconut oil with the cocoa powder, the cream, and the other ingredients, pulse well, divide into bowls and serve cold.

Nutrition:

Calories 514, Fat 56, Fiber 3.9, Carbs 7.8, Protein 3

615. Cranberries Cake

Preparation Time: 10 minutes | **Cooking Time:** 30 minutes | **Servings:** 6

Ingredients:

2 cups coconut flour	2 tablespoon coconut oil, melted
3 tablespoons stevia	1 tablespoon cocoa powder, unsweetened
2 tablespoons flaxseed mixed with 3 tablespoons water	1 cup cranberries
1 cup coconut cream	¼ teaspoon vanilla extract
½ teaspoon baking powder	

Directions:

In a bowl, combine the coconut flour with the coconut oil, the stevia, and the other ingredients, and whisk well.

Pour this into a cake pan lined with parchment paper, introduce it to the oven and cook at 360 degrees F for 30 minutes.

Cool down, slice, and serve.

Nutrition:

Calories 244, Fat 16.7, Fiber 11.8, Carbs 21.3, Protein 4.4

616. Sweet Zucchini Buns

Preparation Time: 10 minutes | **Cooking Time:** 30 minutes | **Servings:** 8

Ingredients:

1 cup almond flour	1/3 cup coconut flesh, unsweetened and shredded
1 cup zucchinis, grated	2 tablespoons stevia
1 teaspoon baking soda	½ teaspoon cinnamon powder
3 tablespoons flaxseed mixed with 4 tablespoons water	1 cup coconut cream

Directions:

In a bowl, mix the almond flour with the coconut flesh, the zucchinis, and the other ingredients, stir well until you obtain a dough, shape 8 buns, and arrange them on a baking sheet lined with parchment paper.
Introduce it in the oven at 350 degrees and bake for 30 minutes.
Serve these sweet buns warm.

Nutrition:

Calories 169, Fat 15.3, Fiber 3.9, Carbs 6.4, Protein 3.2

617. Lime Custard

Preparation Time: 10 minutes | **Cooking Time:** 20 minutes | **Servings:** 6

Ingredients:

1-pint almond milk	4 tablespoons lime zest, grated
3 tablespoons lime juice	3 tablespoons flaxseed mixed with 4 tablespoons water
tablespoons stevia	2 teaspoons vanilla extract

Directions:

In a bowl, combine the almond milk with the lime zest, lime juice, and the other ingredients, whisk well and divide into 4 ramekins.
Bake in the oven at 360 degrees F for 30 minutes.
Cool the custard down and serve.

Nutrition:

Calories 234, Fat 21.6, Fiber 4.3, Carbs 9, Protein 3.5

618. Chocolate Fudge

Preparation Time: 10 minutes | **Cooking Time:** 0 minute | **Servings:** 12

Ingredients:

4 oz unsweetened dark chocolate	3/4 cup coconut butter
15 drops liquid stevia	1 tsp vanilla extract

Directions:

Melt coconut butter and dark chocolate.
Add ingredients to the large bowl and combine well.
Pour mixture into a silicone loaf pan and place in the refrigerator until set.
Cut into pieces and serve.

Nutrition:

Calories: 283 Total Carbohydrate: 10 g Cholesterol: 3 mg Total Fat: 8 g Fiber: 2 g Protein: 9 g Sodium: 271 mg

619. Chocó Chia Pudding

Preparation Time: 10 minutes | **Cooking Time:** 0 minutes | **Servings:** 6

Ingredients:

2 1/2 cups coconut milk	2 scoops stevia extract powder
6 tbsp cocoa powder	1/2 cup chia seeds
1/2 tsp vanilla extract	1/8 cup xylitol
1/8 tsp salt	

Directions:

Add all ingredients into the blender and blend until smooth.
Pour mixture into the glass container and place in the refrigerator.
Serve chilled and enjoy.

Nutrition: Calories: 178 Total Carbohydrate: 3 g Cholesterol: 3 mg Total Fat: 17 g Fiber: g Protein: 9 g Sodium: 297 mg

620. Raspberry Chia Pudding

Preparation Time: 3 hours 10 minutes | **Cooking Time:** 0 minute | **Servings:** 2

Ingredients:
- 4 tbsp chia seeds
- 1/2 cup raspberries
- 1 cup of coconut milk

Directions:
Add raspberry and coconut milk in a blender and blend until smooth.
Pour mixture into the Mason jar.
Add chia seeds in a jar and stir well.
Close the jar tightly with the lid and shake well.
Place in the refrigerator for 3 hours.
Serve chilled and enjoy.

Nutrition:
Calories: 189 Total Carbohydrate: 6 g Cholesterol: 3 mg Total Fat: 7 g Fiber: 4 g Protein: 12 g Sodium: 293 mg

621. Lemon Mousse

Preparation Time: 10 minutes | **Cooking Time:** 0 minute | **Servings:** 2

Ingredients:
- 14 oz coconut milk
- 1/2 tsp lemon extract
- 12 drops liquid stevia
- 1/4 tsp turmeric

Directions:
Place coconut milk in the refrigerator overnight.
Scoop out thick cream into a mixing bowl.
Add remaining ingredients to the bowl and whip using a hand mixer until smooth.
Transfer mousse mixture to a zip-lock bag and pipe into small serving glasses. Place in the refrigerator.
Serve chilled and enjoy.

Nutrition:
Calories: 189 Total Carbohydrate: 2 g Cholesterol: 13 mg Total Fat: 7 g Fiber: 2 g Protein: 15 g Sodium: 321 mg

622. Almond Butter Brownies

Preparation Time: 10 minutes | **Cooking Time:** 20 minutes | **Servings:** 4

Ingredients:
- 1 scoop protein powder
- 1/2 cup almond butter, melted
- 2 tbsp cocoa powder
- 1 cup bananas, overripe

Directions:
Preheat the oven to 350 F/ 176 C.
Spray brownie tray with cooking spray.
Add all ingredients into the blender and blend until smooth.
Pour batter into the prepared dish and bake in a preheated oven for 20 minutes.
Serve and enjoy.

Nutrition:
Calories: 214 Total Carbohydrate: 2 g Cholesterol: 73 mg Total Fat: 7 g Fiber: 2g Protein: 19 g Sodium: 308 g

623. Coconut Peanut Butter Fudge

Preparation Time: 1 hour 15 minutes | **Cooking Time:** 0 minute | **Servings:** 20

Ingredients:
- 12 oz smooth peanut butter
- 4 tbsp coconut cream
- Pinch of salt
- 3 tbsp coconut oil
- 15 drops liquid stevia

Directions:
Line a baking tray with parchment paper.
Melt coconut oil in a saucepan over low heat.
Add peanut butter, coconut cream, stevia, and salt in a saucepan. Stir well.
Pour fudge mixture into the prepared baking tray and place in the refrigerator for 1 hour.
Cut into pieces and serve.

Nutrition:
Calories: 189 Total Carbohydrate: 2 g Cholesterol: 13 mg Total Fat: 7 g Fiber: 2 g Protein: 10 g Sodium: 301 mg

624. Simple Almond Butter Fudge

Preparation Time: 15 minutes | **Cooking Time:** 0 minutes | **Servings:** 8

Ingredients:
  1/2 cup almond butter 15 drops liquid stevia
  2 1/2 tbsp coconut oil

Directions:
Combine almond butter and coconut oil in a saucepan. Gently warm until melted.
Add stevia and stir well.
Pour mixture into the candy container and place in the refrigerator until set.
Serve and enjoy.

Nutrition:
Calories: 198 Total Carbohydrate: 5 g
Cholesterol: 12 mg Total Fat: 10 g Fiber: 2 g
Protein: 6 g Sodium: 257 mg

625. Quick Chocó Brownie

Preparation Time: 10 minutes | **Cooking Time:** 2 minutes | **Servings:** 1

Ingredients:
  1/4 cup almond milk   1 tbsp cocoa powder
  1 scoop chocolate   1/2 tsp baking powder
  protein powder

Directions:
In a microwave-safe mug blend together baking powder, protein powder, and cocoa.
Add almond milk to the mug and stir well.
Place the mug in the microwave and microwave for 30 seconds.
Serve and enjoy.

Nutrition:
Calories: 231   Total Carbohydrate: 2 g
Cholesterol: 13 mg Total Fat: 15 g Fiber: 2 g
Protein: 8 g Sodium: 298 mg

626. Avocado Pudding

Preparation Time: 10 minutes | **Cooking Time:** 0 minute | **Servings:** 8

Ingredients:
  2 ripe avocados,   1 tbsp fresh lime juice
  peeled, pitted, and cut
  into pieces

  14 oz can coconut   80 drops of liquid
  milk   stevia
  2 tsp vanilla extract

Directions:
Add all ingredients into the blender and blend until smooth.
Serve and enjoy.

Nutrition:
Calories: 209   Total Carbohydrate: 6 g
Cholesterol: 13 mg Total Fat: 7 g Fiber: 2 g
Protein: 17 g Sodium: 193 mg

627. Walnut & Chocolate Bars

Preparation Time: 15-30 minutes | **Cooking Time:** 60 minutes | **Servings:** 4

Ingredients:
  1 cup walnuts   3 tbsp sunflower seeds
  2 tbsp unsweetened   1 tbsp unsweetened
  chocolate chips   cocoa powder
  1 ½ tsp vanilla extract ¼ tsp cinnamon
                         powder
  2 tbsp melted coconut 2 tbsp toasted almond
  oil   meal
  2 tsp pure maple
  syrup

Directions:
In a food processor, add the walnuts, sunflower seeds, chocolate chips, cocoa powder, vanilla extract, cinnamon powder, coconut oil, almond meal, maple syrup, and blitz a few times until coarsely combined.
Line a flat baking sheet with plastic wrap, pour the mixture onto the sheet and place another plastic wrap on top. Use a rolling pin to flatten the mixture and then remove the top plastic wrap.
Freeze the snack until firm, 1 hour.
Remove from the freezer, cut into 1 ½-inch bars and enjoy immediately.

Nutrition:
Calories 302 Fats 23. 9g Carbs 20. 2g Protein 5. 2g

628. Nectarine Chia Pudding

Preparation Time: 5-15 minutes | **Cooking Time:** 5 minutes + 4 hour refrigeration | **Servings:** 4

Ingredients:

1 cup of coconut milk
3 tbsp chia seeds
2/3 cup chopped sweet nectarine
½ tsp vanilla extract
½ cup granola

Directions:

In a medium bowl, mix the coconut milk, vanilla, and chia seeds until well combined.

Divide the mixture between 4 breakfast cups and refrigerate for at least 4 hours to allow the mixture to gel.

After, top with the granola and nectarine. Enjoy immediately.

Nutrition:

Calories 72 Fats 3. 4g Carbs 7. 8g Protein 2. 6g

Chapter 7: Drinks

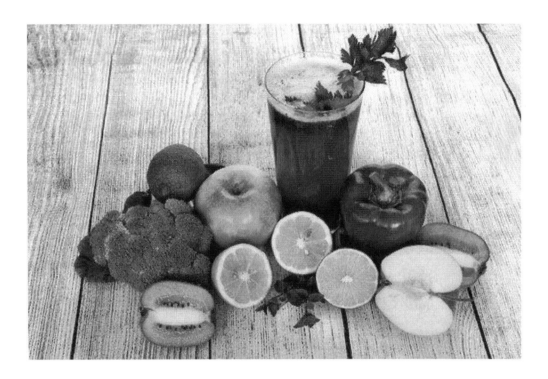

629. Energizing Cinnamon Detox Tonic

Preparation Time: 15-30 minutes | **Cooking Time:** 15 minutes | **Servings:** 2

Ingredients:

4 sticks of cinnamon 2 inches each	1 small lemon slice
1/8 teaspoon of cayenne pepper	1/8 teaspoon of ground turmeric
1 teaspoon of maple syrup	1 teaspoon of apple cider vinegar
2 cups of boiling water	

Directions:
Pour the boiling water into a small saucepan, add and stir the cinnamon sticks, then let it rest for 8 to 10 minutes, before covering the pan.
Pass the mixture through a strainer and into the liquid, add the cayenne pepper, turmeric, cinnamon and stir properly.
Add the maple syrup, vinegar, and lemon slice.
Add and stir an infused lemon and serve immediately.

Nutrition:
Calories:80 Cal, Carbohydrates:0g, Protein:0g, Fats:0g, Fiber:0g.

Cinnamon Cherry Cider | **Servings:** 16
Preparation Time: 15-30 minutes | **Cooking Time:** 4 hours and 5 minutes

Ingredients:

2 cinnamon sticks, each about 3 inches long	6-ounce of cherry gelatin
4 quarts of apple cider	

Directions:
Using a 6-quarts slow cooker, pour the apple cider and add the cinnamon stick.
Stir, then cover the slow cooker with its lid. Plug the cooker and let it cook for 3 hours at the high heat setting or until it is heated thoroughly.
Then add and stir the gelatin properly, then continue cooking for another hour.
When done, remove the cinnamon sticks and serve the drink hot or cold.

Nutrition:
Calories:100 Cal, Carbohydrates:0g, Protein:0g, Fats:0g, Fiber:0g.

630. Warm Pomegranate Punch

Preparation Time: 15-30 minutes | **Cooking Time:** 2 hours and 15 minutes | **Servings:** 10

Ingredients:
3 cinnamon sticks, each about 3 inches long
12 whole cloves
1/2 cup of coconut sugar
1/3 cup of lemon juice
32 fluid ounce of pomegranate juice
32 fluid ounce of apple juice, unsweetened
16 fluid ounce of brewed tea

Directions:
Using a 4-quart slow cooker, pour the lemon juice, pomegranate, juice apple juice, tea, and then sugar.

Wrap the whole cloves and cinnamon stick in a cheesecloth, tie its corners with a string, and immerse it in the liquid present in the slow cooker.

Then cover it with the lid, plug in the slow cooker and let it cook at the low heat setting for 3 hours or until it is heated thoroughly.

When done, discard the cheesecloth bag and serve it hot or cold.

Nutrition:
Calories:253 Cal, Carbohydrates:58g, Protein:7g, Fats:2g, Fiber:3g.

631. Rich Truffle Hot Chocolate

Preparation Time: 15-30 minutes | **Cooking Time:** 1 hour and 10 minutes | **Servings:** 4

Ingredients:

1/3 cup of cocoa powder, unsweetened	1/3 cup of coconut sugar
1/8 teaspoon of salt	1/8 teaspoon of ground cinnamon
1 teaspoon of vanilla extract, unsweetened	32 fluid ounce of coconut milk

Directions:
Using a 2 quarts slow cooker, add all the ingredients, and stir properly.

Cover it with the lid, then plug in the slow cooker and cook it for 2 hours on the high heat setting or until it is heated thoroughly.

When done, serve right away.

Nutrition:
Calories:67 Cal, Carbohydrates:13g, Protein:2g, Fats:2g, Fiber:2. 3g.

632. Warm Spiced Lemon Drink

Preparation Time: 15-30 minutes | **Cooking Time:** 2 hours and 10 minutes | **Servings:** 12

Ingredients:

1 cinnamon stick, about 3 inches long	1/2 teaspoon of whole cloves
2 cups of coconut sugar	4 fluid of ounce pineapple juice
1/2 cup and 2 tablespoons of lemon juice	12 fluid ounce of orange juice
2 1/2 quarts of water	

Directions:
Pour water into a 6-quarts slow cooker and stir the sugar and lemon juice properly.

Wrap the cinnamon, the whole cloves in cheesecloth, and tie its corners with string.

Immerse this cheesecloth bag in the liquid present in the slow cooker and cover it with the lid.

Then plug in the slow cooker and let it cook on a high heat setting for 2 hours or until it is heated thoroughly.

When done, discard the cheesecloth bag and serve the drink hot or cold.

Nutrition:
Calories:15 Cal, Carbohydrates:3. 2g, Protein:0. 1g, Fats:0g, Fiber:0g.

633. Ultimate Mulled Wine

Preparation Time: 15-30 minutes | **Cooking Time:** 35 minutes | **Servings:** 6

Ingredients:

1 cup of cranberries, fresh	2 oranges, juiced
1 tablespoon of whole cloves	2 cinnamon sticks, each about 3 inches long
1 tablespoon of star anise	1/3 cup of honey
8 fluid ounce of apple cider	8 fluid ounce of cranberry juice

24 fluid ounce of red wine

Directions:

Using a 4 quarts slow cooker, add all the ingredients, and stir properly.

Cover it with the lid, then plug in the slow cooker and cook it for 30 minutes on the high heat setting or until it gets warm thoroughly.

When done, strain the wine and serve right away.

Nutrition:

Calories:202 Cal, Carbohydrates:25g, Protein:0g, Fats:0g, Fiber:0g.

634. Pleasant Lemonade

Preparation Time: 15-30 minutes | **Cooking Time:** 3 hours and 15 minutes | **Servings:** 10 servings

Ingredients:

Cinnamon sticks for serving	2 cups of coconut sugar
1/4 cup of honey	3 cups of lemon juice. fresh
32 fluid ounce of water	

Directions:

Using a 4-quarts slow cooker, place all the ingredients except for the cinnamon sticks and stir properly.

Cover it with the lid, then plug in the slow cooker and cook it for 3 hours on the low heat setting or until it is heated thoroughly.

When done, stir properly and serve with the cinnamon sticks.

Nutrition:

Calories:146 Cal, Carbohydrates:34g, Protein:0g, Fats:0g, Fiber:0g.

635. Pumpkin Spice Frappuccino

Preparation Time: 5 minutes | **Cooking Time:** 0 minute | **Servings:** 2

Ingredients:

½ teaspoon ground ginger	1/8 teaspoon allspice
½ teaspoon ground cinnamon	2 tablespoons coconut sugar
1/8 teaspoon nutmeg	¼ teaspoon ground cloves
1 teaspoon vanilla extract, unsweetened	2 teaspoons instant coffee
2 cups almond milk, unsweetened	1 cup of ice cubes

Directions:

Place all the ingredients in the order in a food processor or blender and then pulse for 2 to 3 minutes at high speed until smooth.

Pour the Frappuccino into two glasses and then serve.

Nutrition:

Calories: 490 Fat: 9g Protein: 12g Sugar: 11g

636. Cookie Dough Milkshake

Preparation Time: 5 minutes | **Cooking Time:** 0 minute | **Servings:** 2

Ingredients:

2 tablespoons cookie dough	5 dates, pitted
2 teaspoons chocolate chips	1/2 teaspoon vanilla extract, unsweetened
1/2 cup almond milk, unsweetened	1 ½ cup almond milk ice cubes

Directions:

Place all the ingredients in the order in a food processor or blender and then pulse for 2 to 3 minutes at high speed until smooth.

Pour the milkshake into two glasses and then serve with some cookie dough balls.

Nutrition:

Calories: 240 Fat: 13g Protein: 21g Sugar: 9g

637. Strawberry and Hemp Smoothie

Preparation Time: 5 minutes | **Cooking Time:** 0 minute | **Servings:** 2

Ingredients:

3 cups fresh strawberries	2 tablespoons hemp seeds
1/2 teaspoon vanilla extract, unsweetened	1/8 teaspoon sea salt
2 tablespoons maple syrup	1 cup vegan yogurt

1 cup almond milk, unsweetened
2 tablespoons hemp protein

1 cup of ice cubes

Directions:
Place all the ingredients in the order in a food processor or blender, except for protein powder, and then pulse for 2 to 3 minutes at high speed until smooth.
Pour the smoothie into two glasses and then serve.

Nutrition:
Calories: 510 Fat: 18g Protein: 26g Sugar: 12g

638. Blueberry, Hazelnut, and Hemp Smoothie

Preparation Time: 5 minutes | **Cooking Time:** 0 minute | **Servings:** 2

Ingredients:

2 tablespoons hemp seeds	1 ½ cups frozen blueberries
2 tablespoons chocolate protein powder	1/2 teaspoon vanilla extract, unsweetened
2 tablespoons chocolate hazelnut butter	1 small frozen banana
3/4 cup almond milk	

Directions:
Place all the ingredients in the order in a food processor or blender and then pulse for 2 to 3 minutes at high speed until smooth.
Pour the smoothie into two glasses and then serve.

Nutrition:
Calories: 195 Fat: 14g Protein: 36g Sugar: 10g

639. Mango Lassi

Preparation Time: 5 minutes | **Cooking Time:** 0 minute | **Servings:** 2

Ingredients:

1 ¼ cup mango pulp	1 tablespoon coconut sugar
1/8 teaspoon salt	1/2 teaspoon lemon juice

1/4 cup almond milk, unsweetened
1 cup cashew yogurt

1/4 cup chilled water

Directions:
Place all the ingredients in the order in a food processor or blender and then pulse for 2 to 3 minutes at high speed until smooth.
Pour the lassi into two glasses and then serve.

Nutrition:
Calories: 420 Fat: 12g Protein: 23g Sugar: 13g

640. Mocha Chocolate Shake

Preparation Time: 5 minutes | **Cooking Time:** 0 minute | **Servings:** 2

Ingredients:

1/4 cup hemp seeds	2 teaspoons cocoa powder, unsweetened
1/2 cup dates, pitted	1 tablespoon instant coffee powder
2 tablespoons flax seeds	2 1/2 cups almond milk, unsweetened
1/2 cup crushed ice	

Directions:
Place all the ingredients in the order in a food processor or blender and then pulse for 2 to 3 minutes at high speed until smooth.
Pour the smoothie into two glasses and then serve.

Nutrition:
Calories: 432 Fat: 18g Protein: 14g Sugar: 12g

641. Chard, Lettuce, and Ginger Smoothie

Preparation Time: 5 minutes | **Cooking Time:** 0 minute | **Servings:** 2

Ingredients:

10 Chard leaves, chopped	1-inch piece of ginger, chopped
10 lettuce leaves, chopped	½ teaspoon black salt
2 pear, chopped	2 teaspoons coconut sugar
¼ teaspoon ground black pepper	¼ teaspoon salt
2 tablespoons lemon juice	2 cups of water

Directions:

Place all the ingredients in the order in a food processor or blender and then pulse for 2 to 3 minutes at high speed until smooth.

Pour the smoothie into two glasses and then serve.

Nutrition:

Calories: 240 Fat: 4g Protein: 16g Sugar: 3g

642. Red Beet, Pear, and Apple Smoothie

Preparation Time: 5 minutes | **Cooking Time:** 0 minute | **Servings:** 2

Ingredients:

1/2 of medium beet, peeled, chopped	1 tablespoon chopped cilantro
1 orange, juiced	1 medium pear, chopped
1 medium apple, cored, chopped	1/4 teaspoon ground black pepper
1/8 teaspoon rock salt	1 teaspoon coconut sugar
1/4 teaspoons salt	1 cup of water

Directions:

Place all the ingredients in the order in a food processor or blender and then pulse for 2 to 3 minutes at high speed until smooth.

Pour the smoothie into two glasses and then serve.

Nutrition:

Calories: 240 Fat: 4g Protein: 16g Sugar: 3g

643. Berry and Yogurt Smoothie

Preparation Time: 5 minutes | **Cooking Time:** 0 minute | **Servings:** 2

Ingredients:

2 small bananas	3 cups frozen mixed berries
1 ½ cup cashew yogurt	1/2 teaspoon vanilla extract, unsweetened
1/2 cup almond milk, unsweetened	

Directions:

Place all the ingredients in the order in a food processor or blender and then pulse for 2 to 3 minutes at high speed until smooth.

Pour the smoothie into two glasses and then serve.

Nutrition:

Calories: 291 Fat: 9g Protein: 17g Sugar: 5g

644. Chocolate and Cherry Smoothie

Preparation Time: 5 minutes | **Cooking Time:** 0 minute | **Servings:** 2

Ingredients:

4 cups frozen cherries	2 tablespoons cocoa powder
1 scoop of protein powder	1 teaspoon maple syrup
2 cups almond milk, unsweetened	

Directions:

Place all the ingredients in the order in a food processor or blender and then pulse for 2 to 3 minutes at high speed until smooth.

Pour the smoothie into two glasses and then serve.

Nutrition:

Calories: 247 Fat: 3g Protein: 18g Sugar: 3g

645. Banana Weight Loss Juice

Preparation Time: 10 minutes | **Cooking Time:** 0 minutes | **Servings:** 1

Ingredients:

Water (1/3 C.)	Apple (1, Sliced)
Orange (1, Sliced)	Banana (1, Sliced)
Lemon Juice (1 T.)	

Directions:

Simply place everything into your blender, blend on high for twenty seconds, and then pour into your glass.

Nutrition:

Calories: 289 Total Carbohydrate: 2 g Cholesterol: 3 mg Total Fat: 17 g Fiber: 2 g Protein: 7 g Sodium: 163 mg

646. Vitamin Green Smoothie

Preparation Time: 5 minutes | **Cooking Time:** 5 minutes | **Servings:** 2

Ingredients:

1 cup milk or juice	1 cup spinach or kale
½ cup plain yogurt	1 kiwi
1 Tbsp chia or flax	1 tsp vanilla

Directions:
Mix the milk or juice and greens until smooth. Add the remaining ingredients and continue blending until smooth again.
Enjoy your delicious drink!

Nutrition:
Calories 397 Fat 36.4 g Carbohydrates 4 g Sugar 1 g Protein 14.7 g Cholesterol 4 mg

647. Strawberry Grapefruit Smoothie

Preparation Time: 5 minutes | **Cooking Time:** 5 minutes | **Servings:** 2

Ingredients:

1 banana	½ cup strawberries, frozen
1 grapefruit	¼ cup milk
¼ cup plain yogurt	2 Tbsp honey
½ tsp ginger, chopped	

Directions:
Using a mixer, blend all the ingredients.
When smooth, top your drink with a slice of grapefruit and enjoy it!

Nutrition:
Calories 233 Fat 7.9 g Carbohydrates 3.2 g Sugar 0.1 g Protein 35.6 g Cholesterol 32 mg

648. Spiced Buttermilk

Preparation Time: 5 minutes | **Cooking Time:** 0 minute | **Servings:** 2

Ingredients:

3/4 teaspoon ground cumin	1/4 teaspoon sea salt
1/8 teaspoon ground black pepper	2 mint leaves
1/8 teaspoon lemon juice	1/4 cup cilantro leaves
1 cup of chilled water	1 cup vegan yogurt, unsweetened
Ice as needed	

Directions:
Place all the ingredients in the order in a food processor or blender, except for cilantro and ¼ teaspoon cumin, and then pulse for 2 to 3 minutes at high speed until smooth.
Pour the milk into glasses, top with cilantro and cumin, and then serve.

Nutrition:
Calories: 211 Total Carbohydrate: 7 g Cholesterol: 13 mg Total Fat: 18 g Fiber: 3 g Protein: 17 g Sodium: 289 mg

649. Turmeric Lassi

Preparation Time: 5 minutes | **Cooking Time:** 0 minute | **Servings:** 2

Ingredients:

1 teaspoon grated ginger	1/8 teaspoon ground black pepper
1 teaspoon turmeric powder	1/8 teaspoon cayenne
1 tablespoon coconut sugar	1/8 teaspoon salt
1 cup vegan yogurt	1 cup almond milk

Directions:
Place all the ingredients in the order in a food processor or blender and then pulse for 2 to 3 minutes at high speed until smooth.
Pour the lassi into two glasses and then serve.

Nutrition:
Calories: 392 Fat: 10g Protein: 18g Sugar: 8g

650. Brownie Batter Orange Chia Shake

Preparation Time: 5 minutes | **Cooking Time:** 0 minute | **Servings:** 2

Ingredients:

2 tablespoons cocoa powder	3 tablespoons chia seeds
¼ teaspoon salt	4 tablespoons chocolate chips
4 teaspoons coconut sugar	½ teaspoon orange zest

½ teaspoon vanilla extract, unsweetened   2 cup almond milk

Directions:

Place all the ingredients in the order in a food processor or blender and then pulse for 2 to 3 minutes at high speed until smooth.

Pour the smoothie into two glasses and then serve.

Nutrition:

Calories: 290 Fat: 11g Protein: 20g Sugar: 9g

651. Saffron Pistachio Beverage

Preparation Time: 5 minutes | **Cooking Time:** 0 minute | **Servings:** 2

Ingredients:

8 strands of saffron	1 tablespoon cashews
1/4 teaspoon ground ginger	2 tablespoons pistachio
1/8 teaspoon cloves	1/4 teaspoon ground black pepper
1/4 teaspoon cardamom powder	3 tablespoons coconut sugar
1/4 teaspoon cinnamon	1/8 teaspoon fennel seeds
1/4 teaspoon poppy seeds	

Directions:

Place all the ingredients in the order in a food processor or blender and then pulse for 2 to 3 minutes at high speed until smooth.

Pour the smoothie into two glasses and then serve.

Nutrition:

Calories: 394 Fat: 5g Protein: 12g Sugar: 4g

652. Mexican Hot Chocolate Mix

Preparation Time: 5 minutes | **Cooking Time:** 0 minute | **Servings:** 2

Ingredients:

For the Hot Chocolate Mix:

1/3 cup chopped dark chocolate	1/8 teaspoon cayenne
1/8 teaspoon salt	1/2 teaspoon cinnamon
1/4 cup coconut sugar	1 teaspoon cornstarch
3 tablespoons cocoa powder	1/2 teaspoon vanilla extract, unsweetened

For servings:
2 cups milk, warmed

Directions:

Place all the ingredients of the hot chocolate mix in the order in a food processor or blender and then pulse for 2 to 3 minutes at high speed until ground.

Stir 2 tablespoons of the chocolate mix into a glass of milk until combined and then serve.

Nutrition:

Calories: 160 Fat: 6g Protein: 26g Sugar: 7g

653. Inspirational Orange Smoothie

Preparation Time: 5 minutes | **Cooking Time:** 5 minutes | **Servings:** 1

Ingredients:

4 mandarin oranges, peeled	1 banana, sliced and frozen
½ cup non-fat Greek yogurt	¼ cup of coconut water
1 tsp vanilla extract	5 ice cubes

Directions:

Using a mixer, whisk all the ingredients.

Enjoy your drink!

Nutrition:

Calories 256 Fat 13.3 g Carbohydrates 0 g Sugar 0 g Protein 34.5 g Cholesterol 78 mg

654. High Protein Blueberry Banana Smoothie

Preparation Time: 5 minutes | **Cooking Time:** 5 minutes | **Servings:** 2

Ingredients:

1 cup blueberries, frozen	2 ripe bananas
1 cup of water	1 tsp vanilla extract
2 Tbsp chia seeds	½ cup cottage cheese
1 tsp lemon zest	

Directions:

Put all the smoothie ingredients into the blender and whisk until smooth.

Enjoy your wonderful smoothie!

Nutrition:
Calories 358 Fat 19.8 g Carbohydrates 1.3 g Sugar 0.4 g Protein 41.9 g Cholesterol 131 mg

655. Citrus Detox Juice

Preparation Time: 10 minutes | **Cooking Time:** 0 minutes | **Servings:** 4

Ingredients:

Water (3 C.)	Lemon (1, Sliced)
Grapefruit (1, Sliced)	Orange (1, Sliced)

Directions:
Begin by peeling and slicing up your fruit. Once this is done, place it in a pitcher of water and infuse the water overnight.

Nutrition:
Calories: 269 Total Carbohydrate: 2 g Cholesterol: 3 mg Total Fat: 14 g Fiber: 2 g Protein: 7 g Sodium: 183 mg

656. Metabolism Water

Preparation Time: 10 minutes | **Cooking Time:** 0 minutes | **Servings:** 1

Ingredients:

Water (3 C.)	Cucumber (1, Sliced)
Lemon (1, Sliced)	Mint (2 Leaves)
Ice	

Directions:
All you will have to do is get out a pitcher, place all of the ingredients in, and allow the ingredients to soak overnight for maximum benefits!

Nutrition:
Calories: 301 Total Carbohydrate: 2 g Cholesterol: 13 mg Total Fat: 17 g Fiber: 4 g Protein: 8 g Sodium: 201 mg

657. Stress Relief Detox Drink

Preparation Time: 5 minutes | **Cooking Time:** 0 minutes | **Servings:** 1

Ingredients:

Water (1 Pitcher)	Mint
Lemon (1, Sliced)	Basil
Strawberries (1 C., Sliced)	Ice

Directions:
When you are ready, take all of the ingredients and place them into a pitcher of water overnight and enjoy the next day.

Nutrition:
Calories: 189 Total Carbohydrate: 2 g Cholesterol: 73 mg Total Fat: 17 g Fiber: 0 g Protein: 7 g Sodium: 163 mg

658. Strawberry Pink Drink

Preparation Time: 10 minutes | **Cooking Time:** 5 minutes | **Servings:** 4

Ingredients:

Water (1 C., Boiling)	Sugar (2 T.)
Acai Tea Bag (1)	Coconut Milk (1 C.)
Frozen Strawberries (1/2 C.)	

Directions:
You will begin by boiling your cup of water and steep the teabag in for at least five minutes.
When the tea is set, add in the sugar and coconut milk. Be sure to stir well to spread the sweetness throughout the tea.
Finally, add in your strawberries, and you can enjoy your freshly made pink drink!

Nutrition:
Calories: 321 Total Carbohydrate: 2 g Cholesterol: 13 mg Total Fat: 17 g Fiber: 2 g Protein: 9 g Sodium: 312 mg

659. Lavender and Mint Iced Tea

Preparation Time: 5 minutes | **Cooking Time:** 10 minutes | **Servings:** 8 servings

Ingredients:

8 cups of water	1/3 cup of dried lavender buds
¼ cup of mint	

Directions:
Add the mint and lavender to a pot and set this aside.
Add eight cups of boiling water to the pot. Sweeten to taste, cover, and let steep for ten minutes. Strain, chill and serve.
Tips:
Use a sweetener of your choice when making this iced tea.

Add spirits to turn this iced tea into a summer cocktail.

Nutrition:
Calories 266 Carbs: 9.3g Protein: 20.9g Fat: 16.1g

660. Pear Lemonade

Preparation Time: 5 minutes | **Cooking Time:** 30 minutes | **Servings:** 2 servings

Ingredients:

½ cup of pear, peeled and diced

½ cup of chilled water

1 cup of freshly squeezed lemon juice

Directions:
Add all the ingredients into a blender and pulse until it has all been combined. The pear does make the lemonade frothy, but this will settle.
Place in the refrigerator to cool and then serve.
Tips:
Keep stored in a sealed container in the refrigerator for up to four days.
Pop the fresh lemon in the microwave for ten minutes before juicing, you can extract more juice if you do this.

Nutrition:
Calories: 160 Carbs: 6.3g Protein: 2.9g Fat: 13.6g

661. Energizing Ginger Detox Tonic

Preparation Time: 15 minutes | **Cooking Time:** 10 minutes | **Servings:**

Ingredients:

1/2 teaspoon of grated ginger, fresh

1/8 teaspoon of cayenne pepper

1/8 teaspoon of ground cinnamon

1 teaspoon of apple cider vinegar

1 small lemon slice

1/8 teaspoon of ground turmeric

1 teaspoon of maple syrup

2 cups of boiling water

Directions:
Pour the boiling water into a small saucepan, add and stir the ginger, then let it rest for 8 to 10 minutes, before covering the pan.

Pass the mixture through a strainer and into the liquid, add the cayenne pepper, turmeric, cinnamon and stir properly.
Add the maple syrup, vinegar, and lemon slice.
Add and stir an infused lemon and serve immediately.

Nutrition:
Calories 443 Carbs:9.7 g Protein: 62.8g Fat: 16.9g

662. Strawberry Shake

Preparation Time: 10 minutes | **Cooking Time:** 10 minutes | **Servings:** 2

Ingredients:

1½ cups fresh strawberries, hulled

2 scoops unsweetened vegan vanilla protein powder

2 cups unsweetened hemp milk

1 large frozen banana, peeled

2 tablespoons hemp seeds

Directions:
In a high-speed blender, place all the ingredients and pulse until creamy.
Pour into two glasses and serve immediately.

Nutrition:
Calories: 259 Fat: 3g Protein: 10g Sugar: 2g

663. Chocolatey Banana Shake

Preparation Time: 10 minutes | **Cooking Time:** 10 minutes | **Servings:** 2

Ingredients:

2 medium frozen bananas, peeled

4 tablespoons peanut butter

2 tablespoons cacao powder

2 cups unsweetened soymilk

4 dates, pitted

4 tablespoons rolled oats

2 tablespoons chia seeds

Directions:
Place all the ingredients in a high-speed blender and pulse until creamy.
Pour into two glasses and serve immediately.

Nutrition:
Calories: 502 Fat: 4g Protein: 11g Sugar: 9g

664. Fruity Tofu Smoothie

Preparation Time: 10 minutes | **Cooking Time:** 10 minutes | **Servings:** 2

Ingredients:
12 ounces silken tofu, pressed and drained
2 medium bananas, peeled
1½ cups fresh blueberries
1 tablespoon maple syrup
1½ cups unsweetened soymilk
¼ cup of ice cubes

Directions:
Place all the ingredients in a high-speed blender and pulse until creamy.
Pour into two glasses and serve immediately.

Nutrition:
Calories 235 Carbohydrates: 1.9g Protein: 14.3g Fat: 18.9g

665. Green Fruity Smoothie

Preparation Time: 10 minutes | **Cooking Time:** 10 minutes | **Servings:** 2

Ingredients:

1 cup of frozen mango, peeled, pitted, and chopped	1 large frozen banana, peeled
2 cups fresh baby spinach	1 scoop unsweetened vegan vanilla protein powder
¼ cup pumpkin seeds	2 tablespoons hemp hearts
1½ cups unsweetened almond milk	

Directions:
In a high-speed blender, place all the ingredients and pulse until creamy.
Pour into two glasses and serve immediately.

Nutrition:
Calories 206 Carbohydrates: 1.3g Protein: 23.5g Fat: 11.9g

666. Protein Latte

Preparation Time: 10 minutes | **Cooking Time:** 10 minutes | **Servings:** 2

Ingredients:

2 cups hot brewed coffee	1¼ cups coconut milk
2 teaspoons coconut oil	2 scoops unsweetened vegan vanilla protein powder

Directions:
Place all the ingredients in a high-speed blender and pulse until creamy.
Pour into two serving mugs and serve immediately.

Nutrition:
Calories 483 Carbs: 5.2g Protein: 45.2g Fat: 31.2g

667. Health Boosting Juices

Preparation Time: 10 minutes | **Cooking Time:** 15 minutes | **Servings:** 2

Ingredients:
For a red juice:

4 beetroots, quartered	2 cups of strawberries
2 cups of blueberries	

For an orange juice:

4 green or red apples, halved	10 carrots
½ lemon, peeled	1" of ginger

For a yellow juice:

2 green or red apples, quartered	4 oranges, peeled and halved
½ lemon, peeled	1" of ginger

For lime juice:

6 stalks of celery	1 cucumber
2 green apples, quartered	2 pears, quartered

For a green juice:

½ a pineapple, peeled and sliced	8 leaves of kale
2 fresh bananas, peeled	

Directions:
Juice all ingredients in a juicer, chill, and serve.

Nutrition:
Calories 316 Carbs: 13.5g Protein: 37.8g Fat: 12.2g

668. Thai Iced Tea

Preparation Time: 5 minutes | **Cooking Time:** 10 minutes | **Servings:** 4

Ingredients:

4 cups of water	1 can of light coconut milk (14 oz.)
¼ cup of maple syrup	¼ cup of muscovado sugar
1 teaspoon of vanilla extract	2 tablespoons of loose-leaf black tea

Directions:
In a large saucepan, over medium heat bring the water to a boil.

Turn off the heat and add in the tea, cover and let steep for five minutes.

Strain the tea into a bowl or jug. Add the maple syrup, muscovado sugar, and vanilla extract. Give it a good whisk to blend all the ingredients. Set in the refrigerator to chill. Upon serving, pour ¾ of the tea into each glass, top with coconut milk, and stir.

Tips:
Add a shot of dark rum to turn this iced tea into a cocktail.

You could substitute the coconut milk for almond or rice milk too.

Nutrition:
Calories 844 Carbohydrates: 2.3g Protein: 21.6g Fat: 83.1g

669. Hot Chocolate

Preparation Time: 5 minutes | **Cooking Time:** 15 minutes | **Servings:** 2

Ingredients:

Pinch of brown sugar	2 cups of milk, soy or almond, unsweetened
2 tablespoons of cocoa powder	½ cup of vegan chocolate

Directions:
In a medium saucepan, over medium heat gently bring the milk to a boil. Whisk in the cocoa powder.

Remove from the heat, add a pinch of sugar and chocolate. Give it a good stir until smooth, serve, and enjoy.

Tips:
You may substitute the almond or soy milk for coconut milk too.

Nutrition:
Calories 452 Carbs: 29.8g Protein: 15.2g Fat: 30.2g

670. Chai and Chocolate Milkshake

Preparation Time: 5 minutes | **Cooking Time:** 15 minutes | **Servings:** 2 servings

Ingredients:

1 and ½ cups of almond milk, sweetened or unsweetened	3 bananas, peeled and frozen 12 hours before use
4 dates, pitted	1 and ½ teaspoons of chocolate powder, sweetened or unsweetened
½ teaspoon of vanilla extract	½ teaspoon of cinnamon
¼ teaspoon of ground ginger	Pinch of ground cardamom
Pinch of ground cloves	Pinch of ground nutmeg
½ cup of ice cubes	

Directions:
Add all the ingredients to a blender except for the ice-cubes. Pulse until smooth and creamy, add the ice-cubes, pulse a few more times and serve.

Tips:
The dates provide enough sweetness to the recipe, however, you are welcome to add maple syrup or honey for a sweeter drink.

Nutrition:
Calories 452 Carbs: 29.8g Protein: 15.2g Fat: 30.2g

671. Lemon Infused Water

Preparation Time: 10 minutes | **Cooking Time:** 2 hours | **Servings:** 12

Ingredients:

2 cups of coconut sugar

2 cups of lemon juice

3 quarts of water

Directions:

Pour water into a 6-quarts slow cooker and stir the sugar and lemon juice properly.

Then plug in the slow cooker and let it cook on a high heat setting for 2 hours or until it is heated thoroughly.

Serve the drink hot or cold.

Nutrition:

Calories 523 Carbohydrates: 4.6g Protein: 47.9g Fat: 34.8g

672. Soothing Ginger Tea Drink

Preparation Time: 5 minutes | **Cooking Time:** 2 hours 20 minutes | **Servings:** 8

Ingredients:

1 tablespoon of minced ginger root

2 tablespoons of honey

15 green tea bags

32 fluid ounce of white grape juice

2 quarts of boiling water

Directions:

Pour water into a 4-quarts slow cooker, immerse tea bags, cover the cooker, and let stand for 10 minutes.

After 10 minutes, remove and discard tea bags and stir in the remaining ingredients.

Return cover to the slow cooker, let cook at high heat setting for 2 hours or until heated through.

When done, strain the liquid and serve hot or cold.

Nutrition:

Calories 232 Carbs: 7.9g Protein: 15.9g Fat: 15.1g

673. Ginger Cherry Cider

Preparation Time: 1 hour 5 minutes | **Cooking Time:** 3 hours | **Servings:** 16

Ingredients:

2 knobs of ginger, each about 2 inches

6-ounce of cherry gelatin

4 quarts of apple cider

Directions:

Using a 6-quarts slow cooker, pour the apple cider and add the ginger.

Stir, then cover the slow cooker with its lid. let it cook for 3 hours at the high heat setting or until it is heated thoroughly.

Then add and stir the gelatin properly, then continue cooking for another hour.

When done, remove the ginger and serve the drink hot or cold.

Nutrition:

Calories 78 Carbs: 13.2g Protein: 2.8g Fat: 1.5g

674. Colorful Infused Water

Preparation Time: 5 minutes | **Cooking Time:** 1 hour | **Servings:** 8 servings

Ingredients:

1 cup of strawberries, fresh or frozen

1 cup of blueberries, fresh or frozen

1 tablespoon of baobab powder

1 cup of ice cubes

4 cups of sparkling water

Directions:

In a large water jug, add in the sparkling water, ice cubes, and baobab powder. Give it a good stir.

Add in the strawberries and blueberries and cover the infused water, store in the refrigerator for one hour before serving.

Tips:

Store for 12 hours for optimum taste and nutritional benefits.

Instead of using strawberries and blueberries, add slices of lemon and six mint leaves, one cup of mangoes or cherries, or half a cup of leafy greens such as kale and/or spinach.

Nutrition:

Calories 163 Carbs: 4.1g Protein: 1.7g Fat: 15.5g

675. Hibiscus Tea

Preparation Time: 1 Minute | **Cooking Time:** 5 minutes | **Servings:** 2 servings

Ingredients:

1 tablespoon of raisins, diced	6 Almonds, raw and unsalted
½ teaspoon of hibiscus powder	2 cups of water

Directions:

Bring the water to a boil in a small saucepan, add in the hibiscus powder and raisins. Give it a good stir, cover, and let simmer for a further two minutes.

Strain into a teapot and serve with a side helping of almonds.

Tips:

As an alternative to this tea, do not strain it and serve with the raisin pieces still swirling around in the teacup.

You could also serve this tea chilled for those hotter days.

Double or triple the recipe to provide you with iced-tea to enjoy during the week without having to make a fresh pot each time.

Nutrition:

Calories 139 Carbohydrates: 2.7g Protein: 8.7g Fat: 10.3

676. Lemon and Rosemary Iced Tea

Preparation Time: 5 minutes | **Cooking Time:** 10 minutes | **Servings:** 4 servings

Ingredients:

4 cups of water	4 earl grey tea bags
¼ cup of sugar	2 lemons
1 sprig of rosemary	

Directions:

Peel the two lemons and set the fruit aside.

In a medium saucepan, over medium heat combine the water, sugar, and lemon peels. Bring this to a boil.

Remove from the heat and place the rosemary and tea into the mixture. Cover the saucepan and steep for five minutes.

Add the juice of the two peeled lemons to the mixture, strain, chill, and serve.

Tips: Skip the sugar and use honey to taste.
Do not squeeze the tea bags as they can cause the tea to become bitter.

Nutrition:

Calories 229 Carbs: 33.2g Protein: 31.1g Fat: 10.2g

677. Fragrant Spiced Coffee

Preparation Time: 10 minutes | **Cooking Time:** 3 hours | **Servings:** 8

Ingredients:

4 cinnamon sticks, each about 3 inches long	1 1/2 teaspoons of whole cloves
1/3 cup of honey	2-ounce of chocolate syrup
1/2 teaspoon of anise extract	8 cups of brewed coffee

Directions:

Pour the coffee into a 4-quarts slow cooker and pour in the remaining ingredients except for cinnamon and stir properly.

Wrap the whole cloves in cheesecloth and tie its corners with strings.

Immerse this cheesecloth bag in the liquid present in the slow cooker and cover it with the lid.

Then plug in the slow cooker and let it cook on the low heat setting for 3 hours or until heated thoroughly.

When done, discard the cheesecloth bag and serve.

Nutrition:

Calories 136 Fat 12.6 g Carbohydrates 4.1 g Sugar 0.5 g Protein 10.3 g Cholesterol 88 mg

678. Bracing Coffee Smoothie

Preparation Time: 5 minutes | **Cooking Time:** 5 minutes | **Servings:** 1

Ingredients:

1 banana, sliced and frozen	½ cup strong brewed coffee
½ cup milk	¼ cup rolled oats
1 tsp nut butter	

Directions:

Mix all the ingredients until smooth.

Enjoy your morning drink!

Nutrition:
Calories 414 Fat 20.6 g Carbohydrates 5.6 g Sugar 1.3 g Protein 48.8 g Cholesterol 58 mg

679. Ginger Smoothie with Citrus and Mint

Preparation Time: 5 minutes | **Cooking Time:** 3 minutes | **Servings:** 3

Ingredients:

1 head Romaine lettuce, chopped into 4 chunks	2 Tbsp hemp seeds
5 mandarin oranges, peeled	1 banana, frozen
1 carrot	2-3 mint leaves
½ piece of ginger root, peeled	1 cup of water
¼ lemon, peeled	½ cup ice

Directions:
Put all the smoothie ingredients in a blender and blend until smooth.
Enjoy!

Nutrition:
Calories 101 Fat 4 g Carbohydrates 14 g Sugar 1 g Protein 2 g Cholesterol 3 mg

680. Strawberry Beet Smoothie

Preparation Time: 5 minutes | **Cooking Time:** 50 minutes | **Servings:** 2

Ingredients:

1 red beet, trimmed, peeled, and chopped into cubes	1 cup strawberries, quartered
1 ripe banana	½ cup strawberry yogurt
1 Tbsp honey Milk, to taste	1 Tbsp water

Directions:
Sprinkle the beet cubes with water, place them on aluminum foil, and put them in the oven (preheated to 204°C). Bake for 40 minutes.
Let the baked beet cool.
Combine all the smoothie ingredients.
Enjoy your fantastic drink.

Nutrition:
Calories 184 Fat 9.2 g
Carbohydrates 1 g
Sugar 0.4 g
Protein 24.9 g
Cholesterol 132 mg

681. Peanut Butter Shake

Preparation Time: 5 minutes | **Cooking Time:** 5 minutes | **Servings:** 2

Ingredients:

1 cup plant-based milk	1 handful kale
2 bananas, frozen	2 Tbsp peanut butter
½ tsp ground cinnamon	¼ tsp vanilla powder

Directions:
Use a blender to combine all the ingredients for your shake. Enjoy it!

Nutrition:
Calories 184 Fat 9.2 g Carbohydrates 1 g Sugar 0.4 g Protein 24.9 g Cholesterol 132 mg

682. Creamy Avocado Drink

Preparation Time: 5minutes | **Cooking Time:** 30-120 minutes | **Servings:** 4

Ingredients:

4 large ripe avocados, halved and pitted	4 tbsp swerve sugar
¼ cup cold almond milk	1 tsp vanilla extract
1 tbsp cold heavy cream	

Directions:
In a blender, add the avocado pulp, swerve sugar, almond milk, vanilla extract, and heavy cream. Process until smooth.
Pour the mixture into 2 tall serving glasses, garnish with strawberries, and serve immediately.

Nutrition:
Calories: 193, Total Fat: 20.1g, Saturated Fat12,5g, Total Carbs: 3g, Dietary Fiber: 0g, Sugar: 2 g, Protein: 1g, Sodium: 100 mg

Chapter 8: Dressings, Dips, and Sauces

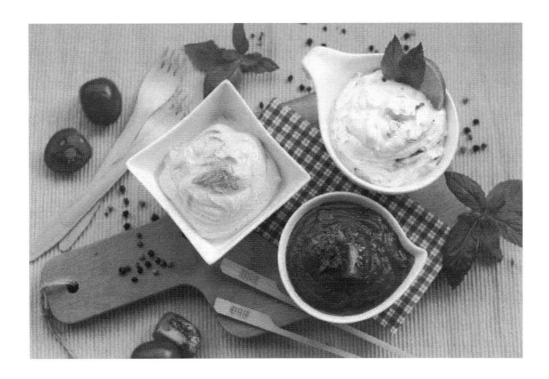

683. Red Salsa

Preparation Time: 10 minutes | **Cooking Time:** 0 minute | **Servings:** 8

Ingredients:

30 ounces diced fire-roasted tomatoes

1 medium jalapeño pepper, deseeded

1 cup chopped cilantro

½ teaspoon of sea salt

¼ teaspoon stevia

4 tablespoons diced green chilies

1/2 cup chopped green onion

1 teaspoon minced garlic

1 teaspoon ground cumin

3 tablespoons lime juice

Directions:

Place all the ingredients in a food processor and process for 2 minutes until smooth.

Tip the salsa in a bowl, taste to adjust seasoning, and then serve.

Nutrition:

Calories: 71 Cal Fat: 0.2 g Carbs: 19 g Protein: 2 g Fiber: 4.1 g

684. Tomato Hummus

Preparation Time: 5 minutes | **Cooking Time:** 0 minute | **Servings:** 4

Ingredients:

1/4 cup sun-dried tomatoes, without oil

1 teaspoon minced garlic

2 tablespoons sesame oil

1 tablespoon olive oil

1 ½ cups cooked chickpeas

1/2 teaspoon salt

1 tablespoon lemon juice

1/4 cup of water

Directions:

Place all the ingredients in a food processor and process for 2 minutes until smooth.

Tip the hummus in a bowl, drizzle with more oil, and then serve straight away.

Nutrition:

Calories: 122.7 Cal Fat: 4.1 g Carbs: 17.8 g Protein: 5.1 g Fiber: 3.5 g

685. Black Bean Lime Dip

Preparation Time: 5 minutes | **Cooking Time:** 6 minutes | **Servings:** 4

Ingredients:

15.5 ounces cooked black beans	1 teaspoon minced garlic
½ of a lime, juiced	1 inch of ginger, grated
1/3 teaspoon salt	1/3 teaspoon ground black pepper
1 tablespoon olive oil	

Directions:

Take a frying pan, add oil and when hot, add garlic and ginger and cook for 1 minute until fragrant.

Then add beans, splash with some water and fry for 3 minutes until hot.

Season beans with salt and black pepper, drizzle with lime juice, then remove the pan from heat and mash the beans until smooth pasta comes together.

Serve the dip with whole-grain breadsticks or vegetables.

Nutrition:

Calories: 374 Cal Fat: 14 g Carbs: 46 g Protein: 15 g Fiber: 17 g

686. Beetroot Hummus

Preparation Time: 10 minutes | **Cooking Time:** 60 minutes | **Servings:** 4

Ingredients:

15 ounces cooked chickpeas	3 small beets
1 teaspoon minced garlic	1/2 teaspoon smoked paprika
1 teaspoon of sea salt	1/4 teaspoon red chili flakes
2 tablespoons olive oil	1 lemon, juiced
2 tablespoon tahini	1 tablespoon chopped almonds
1 tablespoon chopped cilantro	

Directions:

Drizzle oil over beets, season with salt, then wrap beets in a foil and bake for 60 minutes at 425 degrees F until tender.

When done, let beet cool for 10 minutes, then peel and dice them and place them in a food processor.

Add remaining ingredients and pulse for 2 minutes until smooth, tip the hummus in a bowl, drizzle with some more oil, and then serve straight away.

Nutrition:

Calories: 50.1 Cal Fat: 2.5 g Carbs: 5 g Protein: 2 g Fiber: 1 g

687. Zucchini Hummus

Preparation Time: 5 minutes | **Cooking Time:** 0 minute | **Servings:** 8

Ingredients:

1 cup diced zucchini	1/2 teaspoon sea salt
1 teaspoon minced garlic	2 teaspoons ground cumin
3 tablespoons lemon juice	1/3 cup tahini

Directions:

Place all the ingredients in a food processor and pulse for 2 minutes until smooth.

Tip the hummus in a bowl, drizzle with oil, and serve.

Nutrition:

Calories: 65 Cal Fat: 5 g Carbs: 3 g Protein: 2 g Fiber: 1 g

688. Coleslaw Dressing

Preparation Time: 5 minutes | **Cooking Time:** 0 minutes | **Servings:** 12

Ingredients:

Celery seed, one teaspoon
Onion powder, one teaspoon
Agave nectar, one tablespoon
Dijon mustard, one tablespoon
Apple cider vinegar, two tablespoons
Vegenaise (vegan mayo), one half cup

Directions:

Mix well and store in the refrigerator.

Nutrition:

Calories: 47 Fat: 0.3 Fiber: 1.5 Carbs: 0.4 Protein: 0.4

689. Walnut Basil Dressing

Preparation Time: 10 minutes | **Cooking Time:** 0 minutes | **Servings:** 12

Ingredients:

Water, two to four tablespoons as needed

Salt, one quarter teaspoon

Garlic, minced, one tablespoon

Lemon juice, three tablespoons

Nutritional yeast, one quarter cup

Olive oil, one quarter cup

Walnuts, one-half cup crushed

Basil leaves, one cup packed loosely, chopped fine

Directions:

Mix all of the ingredients in a food processor or blender until smooth. Add spoons of water as needed to maintain a thick but workable consistency.

The finished product should resemble a pesto sauce.

Nutrition:

Calories: 89 Fat: 0.3 Fiber: 1.5 Carbs: 0.4 Protein: 0.4

690. Beer "Cheese" Dip

Preparation Time: 10 minutes | **Cooking Time:** 7 minutes | **Servings:** 3

Ingredients:

¾ cup of water

¾ cup brown ale

½ cup raw walnuts, soaked in hot water for at least 15 minutes, then drained

½ cup raw cashews, soaked in hot water for at least 15 minutes, then drained

2 tablespoons tomato paste

2 tablespoons fresh lemon juice

1 tablespoon apple cider vinegar

½ cup nutritional yeast

½ teaspoon sweet or smoked paprika

1 tablespoon arrowroot powder

1 tablespoon red miso

Directions:

Place the water, brown ale, walnuts, cashews, tomato paste, lemon juice, and apple cider vinegar into a high-speed blender, and purée until thoroughly mixed and smooth.

Transfer the mixture to a saucepan over medium heat. Add the nutritional yeast, paprika, and arrowroot powder, and whisk well. Bring to a simmer for about 7 minutes, stirring frequently, or until the mixture begins to thicken and bubble.

Remove from the heat and whisk in the red miso. Let the dip cool for 10 minutes and refrigerate in an airtight container for up to 5 days.

Nutrition:

Calories: 113 Fat: 5.1g Carbs: 10.4g Protein: 6.3g Fiber: 3.8g

691. Creamy Black Bean Dip

Preparation Time: 10 minutes | **Cooking Time:** 0 minutes | **Servings:** 3

Ingredients:

4 cups cooked black beans, rinsed and drained

2 tablespoons Italian seasoning

2 tablespoons minced garlic

2 tablespoon low-sodium vegetable broth

2 tablespoons onion powder

1 tablespoon lemon juice, or more to taste

¼ teaspoon salt (optional)

Directions:

In a large bowl, mash the black beans with a potato masher or the back of a fork until mostly smooth.

Add the remaining ingredients to the bowl and whisk to combine.

Taste and add more lemon juice or salt, if needed. Serve immediately, or refrigerate for at least 30 minutes to better incorporate the flavors.

Nutrition:

Calories: 387 Fat: 6.5g Carbs: 63.0g Protein: 21.2g Fiber: 16.0g

692. Moroccan Carrot Dip

Preparation Time: 15 minutes | **Cooking Time:** 0 minutes | **Servings:** 1

Ingredients:

Water, one half cup

Black pepper, one quarter teaspoon

Salt, one half teaspoon	Fennel, one quarter teaspoon
Coriander, ground, one half teaspoon	Cumin, ground, one half teaspoon
Cinnamon, one teaspoon	Ginger, ground, one teaspoon
Garlic, minced, one tablespoon	Apple cider vinegar, two teaspoons
Cashews, raw, one third cup	Carrot, raw, one cup cut into small chunks

Directions:
Puree all of the listed ingredients until everything is smooth and creamy.

Nutrition:
Calories: 110 Fat: 0.3 Fiber: 1.5 Carbs: 0.4 Protein: 0.4

693. Tahini Citrus Dressing

Preparation Time: 15 minutes | **Cooking Time:** 0 minutes | **Servings:** 1 cup

Ingredients:

Black pepper, one half teaspoon	Salt, one half teaspoon
Garlic, minced, one tablespoon	Ginger, ground, one teaspoon
Dijon mustard, two teaspoons	Agave nectar, two tablespoons
Apple cider vinegar, one tablespoon	Tahini, two tablespoons
Lemon juice, one tablespoon	Orange juice, three tablespoons

Directions:
Mix all of the ingredients that are listed in a blender until they are creamy and smooth.

Nutrition:
Calories: 98 Fat: 0.3 Fiber: 1.5 Carbs: 0.4 Protein: 0.4

694. Curried Almond Dressing

Preparation Time: 15 minutes | **Cooking Time:** 8 minutes | **Servings:** 1 cup

Ingredients:

Curry powder, one eighth teaspoon	Black pepper, one eighth teaspoon
Salt, one half teaspoon	Dijon mustard, one half teaspoon

Ginger, ground, one teaspoon	Garlic, minced, one tablespoon
Water, two-thirds cup	Agave nectar, two tablespoons
Apple cider vinegar, two tablespoons	Almonds, raw, one half cup

Directions:
Puree well all of the ingredients in a blender until they are creamy and smooth.

Nutrition:
Calories: 85 Fat: 0.3 Fiber: 1.5 Carbs: 0.4 Protein: 0.4

695. Keto Vegan Raw Cashew Cheese Sauce

Preparation Time: 5 minutes | **Cooking Time:** 5 minutes | **Servings:** 6

Ingredients:

1 cup raw cashews, soaked in water for at least 3 hours before making the recipe	2 tablespoon olive oil
2 tablespoon nutritional yeast	1/4 teaspoon garlic powder
2 tablespoon fresh lemon juice	1/2 cup water
Salt to taste	

Directions:
To prepare cashews before making the sauce, boil 2 cups of water, turn off the heat and add cashews. This can be allowed to soak overnight. Rinse and strained cashews. Discard water.
Add all ingredients to a food processor and blend until a smooth consistency is achieved. Can be used to make pizzas, over roasted veggies, in lasagna, as a dip, and more.

Nutrition:
Total fat: 15.5g
Sodium: 34mg
Total carbohydrates: 9.23g
Protein: 5.1g

696. Spicy Avocado Mayonnaise

Preparation Time: 10 minutes | **Cooking Time:** 10 minutes | **Servings:** 8

Ingredients:

2 ripe avocados, pitted and peeled	1/4 jalapeno pepper, minced
2 tablespoon lemon juice	1/2 teaspoon onion powder
2 tablespoon fresh cilantro, chopped	Salt to taste

Directions:

Add all ingredients to a food processor and blender until a smooth creamy consistency is achieved.

The jalapeno peppers can be foregone if you prefer a cooler mayo. Can be enjoyed in sandwiches, on toast, as a topping, in veggie wraps, and salads

Nutrition:

Total fat: 9.8g
Cholesterol: 0mg
Sodium: 23mg
Total carbohydrates: 4.6g
Dietary fiber: 3.4g
Protein: 1g

697. Green Coconut Butter

Preparation Time: 10 minutes | **Cooking Time:** 10 minutes | **Servings:** 8

Ingredients:

2 cups unsweetened shredded coconut	2 teaspoon matcha powder
1 tablespoon coconut oil	

Directions:

Add shredded coconut to a food processor and blend for 5 minutes or until a smooth but runny consistency is achieved.

Add matcha powder and olive oil. Blend for 1 more minute.

Can be stored in an airtight container at room temperature for up to 2 weeks. Makes a delicious fruit dip and can be added to smoothies, on pancakes, and toast.

Nutrition:

Total fat: 5.2g

Cholesterol: 0mg
Sodium: 3mg
Total carbohydrates: 1.7g
Dietary fiber: 1.2g
Protein: 0.7g

698. Spiced Almond Butter

Preparation Time: 10 minutes | **Cooking Time:** 5 minutes | **Servings:** 10

Ingredients:

2 cups raw almond	1/8 teaspoon allspice
1/8 teaspoon cinnamon	1/8 teaspoon cardamom
1/8 teaspoon ground ginger	1/8 teaspoon ground cloves
1/2 teaspoon salt	

Directions:

Place all ingredients in a food processor and blend until a smooth consistency is achieved. Makes a delicious fruit and veggie dip and can be added to smoothies, on toast, on pancakes, and on waffles.

Nutrition:

Total fat: 9.5g
Cholesterol: 0mg
Sodium: 117mg
Total carbohydrates: 4.1g
Dietary fiber: 2.4g
Protein: 4g

699. Tangy Cashew Mustard Dressing

Preparation Time: 20 minutes | **Cooking Time:** 0 minutes | **Servings:** 1

Ingredients:

2 ounces (57 g) raw, unsalted cashews (about ½ cup)	½ cup of water
3 tablespoons lemon juice	2 teaspoons apple cider vinegar
2 tablespoons Dijon mustard	1 medium clove garlic

Directions:

Put all the ingredients in a food processor and keep it aside for at least 15 minutes.

Purée until the ingredients are combined into a smooth and creamy mixture. Thin the dressing with a little extra water as needed to achieve your preferred consistency.

Store in an airtight container in the refrigerator for up to 5 days.

Nutrition:
Calories: 187 Fat: 13.0g Carbs: 11.5g Protein: 5.9g Fiber: 1.7g

700. Avocado-dill Dressing

Preparation Time: 20 minutes | **Cooking Time:** 0 minutes | **Servings:** 1

Ingredients:

2 ounces (57 g) raw, unsalted cashews (about ½ cup)	½ cup of water
3 tablespoons lemon juice	½ medium, ripe avocado, chopped
1 medium clove garlic	2 tablespoons chopped fresh dill
2 green onions, white and green parts, chopped	

Directions:
Put the cashews, water, lemon juice, avocado, and garlic into a blender. Keep it aside for at least 15 minutes to soften the cashews.

Blend until everything is fully mixed. Fold in the dill and green onions, and blend briefly to retain some texture.

Store in an airtight container in the fridge for up to 3 days and stir well before serving.

Nutrition:
Calories: 312 Fat: 21.1g Carbs: 22.6g Protein: 8.0g Fiber: 7.1g

701. Easy Lemon Tahini Dressing

Preparation Time: 5 minutes | **Cooking Time:** 0 minutes | **Servings:** 1

Ingredients:

½ cup tahini	¼ cup fresh lemon juice (about 2 lemons)
1 teaspoon maple syrup	1 small garlic clove, chopped
1/8 teaspoon black pepper	¼ teaspoon salt (optional)
¼ to ½ cup of water	

Directions:
Process the tahini, lemon juice, maple syrup, garlic, black pepper, and salt (if desired) in a blender (high-speed blenders work best for this). Gradually add the water until the mixture is completely smooth.

Store in an airtight container in the fridge for up to 5 days.

Nutrition:
Calories: 128 Fat: 9.6g Carbs: 6.8g Protein: 3.6g Fiber: 1.9g

702. Catalina Dressing

Preparation Time: 5 minutes | **Cooking Time:** 0 minutes | **Servings:** 12

Ingredients:
Dry mustard, one half teaspoon
Chili powder, one half teaspoon
Onion powder, one half teaspoon
Apple cider vinegar, three tablespoons
Olive oil, one quarter cup
Tomato sauce, one quarter cup

Directions:
Mix well and store in the refrigerator.

Nutrition:
Calories: 47 Fat: 4.3 Fiber: 1.5 Carbs: 2.4 Protein: 2.4

703. Applesauce Salad Dressing

Preparation Time: 5 minutes | **Cooking Time:** 8 minutes | **Servings:** 12

Ingredients:

Black pepper, one eighth teaspoon	Salt, one quarter teaspoon
Cinnamon, one teaspoon	Cumin, one quarter teaspoon
Dijon mustard, one teaspoon	Chickpea miso, one teaspoon
Balsamic vinegar, one tablespoon	Apple cider vinegar, two tablespoons
Applesauce, unsweetened, one quarter cup	

Directions:
Mix well in a blender.

Nutrition:
Calories: 105 Fat: 0.3 Fiber: 1.5 Carbs: 0.4 Protein: 0.4

704. Satay Sauce

Preparation Time: 5 minutes | **Cooking Time:** 8 minutes | **Servings:** 2

Ingredients:

½ yellow onion, diced	3 garlic cloves, minced
1 fresh red chile, thinly sliced (optional)	1-inch (2.5-cm) piece fresh ginger, peeled and minced
¼ cup smooth peanut butter	2 tablespoons coconut aminos
1 (13.5-ounce / 383-g) can unsweetened coconut milk	¼ teaspoon freshly ground black pepper
¼ teaspoon salt (optional)	

Directions:
Heat a large nonstick skillet over medium-high heat until hot.
Add the onion, garlic cloves, chile (if desired), and ginger to the skillet, and sauté for 2 minutes. Pour in the peanut butter and coconut aminos and stir well. Add the coconut milk, black pepper, and salt (if desired) and continue whisking, or until the sauce is just beginning to bubble and thicken.
Remove the sauce from the heat to a bowl. Taste and adjust the seasoning if necessary.

Nutrition:
Calories: 322 Fat: 28.8g Carbs: 9.4gProtein: 6.3gFiber: 1.8g

705. Tahini BBQ Sauce

Preparation Time: 10 minutes | **Cooking Time:** 0 minutes | **Servings:** 4

Ingredients:

½ cup of water	¼ cup red miso
3 cloves garlic, minced	1-inch (2.5 cm) piece ginger, peeled and minced

2 tablespoons rice vinegar	2 tablespoons tahini
2 tablespoons chili paste or chili sauce	1 tablespoon date sugar
½ teaspoon crushed red pepper (optional)	

Directions:
Place all the ingredients in a food processor, and purée until thoroughly mixed and smooth. You can thin the sauce out by stirring in ½ cup of water or keep it thick.
Transfer to the refrigerator to chill until ready to serve.

Nutrition:
Calories: 206 Fat: 10.2g Carbs: 21.3g Protein: 7.2gFiber: 4.4g

706. Tamari Vinegar Sauce

Preparation Time: 10 minutes | **Cooking Time:** 0 minutes | **Servings:** 1

Ingredients:

¼ cup tamari	½ cup nutritional yeast
2 tablespoons balsamic vinegar	2 tablespoons apple cider vinegar
2 tablespoons Worcestershire sauce	2 teaspoons Dijon mustard
1 tablespoon plus 1 teaspoon maple syrup	½ teaspoon ground turmeric
¼ teaspoon black pepper	

Directions:
Place all the ingredients in an airtight container, and whisk until everything is well incorporated. Store in the refrigerator for up to 3 weeks.

Nutrition:
Calories: 216 Fat: 9.9g Carbs: 18.0g Protein: 13.7g Fiber: 7.7g

707. Sweet and Tangy Ketchup

Preparation Time: 5 minutes | **Cooking Time:** 15 minutes | **Servings:** 2

Ingredients:

1 cup of water	¼ cup maple syrup
1 cup tomato paste	3 tablespoons apple cider vinegar

| 1 teaspoon onion powder | 1 teaspoon garlic powder |

Directions:

Add the water to a medium saucepan and bring to a rolling boil over high heat.

Reduce the heat to low, stir in the maple syrup, tomato paste, vinegar, onion powder, and garlic powder. Cover and bring to a gentle simmer for about 10 minutes, stirring frequently, or until the sauce begins to thicken and bubble.

Let the sauce rest for 30 minutes until cooled completely. Transfer to an airtight container and refrigerate for up to 1 month.

Nutrition:

Calories: 46 Fat: 5.2g Carbs: 1.0g Protein: 1.1g Fiber: 1.0g

708. Homemade Tzatziki Sauce

Preparation Time: 20 minutes | **Cooking Time:** 0 minutes | **Servings:** 1

Ingredients:

2 ounces (57 g) raw, unsalted cashews (about ½ cup)	2 tablespoons lemon juice
1/3 cup water	1 small clove garlic
1 cup chopped cucumber, peeled	2 tablespoons fresh dill

Directions:

In a blender, add the cashews, lemon juice, water, and garlic. Keep it aside for at least 15 minutes to soften the cashews.

Blend the ingredients until smooth. Stir in the chopped cucumber and dill, and continue to blend until it reaches your desired consistency. It doesn't need to be super smooth. Feel free to add more water if you like a thinner consistency. Transfer to an airtight container and chill for at least 30 minutes for best flavors.

Bring the sauce to room temperature and shake well before serving.

Nutrition:

Calories: 208 Fat: 13.5g Carbs:15.0 g Protein: 6.7g Fiber: 2.8g

709. Balsamic Vinaigrette

Preparation Time: 5 minutes | **Cooking Time:** 8 minutes | **Servings:** 1 cup

Ingredients:

Black pepper, one quarter teaspoon
Salt, one quarter teaspoon
Garlic powder, one quarter teaspoon
Agave nectar, one tablespoon
Dijon mustard, one tablespoon
Balsamic vinegar, one quarter cup
Olive oil, one half cup

Directions:

Mix well in a blender or a shaker jar.

Nutrition:

Calories: 91 Fat: 0.3 Fiber: 1.5 Carbs: 0.4 Protein: 0.4

710. Chipotle Lime Dressing

Preparation Time: 5 minutes | **Cooking Time:** 8 minutes | **Servings:** 1 cup

Ingredients:

Garlic powder, one quarter teaspoon
Paprika, one quarter teaspoon
Agave nectar, one tablespoon
Red pepper, one chopped
Lime juice, three tablespoons
Vegenaise, three tablespoons

Directions:

Mix well in a shaker jar or a blender.

Nutrition:

Calories: 32 Fat: 0.3 Fiber: 1.5 Carbs: 0.4 Protein: 0.4

711. Sweet Mango and Orange Dressing

Preparation Time: 5 minutes | **Cooking Time:** 0 minutes | **Servings:** 1

Ingredients:

| 1 cup (165 g) diced mango, thawed if frozen | ½ cup of orange juice |
| 2 tablespoons rice vinegar | 2 tablespoons fresh lime juice |

¼ teaspoon salt
(optional)
2 tablespoons
chopped cilantro

1 teaspoon date sugar
(optional)

Directions:
Pulse all the ingredients except for the cilantro in a food processor until it reaches the consistency you like. Add the cilantro and whisk well.
Store in an airtight container in the fridge for up to 2 days.

Nutrition:
Calories: 32 Fat: 0.1g Carbs: 7.4g Protein: 0.3g Fiber: 0.5g

712. Creamy Avocado Cilantro Lime Dressing

Preparation Time: 5 minutes | **Cooking Time:** 0 minutes | **Servings:** 2

Ingredients:
1 avocado, diced
¼ cup cilantro leaves

½ cup of water
¼ cup fresh lime or lemon juice (about 2 limes or lemons)
½ teaspoon ground cumin
¼ teaspoon salt (optional)

Directions:
Put all the ingredients in a blender (high-speed blenders work best for this), and pulse until well combined. Taste and adjust the seasoning as needed. It is best served within 1 day.

Nutrition:
Calories: 94 Fat: 7.4g Carbs: 5.7g Protein: 1.1g Fiber: 3.5g

713. Maple Dijon Dressing

Preparation Time: 5 minutes | **Cooking Time:** 0 minutes | **Servings:** 1

Ingredients:
¼ cup apple cider vinegar
2 tablespoons maple syrup

2 teaspoons Dijon mustard
2 tablespoons low-sodium vegetable broth
¼ teaspoon black pepper
Salt, to taste (optional)

Directions:
Mix the apple cider vinegar, Dijon mustard, maple syrup, vegetable broth, and black pepper in a resealable container until well incorporated. Season with salt to taste, if desired.
The dressing can be refrigerated for up to 5 days.

Nutrition:
Calories: 82 Fat: 0.3g Carbs: 19.3g Protein: 0.6g Fiber: 0.7g

714. Avocado-chickpea Dip

Preparation Time: 15 minutes | **Cooking Time:** 0 minutes | **Servings:** 2

Ingredients:
1 (15-ounce / 425-g) can cooked chickpeas, drained and rinsed
¼ cup red onion, finely chopped
1 to 2 tablespoons lemon juice
1/2 teaspoon garlic clove, finely chopped

2 large, ripe avocados, chopped
1 tablespoon Dijon mustard
2 teaspoons chopped fresh oregano

Directions:
In a medium bowl, mash the cooked chickpeas with a potato masher or the back of a fork, or until the chickpeas pop open (a food processor works best for this).
Stir in the remaining ingredients and continue to mash until completely smooth.
Place in the refrigerator to chill until ready to serve.

Nutrition:
Calories: 101 Fat: 1.9g Carbs: 16.2g Protein: 4.7g Fiber: 4.6g

715. Spicy and Tangy Black Bean Salsa

Preparation Time: 15 minutes | **Cooking Time:** 0 minutes | **Servings:** 3

Ingredients:
1 (15-ounce / 425-g) can cooked black beans, drained and rinsed

1 cup chopped tomatoes

1 cup corn kernels, thawed if frozen

¼ cup finely chopped red onion

1 tablespoon lime juice

½ teaspoon ground cumin

1 medium clove garlic, finely chopped

½ cup cilantro or parsley, chopped

1 tablespoon lemon juice

1 teaspoon chili powder

½ teaspoon regular or smoked paprika

Directions:
Put all the ingredients in a large bowl and stir with a fork until well incorporated.

Serve immediately, or chill for 2 hours in the refrigerator to let the flavors blend.

Nutrition:
Calories: 83 Fat: 0.5g Carbs: 15.4g Protein: 4.3g Fiber: 4.6g

716. Homemade Chimichurri

Preparation Time: 5 minutes | **Cooking Time:** 0 minutes | **Servings:** 1

Ingredients:

1 cup finely chopped flat-leaf parsley leaves

¼ cup low-sodium vegetable broth

1 teaspoon dried oregano

Zest and juice of 2 lemons

4 garlic cloves

Directions:
Place all the ingredients into a food processor, and pulse until it reaches the consistency you like. Refrigerate the chimichurri in an airtight container for up to 5 days. It's best served within 1 day.

Nutrition:
Calories: 19 Fat: 0.2g Carbs: 3.7g Protein: 0.7g Fiber: 0.7g

717. Cilantro Coconut Pesto

Preparation Time: 5 minutes | **Cooking Time:** 0 minutes | **Servings:** 2

Ingredients:

1 (13.5-ounce / 383-g) can unsweetened coconut milk

2 jalapeños, seeds, and ribs removed

1 bunch cilantro, leaves only

1-inch (2.5 cm) piece ginger, peeled and minced

1 tablespoon white miso

Water, as needed

Directions:
Pulse all the ingredients in a blender until creamy and smooth.

Thin with a little extra water as needed to reach your preferred consistency.

Store in an airtight container in the fridge for up t0 2 days or in the freezer for up to 6 months.

Nutrition:
Calories: 141 Fat: 13.7g Carbs: 2.8g Protein: 1.6g Fiber: 0.3g

718. Fresh Mango Salsa

Preparation Time: 10 minutes | **Cooking Time:** 0 minutes | **Servings:** 6

Ingredients:

2 small mangoes, diced

½ red onion, finely diced

2 tablespoon low-sodium vegetable broth

Freshly ground black pepper, to taste

1 red bell pepper, finely diced

Juice of ½ lime, or more to taste

Handful cilantro, chopped

Salt, to taste (optional)

Directions:
Stir together all the ingredients in a large bowl until well incorporated.

Taste and add more lime juice or salt, if needed. Store in an airtight container in the fridge for up to 5 days.

Nutrition:
Calories: 86 Fat: 1.9g Carbs: 13.3g Protein: 1.2g Fiber: 0.9g

719. Pineapple Mint Salsa

Preparation Time: 10 minutes | **Cooking Time:** 0 minutes | **Servings:** 3

Ingredients:

1 pound (454 g) fresh pineapple, finely diced and juices reserved

1 bunch mint, leaves only, chopped

1 minced jalapeño, (optional)
Salt, to taste (optional)

1 white or red onion, finely diced

1 1/4 cups vegetable broth

Directions:
In a medium bowl, mix the pineapple with its juice, mint, jalapeño (if desired), and onion, and whisk well. Season with salt to taste, if desired. Refrigerate in an airtight container for at least 2 hours to better incorporate the flavors.

Directions:
Take a small saucepan, place it over medium heat, pour in vegetable broth, and bring it to a boil.
Then whisk together flour and yogurt, add to the boiling broth, stir in all the spices, switch heat to medium-low level and cook for 5 minutes until thickened.
Serve straight away.

Nutrition:
Calories: 58 Fat: 0.1g Carbs: 13.7g Protein: 0.5g Fiber: 1.0g

Nutrition:
Calories: 282 Cal Fat: 1 g Carbs: 63 g Protein: 3 g Fiber: 12 g

720. Cashew Dip

Preparation Time: 5 minutes | **Cooking Time:** 0 minute | **Servings:** 6

Ingredients:

1 cup cashews	½ teaspoon minced garlic
1/2 teaspoon salt	1/2 teaspoon ground cumin
1 teaspoon red chili powder	2 tablespoons nutritional yeast
1 tablespoon harissa	1 cup hot water

Directions:
Place all the ingredients in a food processor and pulse for 2 minutes until smooth and well combined.
Transfer the dip in a bowl, taste to adjust seasoning, and then serve.

Nutrition:
Calories: 133 Cal Fat: 9 g Carbs: 8 g Protein: 5 g Fiber: 1 g

721. Nacho Cheese Sauce

Preparation Time: 5 minutes | **Cooking Time:** 10 minutes | **Servings:** 4

Ingredients:

3 tablespoons flour	1/4 teaspoon garlic salt
1/4 teaspoon salt	1/2 teaspoon cumin
1/4 teaspoon paprika	1 teaspoon red chili powder
1/8 teaspoon cayenne powder	1 cup vegan cashew yogurt

722. Guacamole

Preparation Time: 15-30 minutes | **Cooking Time:** 15 minutes | **Servings:** 4

Ingredients:

Avocados: 3 ripe	Fresh jalapeño chilies: 1 finely chopped
Red onion: ¼ finely chopped	Tomatoes: 2 small diced
Garlic: ½ crushed	Lime juice: 2 tbsp
Coriander: ¼ cup finely chopped	Sea salt: 1 tsp
Plain tortilla chips to serve	

Directions:
Take a bowl and add onion, chilies, garlic and lime juice
Add salt from the top, mix and leave for 5 minutes
Add the remaining ingredient and mash using a fork
Add avocados, mix and serve with plain tortilla chips

Nutrition:
Carbs: 21. 7 g Protein: 5. 2 g Fats: 7. 1 g Calories: 256 Kcal

723. Lentil Sandwich Spread

Preparation Time: 15 minutes | **Cooking Time:** 20 minutes | **Servings:** 3

Ingredients:

1 tablespoon water or oil	1 small onion, chopped
2 cloves garlic, minced	1 cup dry lentils
2 cups vegetable stock	1 tablespoon apple cider vinegar
2 tablespoons tomato paste	3 sun-dried tomatoes
2 tablespoons maple	1 teaspoon dried oregano
½ teaspoon ground cumin	1 teaspoon coriander
1 teaspoon turmeric	½ lemon, juiced
1 tablespoon fresh parsley, chopped	

Directions:

Warm a Dutch oven over medium heat and add the water or oil.

Immediately add the onions and sauté for two to three minutes or until softened. Add more water if this starts to stick to the pan.

Add the garlic and sauté for one minute.

Add the lentils, vegetable stock, and vinegar; bring to a boil. Turn down to a simmer and cook for 15 minutes or until the lentils are soft and the liquid is almost completely absorbed.

Ladle the lentils into a food processor and add the tomato paste, sun-dried tomatoes, and syrup; process until smooth.

Add the oregano, cumin, coriander, turmeric, and lemon; process until thoroughly mixed.

Remove the spread to a bowl and apply it to bread, toast, a wrap, or pita. Sprinkle With toppings as desired.

Nutrition:

Calories 360 Carbohydrates 60. 7 g Fats 5. 4 g Protein 17. 5 g Mediterranean Tortilla

Chapter 9: Bonus Recipes

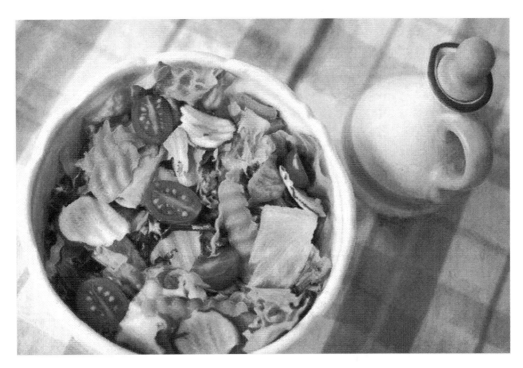

724. Veggie Fried Rice

Preparation Time: 10 minutes | **Cooking Time:** 25 minutes | **Servings:** 4

Ingredients:

2 cups brown rice	2 cups vegetable broth
2 carrots, diced	1 tablespoon olive oil
1 white onion, chopped	2 cloves garlic, minced
½ cup frozen peas	salt and pepper to taste
Diced green scallions for garnish	

Directions:

To the Instant Pot, add the brown rice, broth, and diced carrots. Stir to combine.

Close the lid and set the vent to the Sealing position.

Press the Rice button and cook on low pressure using the pre-set cooking time.

Once the timer goes off, do natural pressure release and open the lid. Fluff the rice and transfer it into a bowl.

Clean the inner pot and place it in the Instant Pot. Press the Sauté button and heat the olive oil.

Sauté the onion and garlic until fragrant.

Add in the peas and stir for 3 minutes.

Stir in the cooked rice and season with salt and pepper to taste. Garnish with green scallions before serving.

Nutrition:

Calories 405, Total Fat 6g, Saturated Fat 1g, Total Carbs 79g, Net Carbs g74, Protein 9g, Sugar: 3g, Fiber: 5g, Sodium: 30mg, Potassium: 385mg, Phosphorus: 338mg

725. Vegetable Lo Mein

Preparation Time: 10 minutes | **Cooking Time:** 15 minutes | **Servings:** 4

Ingredients:

8 ounces of spaghetti noodles	2 cups vegetable broth
1 teaspoon sesame oil	1 teaspoon ginger paste
1 teaspoon minced garlic	1 tablespoon soy sauce
1 tablespoon vinegar	1 teaspoon red chili paste

1 teaspoon brown sugar	1 teaspoon coconut oil
½ cup carrots, thinly sliced	½ cup cabbages, thinly sliced
½ cup broccoli florets	salt and pepper to taste
½ cup green scallions	Toasted sesame seeds for garnish

Directions:

Place the spaghetti noodles and vegetable broth in the Instant Pot.

Close the lid and set the vent to the Sealing position. Press the Pressure Cook or Manual button and adjust the cooking time to 8 minutes. Do quick pressure release and drain the noodles. Set the noodles aside to cool.

Meanwhile, mix the sesame oil, ginger paste, garlic, soy sauce, vinegar, chili paste, and brown sugar. Set aside.

Clean the inner pot and place it in the Instant Pot. Press the Sauté button and heat the oil. Sauté the carrots, cabbages, and broccoli florets. Season with salt and pepper to taste. Stir for 3 minutes. Add in the noodles and the sauce prepared earlier.

Toss to coat the noodles and vegetables.

Press the Cancel button to turn off the cooking. Garnish with scallions and sesame seeds before serving.

Nutrition:

Calories 120, Total Fat 3g, Saturated Fat 1g, Total Carbs 20g, Net Carbs 16g, Protein 4g, Sugar: 3g, Fiber: 4g, Sodium: 75mg, Potassium: 155mg, Phosphorus: 74mg

726. Herb and Vegetable Brown Rice

Preparation Time: 10 minutes | **Cooking Time:** 25 minutes | **Servings:** 6

Ingredients:

1 ½ tablespoon olive oil	1 cup onion, chopped
4 cloves of garlic, minced	½ cup red bell pepper, chopped
½ cup celery, chopped	¼ teaspoon dried oregano
1 ½ cup long-grain brown rice	1 ¾ cup water

salt and pepper to taste	½ cup fresh parsley, minced

Directions:

Press the Sauté button on the Instant Pot and heat the olive oil. Sauté the onion and garlic until fragrant. Stir in the bell pepper, celery, and oregano for 2 minutes until the celery has wilted. Stir in the brown rice, water, salt, and pepper. Stir everything to combine.

Press the Rice button and cook using the pre-set cooking time. Do natural pressure release.

Once the lid is open, fluff the rice and garnish with chopped parsley.

Nutrition:

Calories 233, Total Fat 6g, Saturated Fat 1g, Total Carbs 40g, Net Carbs 37g, Protein 6g, Sugar: 2g, Fiber: 3g, Sodium: 35mg, Potassium: 242mg, Phosphorus: 181mg

727. Kung Pao Brussels Sprouts

Preparation Time: 5 minutes | **Cooking Time:** 4 hours and 5 minutes | **Servings:** 4

Ingredients:

2 pounds Brussels sprouts, halved	½ cup of water
2 tablespoons extra-virgin olive oil	salt and pepper to taste
1 tablespoon sesame oil	2 cloves of garlic, minced
½ cup of soy sauce	2 teaspoons apple cider vinegar
1 tablespoon hoisin sauce	1 tablespoon brown sugar
2 teaspoons garlic chili sauce	1 tablespoon cornstarch + 2 tablespoons water
Sesame seeds for garnish	Green onions for garnish
2 tablespoons chopped roasted peanuts	

Directions:

Place the Brussels sprouts and water in the Instant Pot and drizzle over the olive oil. Season with salt and pepper to taste. Close the lid but do not seal the vent.

Press the Slow Cook button and adjust the cooking time to 4 hours.

Take the broccoli out and set it aside.

To the inner pot, stir in the sesame oil and press the Sauté button. Stir in the garlic for 30 seconds. Add in the water and bring to a boil.

Stir in the soy sauce, apple cider vinegar, hoisin sauce, brown sugar, and garlic sauce. Bring to a boil and add in the cornstarch slurry until the sauce thickens.

Add the slow-cooked broccoli into the sauce.

Garnish with sesame seeds, green onions, and roasted peanuts before serving.

Nutrition:
Calories 343, Total Fat 16g, Saturated Fat 3g, Total Carbs 43g, Net Carbs 32g, Protein 13g, Sugar: 20g, Fiber: 11g, Sodium: 757mg, Potassium: 1151mg, Phosphorus: 257mg

728. Parsnips and Carrots

Preparation Time: 5 minutes | **Cooking Time:** 10 minutes | **Servings:** 4

Ingredients:

1 tablespoon olive oil	2 cloves of garlic, minced
2 pounds carrots, peeled and sliced	2 pounds parsnips, peeled and sliced
½ cup of water	¼ cup maple syrup
Salt and pepper to taste	Fresh parsley, chopped

Directions:
Press the Sauté button on the Instant Pot and heat the oil.

Sauté the garlic for 30 seconds until fragrant.

Stir in the carrots and parsnips for 3 minutes.

Pour in water and maple syrup. Season with salt and pepper to taste.

Close the lid and set the vent to the Sealing position.

Press the Pressure Cooker or Manual button and adjust the cooking time to 6 minutes.

Do natural pressure release.

Once the lid is open, garnish with parsley.

Nutrition:
Calories 356, Total Fat 5g, Saturated Fat 0.7g, Total Carbs 78g, Net Carbs 60g, Protein 6g, Sugar: 34g, Fiber: 18g, Sodium: 192mg, Potassium: 1745mg, Phosphorus: 257mg

729. Vegetarian Pad Thai

Preparation Time: 10 minutes | **Cooking Time:** 9 minutes | **Servings:** 4

Ingredients:

½ cup of soy sauce	1 tablespoon fresh lime juice
2 tablespoons of rice wine vinegar	3 tablespoons coconut aminos
1/3 cup granulated sugar	1 tablespoon vegetable oil
12 ounces extra-firm tofu, sliced	1 onion, chopped
1 clove garlic, minced	10 ounces Pad Thai rice noodles
2 cups vegetable stock	2 tablespoons shredded radish
1 cup bean sprouts	1 medium carrot, peeled and shredded
¼ cup unsalted peanuts, roasted	3 scallions, chopped
1 medium lime, cut into wedges	

Directions:
In a mixing bowl, combine the soy sauce, lime juice, wine vinegar, coconut aminos, and sugar. Set aside.

Press the Sauté button on the Instant Pot and heat the olive. Brown the tofu for 3 minutes on each side. Set aside.

Sauté the onion and garlic for 30 seconds until fragrant.

Add the rice noodles, tofu, and vegetable stock. Close the lid and set the vent to the Sealing position.

Press the Pressure Cooker or Manual button and adjust the cooking time to 6 minutes.

Do quick pressure release. Once the lid is open, drain the noodles and set them aside.

Place the noodles in bowls and top with radish, bean sprouts, carrots, peanuts, scallions, and lime wedges.

Drizzle with the prepared sauce.

Nutrition:
Calories 559, Total Fat 12g, Saturated Fat 4g, Total Carbs 93g, Net Carbs g, Protein 17g, Sugar: 23g, Fiber: 4g, Sodium: 432mg, Potassium: 521mg, Phosphorus: 125mg

730. Red Curry Vegetables

Preparation Time: 5 minutes | **Cooking Time:** 15 minutes | **Servings:** 4

Ingredients:

1 onion, chopped	3 cloves garlic, minced
2 ½ cups chopped cauliflower florets	2 ½ cups cubed sweet potato
1 can coconut milk	1 can diced tomatoes
3 tablespoon red curry paste	2 teaspoons soy sauce
1 teaspoon turmeric	1 cup of water
A bunch of kale leaves	Fresh lime juice
Fresh cilantro leaves	

Directions:

Place the onions and garlic in the Instant Pot. Add a teaspoon of water. Press the Sauté button and do water sauté for 1 minute.

Stir in the cauliflower, sweet potato, milk, tomatoes, red curry paste, soy sauce, and turmeric. Add water.

Close the lid and set the vent to the Sealing position.

Press the Pressure Cooker or Manual button and adjust the cooking time to 10 minutes.

Do quick pressure release.

Once the lid is open, press the Sauté button and add the kale leaves. Cook for 3 more minutes until the kale leaves are wilted.

Serve with lime juice and cilantro leaves.

Nutrition:

Calories 70, Total Fat 1g, Saturated Fat 0g, Total Carbs 14g, Net Carbs 9g, Protein 3g, Sugar: 6g, Fiber:5 g, Sodium: 172mg, Potassium: 615mg, Phosphorus: 84mg

731. Vegetable Chow Mein

Preparation Time: 5 minutes | **Cooking Time:** 10 minutes | **Servings:** 5

Ingredients:

4 cups vegetable broth	2 tablespoon dark soy sauce
1 teaspoon sesame oil	1 tablespoon vinegar
1 tablespoons sriracha sauce	1 tablespoon brown sugar
16 ounces Hakka noodles	1 teaspoon grated ginger
1 teaspoon grated garlic	1 cup cabbage, thinly sliced
½ cup celery, chopped	2 carrots, peeled and julienned
1 cup snow peas, trimmed	1 cup broccoli florets
½ cup green onion, chopped	

Directions:

In a bowl, mix the vegetable broth, soy sauce, sesame oil, sriracha sauce, and brown sugar. Whisk and set aside.

Press the Sauté button on the Instant Pot and pour the prepared sauce. Spread the noodles over the sauce. Top with grated ginger, garlic, cabbage, celery, and carrots.

Close the lid and set the vent to the Sealing position.

Press the Pressure Cooker or Manual button. Adjust the cooking time to 5 minutes.

Do quick pressure release.

Once the lid is open, press the Sauté button and stir in the snow peas and broccoli. Cook for 5 minutes.

Garnish with green onion.

Nutrition:

Calories 172, Total Fat 2g, Saturated Fat 0.4g, Total Carbs 33g, Net Carbs 31g, Protein 5g, Sugar: 5g, Fiber: 2g, Sodium: 295mg, Potassium: 201mg, Phosphorus: 56mg

732. Instant Pot Carrots

Preparation Time: 5 minutes | **Cooking Time:** 8 minutes | **Servings:** 4

Ingredients:

2 pounds fresh carrots, cut into thick strips	1 cup of water
1 tablespoon olive oil	1 teaspoon fresh thyme

Directions:

Place the carrots and water in the Instant Pot.

Lock the lid and set the vent to the Sealing position.

Press the Pressure Cooker or Manual button and adjust the cooking time to 5 minutes.

Once the timer sets off, do a quick pressure release and drain the carrots.

Clean the inner pot.

Press the Sauté button and heat the oil. Stir in the thyme to toast and add in the carrots. Stir fry for 3 minutes.

Nutrition:

Calories 109, Total Fat 4g, Saturated Fat 0.5g, Total Carbs 19g, Net Carbs 12g, Protein 2g, Sugar: 8g, Fiber: 7g, Sodium: 132mg, Potassium: 534mg, Phosphorus: 68mg

733. Instant Pot Carrot Soup

Preparation Time: 10 minutes | **Cooking Time:** 20 minutes | **Servings:** 4

Ingredients:

1 tablespoon olive oil	1 onion, chopped
4 cloves garlic, minced	1 carrot, peeled and diced
1 teaspoon dried oregano	½ teaspoon paprika
½ teaspoon cumin	½ teaspoon chopped mint
½ cup coarse bulgur	salt and pepper to taste
4 cups vegetable stock	2 cups baby spinach
1 lemon juice, freshly squeezed	

Directions:

Press the Sauté button on the Instant Pot and heat the oil.

Sauté the onion and garlic for 30 seconds or until fragrant.

Stir in the carrot, oregano, paprika, cumin, mint, bulgur, and vegetable stock. Season with salt and pepper to taste.

Close the lid and set the vent to the Sealing position.

Press the Pressure Cook or Manual button and adjust the cooking time to 15 minutes.

Do quick pressure release.

Once the lid is open, press the Sauté button and stir in the spinach. Cook for 3 minutes or until the spinach has wilted.

Drizzle with lemon juice before serving.

Nutrition:

Calories 118, Total Fat 6g, Saturated Fat g, Total Carbs 11g, Net Carbs g, Protein 7g, Sugar: 2g, Fiber: 2.5g, Sodium: 33mg, Potassium: 273mg, Phosphorus:79 mg

734. Summer Vegetable Soup

Preparation Time: 10 minutes | **Cooking Time:** 20 minutes | **Servings:** 4

Ingredients:

4 cups vegetable broth	1 14-ounce can diced tomatoes
2 tablespoon tomato paste	1 small yellow onion, diced
1 red bell pepper, diced	1 small zucchini, chopped
2 ears of corn, shucked	1 tablespoon fresh lemon juice
1 tablespoon fresh parsley, chopped	salt and pepper to taste

Directions:

Place all ingredients in the Instant Pot and give a good stir.

Press the Broth/Soup button and adjust the cooking time to 20 minutes. Cook on high pressure.

Do quick pressure release.

Nutrition:

Calories 97, Total Fat 1g, Saturated Fat 0.2g, Total Carbs 22g, Net Carbs 17g, Protein 4g, Sugar: 7g, Fiber: 5g, Sodium: 132mg, Potassium: 547mg, Phosphorus: 100mg

735. Hibachi Mushroom Steak

Preparation Time: minutes | **Cooking Time:** minutes | **Servings:** 2

Ingredients:

1/3 cup soy sauce	2 tablespoons white vinegar
1 tablespoon grated ginger	1 tablespoon minced garlic
1-pound large chestnut mushrooms stems removed	1 zucchini, sliced in rounds
1 yellow onion.	1 tablespoon granulated sugar
Salt and pepper to taste	

Directions:

Place all ingredients in a bowl and allow ingredients to marinate in the fridge for at least 30 minutes.

Pour in the Instant Pot all ingredients.

Close the lid and set the vent to the Sealing position.

Press the Pressure Cook or Manual button and cook on high. Adjust the cooking time to 5 minutes.

Do natural pressure release.

Nutrition:

Calories 208, Total Fat 8g, Saturated Fat 2g, Total Carbs 26g, Net Carbs 22g, Protein 11g, Sugar: 18g, Fiber: 4g, Sodium: 650mg, Potassium: 950mg, Phosphorus: 265mg

736. Lemony Rice and Vegetable Soup

Preparation Time: 10 minutes | **Cooking Time:** 20 minutes | **Servings:** 4

Ingredients:

1 tablespoon extra-virgin olive oil	1 yellow onion, chopped
2 cloves of garlic, minced	2 large carrots, diced
2 stalks celery, diced	½ large fennel bulb, diced
½ teaspoon ground cumin	1 cup brown basmati rice
2 handful spinach	6 cups vegetable broth
salt and pepper to taste	4 tablespoons fresh lemon juice

Directions:

Press the Sauté button on the Instant Pot and heat the oil.

Sauté the onion and garlic for 30 seconds until fragrant.

Stir in the carrots, celery, fennel, and cumin. Stir for 2 minutes until the vegetables are wilted.

Add in the rice, spinach, and broth. Season with salt and pepper to taste.

Stir the ingredients until well-combined.

Close the lid and set the vent to the Sealing position.

Press the Rice button and cook using the preset cooking time.

Do natural pressure release.

Once the lid is open, drizzle with lemon juice then fluff the rice.

Nutrition:

Calories 245, Total Fat 5g, Saturated Fat 0.8g, Total Carbs 45g, Net Carbs 41g, Protein 5g, Sugar: 5g, Fiber: 4g, Sodium: 84mg, Potassium: 418mg, Phosphorus: 196mg

737. Vegetable Pho Soup

Preparation Time: 10 minutes | **Cooking Time:** 40 minutes | **Servings:** 4

Ingredients:

2 tablespoons olive oil	1 onion, quartered
5 whole star anise pods	1 tablespoon fennel seeds
1 tablespoon coriander seeds	1 cinnamon stick
½ tablespoon whole black peppercorns	1 cup dried mushrooms
1 1-inch ginger, peeled	2 kaffir lime leaves
2 bay leaves	2 celery stalks, chopped roughly
1 large carrot, chopped roughly	4 cups of water
salt to taste	2 cup broccoli florets
2 tablespoons cilantro, chopped	1 cup straw mushrooms
8 ounces shiitake mushrooms	1 small zucchini, chopped
1 cup mung bean sprouts	1 cup basil leaves
1 lime, cut into wedges	Sriracha sauce

Directions:

Press the Sauté button and heat the oil. Toast the onion, anise, fennel seeds, coriander, cinnamon stick, black peppercorns, dried mushrooms, ginger, kaffir lime leaves, and bay leaves. Stir for 2 minutes until fragrant.

Add in the celery and carrots and stir for another 3 minutes before pouring in water. Season with salt to taste.

Close the lid and set the vent to the Sealing position.

Press the Broth/Soup button and cook using the preset cooking time. Do quick pressure release once the timer has set off.

Once the lid is open, remove the solids. Add in the broccoli, cilantro, mushrooms, and zucchini.

Close the lid again and set the vent to the Sealing position. Press the Pressure Cook or Manual button and adjust the cooking time to 5 minutes. Do natural pressure release.

Garnish with bean sprouts, basil leaves, and lime wedges before serving. Drizzle with sriracha sauce if desired.

Nutrition:
Calories 171, Total Fat 9g, Saturated Fat 1g, Total Carbs 23g, Net Carbs 17g, Protein 6g, Sugar: 6g, Fiber: 6g, Sodium: 215mg, Potassium: 511mg, Phosphorus: 143mg

738. Veggie Macaroni

Preparation Time: 10 minutes | **Cooking Time:** 20 minutes | **Servings:** 4

Ingredients:

2 cups dry macaroni	2 cups of water
1 ½ cups marinara sauce	½ cup of coconut milk
1 cup frozen veggies of your choice	2 tablespoons nutritional yeast
salt and pepper to taste	

Directions:
Add all ingredients to the Instant Pot and give a good stir.

Close the lid and set the vent to the Sealing position.

Press the Multigrain button and cook on high. Adjust the cooking time to 20 minutes.

Do natural pressure release.

Nutrition:
Calories 330, Total Fat 9g, Saturated Fat 7g, Total Carbs 51g, Net Carbs 56g, Protein 11g, Sugar: 8g, Fiber: 5g, Sodium: 306mg, Potassium: 692mg, Phosphorus: 171mg

739. Instant Pot Broccoli

Preparation Time: 10 minutes | **Cooking Time:** 10 minutes | **Servings:** 4

Ingredients:

2 heads broccoli, cut into florets	2 tablespoons coconut oil
salt and pepper to taste	3 tablespoons nutritional yeast

Directions:
Pour a cup of water into the Instant Pot and place a steamer basket or trivet.

Place the broccoli florets in the steamer basket.

Close the lid and set the vent to the Sealing position.

Press the Steam button and cook for 10 minutes. Do quick pressure release.

Once the lid is open, take the broccoli out and place it in a bowl.

Drizzle with oil and season with salt, pepper, and nutritional yeast.

Toss to combine everything.

Nutrition:
Calories 88, Total Fat 7g, Saturated Fat 4g, Total Carbs 3g, Net Carbs 2g, Protein 4g, Sugar: 0.3g, Fiber: 1g, Sodium: 406mg, Potassium: 323mg, Phosphorus: 29mg

740. Vegan Jambalaya

Preparation Time: 10 minutes | **Cooking Time:** 25 minutes | **Servings:** 4

Ingredients:

1 tablespoon oil	1 onion, diced
1 green bell pepper, seeded and diced	3 ribs of celery, diced
4 cloves of garlic, minced	1 ½ cup long-grain white rice
1 can small diced tomatoes	1 tablespoon Cajun seasoning
2 teaspoons smoked paprika	3 cups vegetable broth
¼ cup chopped parsley	salt and pepper to taste

Directions:
Press the Sauté button on the Instant Pot and heat the oil.

Sauté the onion, green bell pepper, celery, and garlic. Stir for 2 minutes until fragrant.

Add in the rest of the ingredients and give a good stir.

Close the lid and set the vent to the Sealing position.

Press the Rice button and cook on low pressure. Do natural pressure release.

Nutrition:
Calories 319, Total Fat 4g, Saturated Fat 0.7g, Total Carbs 63g, Net Carbs 60g, Protein 6g,

Sugar: 3g, Fiber: 3g, Sodium: 165mg, Potassium: 293mg, Phosphorus: 109mg

741. Instant Pot Veggie Curry

Preparation Time: 5 minutes | **Cooking Time:** 10 minutes | **Servings:** 4

Ingredients:

1 tablespoon coconut oil	1 onion, diced
1 teaspoon mustard seeds	4 cloves of garlic, minced
2 tablespoons Indian curry powder	1 teaspoon grated ginger
1 cup vegetable broth	1 cup light coconut milk
1 butternut squash, seeded and diced	1 red bell pepper, diced
1 14-ounce canned chickpeas, drained and rinsed	2 tablespoons brown sugar
½ teaspoon salt	Chopped cilantro for garnish

Directions:

Set the Instant Pot to the Sauté mode and add oil. Stir in the onion, mustard seeds, garlic, curry powder, and ginger. Keep stirring for 1 minute until fragrant.

Add in the broth, coconut milk, squash, bell pepper, and chickpeas. Season with brown sugar and salt.

Close the lid and set the vent to the Sealing position.

Press the Pressure Cook or Manual button and cook on high. Adjust the cooking time to 10 minutes.

Do quick pressure release.

Garnish with cilantro before serving.

Nutrition:

Calories 353, Total Fat 21g, Saturated Fat 16g, Total Carbs 37g, Net Carbs 27g, Protein 10g, Sugar: 11g, Fiber: 10g, Sodium: 397mg, Potassium: 515mg, Phosphorus: 173mg

742. Potato Curry

Preparation Time: 10 minutes | **Cooking Time:** 30 minutes | **Servings:** 5

Ingredients:

1 teaspoon oil	1 yellow onion, chopped
4 cloves of garlic, minced	5 cups baby potatoes, scrubbed clean
2 tablespoons curry powder	2 cups of water
1 can coconut milk, full fat	Salt and pepper to taste
1 teaspoon chili pepper flakes	2 cups green beans, chopped into inch-thick pieces
3 tablespoons arrowroot powder + 4 tablespoons water	

Directions:

Set the Sauté button on the Instant Pot and heat oil. Sauté the onion and garlic for 30 seconds until fragrant.

Stir in the potatoes and curry powder. Keep stirring for 3 minutes.

Add water and coconut milk. Season with salt, pepper, and chili flakes.

Close the lid and set the vent to the Sealing position.

Press the Pressure Cook or Manual button and cook on high. Adjust the cooking time to 20 minutes.

Do quick pressure release.

Once the lid is open, press the Sauté button and add in the green beans. Cook for 5 minutes.

Stir in the arrowroot slurry and allow to thicken for 5 more minutes.

Nutrition:

Calories 187, Total Fat 4g, Saturated Fat 0.6g, Total Carbs 36g, Net Carbs 29g, Protein 5g, Sugar: 6g, Fiber: 7g, Sodium: 61mg, Potassium: 917mg, Phosphorus: 133mg

743. Vegan Tofu and Little Potato Stew

Preparation Time: 10 minutes | **Cooking Time:** 28 minutes | **Servings:** 5

Ingredients:

2 tablespoons olive oil	1 block (350g) extra-firm tofu, cubed
½ cup chopped yellow onion	2 cloves of garlic
1 ½ cups carrots	1 ½ cup chopped celery
1 ½ pounds baby potatoes, scrubbed	1 cup frozen peas
2 tablespoons soy sauce	6 cups vegetable broth
3 tablespoons tomato paste	1 cup of water
salt and pepper to taste	2 tablespoons cornstarch + 3 tablespoons water

Directions:

Press the Sauté button on the Instant Pot and heat the oil.

Sear the tofu on all sides until lightly golden.

Stir in the onion and garlic until fragrant.

Add the carrots, celery, potatoes, and peas. Stir-fry the vegetables for 2 minutes.

Pour in the water and season with soy sauce, salt, and pepper. Add the tomato paste.

Close the lid and set the vent to the Sealing position.

Press the Meat/Stew button and adjust the cooking time to 20 minutes.

Do quick pressure release.

Once the lid is open, press the Sauté button and stir in the cornstarch slurry and cook for 5 minutes until the sauce thickens.

Nutrition:

Calories 152, Total Fat 7g, Saturated Fat 2g, Total Carbs 17g, Net Carbs 14g, Protein 6g, Sugar: 3g, Fiber: 3g, Sodium: 880mg, Potassium: 975mg, Phosphorus: 436mg

744. Instant Pot Cabbage

Preparation Time: 10 minutes | **Cooking Time:** 9vminutes | **Servings:** 6

Ingredients:

1 onion, diced	2 cups vegetable broth
1 teaspoon oregano	½ teaspoon thyme
1 head of green cabbage, chopped	salt and pepper to taste

Directions:

Press the Sauté button on the Instant Pot and cook the onion with a tablespoon of vegetable broth for 3 minutes. Stir in the oregano and thyme and cook for another minute.

Stir in the remaining broth and cabbages. Season with salt and pepper to taste.

Close the lid and set the vent to the Sealing position.

Press the Pressure Cook or Manual button and cook on high. Adjust the cooking time to 5 minutes.

Do natural pressure release.

Nutrition:

Calories 69, Total Fat 3g, Saturated Fat 0.5g, Total Carbs 11g, Net Carbs 8g, Protein 2g, Sugar: 5g, Fiber: 3g, Sodium: 416mg, Potassium: 340mg, Phosphorus: 57mg

745. Instant Pot Homestyle Veggies

Preparation Time: 5 minutes | **Cooking Time:** 20 minutes | **Servings:** 4

Ingredients:

1 cup vegetable broth	½ pound whole carrots, peeled and roughly chopped
1-pound fresh green beans, trimmed	1 ½ pounds red potatoes, cut in half
salt and pepper to taste	

Directions:

Pour broth into the Instant Pot.

Place the vegetables on a steamer basket or trivet and season with salt and pepper to taste.

Close the lid and set the vent to the Sealing position.

Press the Steam button and cook using the pre-set cooking time.

Do natural pressure release.

Nutrition:
Calories 122, Total Fat 0g, Saturated Fat 0g, Total Carbs 26g, Net Carbs g, Protein 4g, Sugar: 4g, Fiber: 4g, Sodium: 39mg, Potassium: 673mg, Phosphorus: 235mg

746. Instant Pot Steamed Vegetables

Preparation Time: 10 minutes | **Cooking Time:** 5 minutes | **Servings:** 6

Ingredients:

1 cup of water	2 cups raw baby carrots
2 cups raw cauliflower florets	2 cups raw broccoli florets

Directions:
Pour water into the Instant Pot and place a steamer basket or trivet inside.

Place the vegetables in the steamer basket.

Close the lid and set the vent to the Sealing position.

Press the Steam button and cook using the pre-set cooking time.

Do natural pressure release.

Nutrition:
Calories 27, Total Fat 0.3g, Saturated Fat 0g, Total Carbs 6g, Net Carbs 4g, Protein 2g, Sugar: 2g, Fiber:2 g, Sodium: 40mg, Potassium: 250mg, Phosphorus: 38mg

747. Instant Pot Vegetable Korma

Preparation Time: 10 minutes | **Cooking Time:** 27minutes | **Servings:** 4

Ingredients:

1 large sweet onion, chopped	15 raw cashews, soaked in water overnight
1 1-inch ginger, sliced	4 cloves garlic, peeled
2 tablespoons coconut oil	6 whole black peppercorns
4 green cardamoms	4 whole cloves
1 bay leaf	½ cup tomato puree
2 tablespoons garam masala or curry powder	½ teaspoon sugar
1 large potato, peeled and diced	2 medium carrots, peeled and diced
¼ cup of frozen green peas	1 cup of coconut milk
½ cup of water	Juice from half of lemon
salt and pepper to taste	2 tablespoons chopped cilantro

Directions:
Place the onion, cashews, ginger, and garlic in a blender and pulse until smooth. Set aside.

Press the Sauté button on the Instant Pot and heat the oil. Toast the peppercorns, cardamoms, cloves, bay leaf for 2 minutes until fragrant.

Stir in the onion-cashew paste and stir for 3 minutes. Add the tomato puree and stir to remove the brown bits at the bottom.

Add the garam masala and sugar. Stir in the vegetables. Continue stirring for 2 minutes.

Stir in the coconut milk, water, and lemon juice. Season with salt and pepper to taste.

Press the Cancel button and close the lid. Set the vent to the Sealing position.

Press the Meat/Stew button and cook on the lowest pre-set cooking button.

Do natural pressure release.

Serve with chopped cilantro.

Nutrition:
Calories 189, Total Fat 21g, Saturated Fat 11g, Total Carbs 14g, Net Carbs 11g, Protein 4g, Sugar: 4g, Fiber: 3g, Sodium: 341mg, Potassium: 509mg, Phosphorus: 236mg

748. One-Pot Vegetarian Linguine

Preparation Time: 10 minutes | **Cooking Time:** 10 minutes | **Servings:** 6

Ingredients:

1 tablespoon olive oil	2 small onions, chopped
1 clove garlic, minced	½ pound fresh cremini mushrooms, sliced
1 large tomato, chopped	2 medium zucchinis, thinly sliced

4 tablespoons nutritional yeast

salt and pepper

6 ounces uncooked linguine

3 cups of water

2 tablespoons cornstarch + 3 tablespoons water

Directions:

Press the Sauté button on the Instant Pot. Heat the oil and sauté the onions and garlic for 1 minute until fragrant.

Stir in the mushrooms and tomato. Stir for a minute.

Add in the zucchini and season with nutritional yeast, salt, and pepper to taste.

Add the linguine and water. Stir to combine.

Close the lid and set the vent to the Sealing position.

Press the Pressure Cook or Manual button and cook on high. Adjust the cooking time to 6 minutes.

Do quick pressure release once the timer sets off.

Open the lid and press the Sauté button. Stir in the cornstarch slurry and continue to stir until the sauce thickens.

Nutrition:

Calories 239, Total Fat 3g, Saturated Fat 0.4g, Total Carbs 52g, Net Carbs 44g, Protein 8g, Sugar: 18g, Fiber:8 g, Sodium: 366mg, Potassium: 1286mg, Phosphorus: 162mg

749. Creamy Cauliflower and Broccoli Medley

Preparation Time: 5 minutes | **Cooking Time:** 5 minutes | **Servings:** 8

Ingredients:

2 pounds bag of cauliflower and broccoli florets mix

1 can coconut milk

Zest of 1 lemon

Juice from ½ lemon

¼ teaspoon garlic powder

¼ teaspoon oregano

¼ teaspoon dried parsley

¼ teaspoon dried basil

1/8 teaspoon onion powder

salt and pepper to taste

Directions:

Place all ingredients in the Instant Pot.

Stir to combine everything.

Close the lid and set the vent to the Sealing position.

Press the Pressure Cooker or Manual button and cook on high. Adjust the cooking time to 5 minutes.

Do natural pressure release.

Nutrition:

Calories 32, Total Fat 0.6g, Saturated Fat 0g, Total Carbs 5g, Net Carbs 2g, Protein 4g, Sugar: 1g, Fiber:3 g, Sodium: 65mg, Potassium: 299mg, Phosphorus: 89mg

750. Potato and Carrot Medley

Preparation Time: 10 minutes | **Cooking Time:** 19 minutes | **Servings:** 6

Ingredients:

2 tablespoons extra virgin olive oil

1 onion, chopped

3 cloves of garlic, minced

4 pounds Yukon potatoes, cut into chunks

2 pounds carrots, sliced

1 teaspoon Italian seasoning mix

salt and pepper to taste

1 ½ cup vegetable broth

Fresh parsley for garnish

Directions:

Press the Sauté button on the Instant Pot and heat the oil.

Sauté the onion and garlic. Stir for 30 seconds until fragrant.

Stir in the potatoes and carrots. Season with salt, pepper, and Italian seasoning mix. Stir for 3 minutes.

Add in the broth.

Close the lid and set the vent to the Sealing position.

Press the Pressure Cooker or Manual button and cook on high. Adjust the cooking time to 15 minutes.

Do natural pressure release.

Once the lid is open, garnish with parsley before serving.

Nutrition:

Calories 341, Total Fat 4g, Saturated Fat 0.8g, Total Carbs 71g, Net Carbs 60g, Protein 9g,

Sugar: 11g, Fiber: 11g, Sodium: 354mg, Potassium: 1810mg, Phosphorus: 242mg

751. Instant Pot Vegetable Spaghetti

Preparation Time: 5 minutes | **Cooking Time:** 6 minutes | **Servings:** 6

Ingredients:

1 tablespoon olive oil	2 cloves of garlic, minced
4 ounces mushrooms, diced	1 large carrot, chopped
2 zucchinis, chopped	1 green bell pepper, diced
½ cup chopped basil	2 cups of water
8 ounces of spaghetti noodles	24 ounces pasta sauce
salt and pepper to taste	

Directions:

Press the Sauté button on the Instant Pot.

Heat the oil and stir in the garlic once the oil is hot. Add in the mushrooms and sauté for 4 minutes.

Add the carrots, zucchini, and bell pepper. Stir for another 3 minutes. Add the basil.

Deglaze the pot with water to remove the browned bits.

Break the spaghetti pasta into the Instant Pot. Pour over the remaining water and pasta sauce. Season with salt and pepper to taste.

Close the lid and set the vent to the Sealing position.

Press the Pressure Cooker or Manual button and cook on high for 6 minutes.

Do quick pressure release.

Once the lid is open, give the pasta a good mix to combine everything.

Nutrition:

Calories 114, Total Fat 3g, Saturated Fat 0.4g, Total Carbs 21g, Net Carbs 16g, Protein 5g, Sugar: 6g, Fiber: 5g, Sodium: 812mg, Potassium: 491mg, Phosphorus: 102mg

752. Lemon Couscous

Preparation Time: 10 minutes | **Cooking Time:** 24 minutes | **Servings:** 4

Ingredients:

1 cup pearl couscous	1 ¼ cup water
1 tablespoon olive oil	¾ cup sliced scallions
1 clove garlic, minced	¾ teaspoon salt
¼ teaspoon pepper	1 teaspoon lemon zest

Directions:

Place couscous and water in the Instant Pot.

Close the lid and set the vent to the Sealing position. Press the Rice button and cook using the preset cooking time.

Once the timer sets off, open the lid and fluff the couscous. Remove from the Instant Pot and clean the inner pot.

Return the inner pot into the Instant Pot and press the Sauté button. Heat the oil and sauté the scallions and garlic for 30 seconds until fragrant. Stir in the couscous and season with salt, pepper, and lemon zest.

Stir for 3 minutes.

Serve warm.

Nutrition:

Calories 81, Total Fat 3g, Saturated Fat g0.5, Total Carbs 11g, Net Carbs 10g, Protein 2g, Sugar: 0.5g, Fiber: 1g, Sodium: 5mg, Potassium: 79mg, Phosphorus: 17mg

753. Veggie Pasta Shells

Preparation Time: 10 minutes | **Cooking Time:** 10 minutes | **Servings:** 6

Ingredients:

2 tablespoons olive oil	1 small onion, chopped
1 clove garlic, minced	½ bunch broccoli, cut into florets
1 cup shredded carrot	¼ cup basil leaves
½ cup marinara sauce	1 box pasta shells
4 tablespoons nutritional yeast	salt and pepper to taste

Directions:

Press the Sauté button on the Instant Pot and heat the oil.

Sauté the onion and garlic until fragrant. Stir in the rest of the ingredients.

Give a stir to combine.

Close the lid and set the vent to the Sealing position.

Press the Pressure Cook or Manual button and cook on high. Adjust the cooking time to 8 minutes.

Once the timer sets off, do a quick pressure release.

Nutrition:

Calories 98, Total Fat 5g, Saturated Fat 0.7g, Total Carbs 8g, Net Carbs 5g, Protein 5g, Sugar: 3g, Fiber: 3g, Sodium: 396mg, Potassium: 523mg, Phosphorus: 60mg

754. Veggies with Herbed Mushrooms

Preparation Time: 5 minutes | **Cooking Time:** 8 minutes | **Servings:** 6

Ingredients:

1 tablespoon coconut oil	1 onion, chopped
4 cloves garlic, minced	3 ounces shiitake mushrooms, sliced
3 ounces cremini mushrooms, sliced	3 ounces button mushrooms, sliced
1 teaspoon dried thyme	1 teaspoon Italian oregano
salt and pepper to taste	12 ounces of frozen vegetables
1 cup vegetable broth	

Directions:

Press the Sauté button on the Instant Pot and heat the oil. Sauté the onion and garlic for 30 seconds until fragrant.

Stir in the mushrooms and season with thyme, oregano, salt, and pepper. Stir for 2 minutes.

Add in the rest of the ingredients.

Close the lid and set the vent to the Sealing position.

Press the Pressure Cook or Manual button and cook on high. Set the cooking time to 5 minutes.

Do natural pressure release once the timer sets off.

Nutrition:

Calories 159, Total Fat 3g, Saturated Fat 2g, Total Carbs 33g, Net Carbs 26g, Protein 5g, Sugar: 4g, Fiber: 7g, Sodium: 25mg, Potassium: 585mg, Phosphorus: 125mg

755. Simple Steamed Butternut Squash

Preparation Time: 10 minutes | **Cooking Time:** 10minutes | **Servings:** 4

Ingredients:

1 cup of water	1 medium butternut squash, peeled and sliced thickly
2 tablespoons extra virgin olive oil	1 tablespoon vegetable bouillon, cracked into powder
salt and pepper to taste	

Directions:

Place a cup of water in the Instant Pot and place a trivet or steamer basket inside.

In a bowl, season the butternut squash with olive oil, vegetable bouillon, salt, and pepper.

Place in a heat-proof dish that will fit inside the Instant Pot.

Place inside the Instant Pot and close the lid. Set the vent to the Sealing position.

Press the Steam button and cook on high for 10 minutes.

Do natural pressure release.

Nutrition:

Calories 57, Total Fat 6g, Saturated Fat 3g, Total Carbs 1g, Net Carbs 0.5g, Protein 0.01g, Sugar: 0.005g, Fiber: 0.5g, Sodium: 60mg, Potassium: 9mg, Phosphorus:2 mg

756. Summer Squash and Mint Pasta

Preparation Time: 10 minutes | **Cooking Time:** 10 minutes | **Servings:** 5

Ingredients:

2 tablespoons olive oil	1 shallot, minced
1 cup sliced squash	1/3 cup mint, chopped
1 tablespoon lemon juice	12 ounces rigatoni pasta
4 tablespoons nutritional yeast	
salt and pepper to taste	
1 ½ cups water	

Directions:

Press the Sauté button on the Instant Pot. Heat the oil.

Sauté the shallots until fragrant. Add in the squash, mint, and the rest of the ingredients. Give a good stir.

Close the lid and set the vent to the Sealing position.

Press the Pressure Cook or Manual button. Adjust the cooking time to 7 minutes.

Do natural pressure release.

Nutrition:

Calories 183, Total Fat 7g, Saturated Fat 1g, Total Carbs 22g, Net Carbs 18g, Protein 8g, Sugar: 0.3g, Fiber: 4g, Sodium: 432mg, Potassium: 364mg, Phosphorus: 90mg

757. Root Vegetable and Squash Stew

Preparation Time: 5 minutes | **Cooking Time:** 25 minutes | **Servings:** 5

Ingredients:

1 tablespoon olive oil	1 red onion
½ small celeriac, sliced	½ butternut squash, seeded and sliced into chunks
1 sweet potato, peeled and cubed	2 carrots, peeled and cubed
1 teaspoon red wine vinegar	1 teaspoon dried thyme
1 bay leaf	1 tablespoon tomato puree
1 cup plum tomatoes, chopped	salt and pepper to taste
1 tablespoon plain flour + 2 tablespoons cold water	

Directions:

Press the Sauté button on the Instant Pot and heat the oil. Sauté the onion and celeriac. Stir for 3 minutes.

Add in the squash, sweet potato, and carrots. Stir for another minute.

Stir in the red wine vinegar, thyme, bay leaf, tomato puree, and tomatoes. Season with salt and pepper to taste. Add a cup of water.

Close the lid and set the vent to the Sealing position.

Press the Meat/Stew button and adjust the cooking time to 20 minutes.

Do quick pressure release.

Once the lid is open, press the Sauté button and stir in the flour slurry. Cook for another 3 minutes until the sauce thickens.

Nutrition:

Calories 122, Total Fat 3g, Saturated Fat 1g, Total Carbs 24g, Net Carbs 21g, Protein 1g, Sugar: 15g, Fiber: 3g, Sodium: 53mg, Potassium: 323mg, Phosphorus: 55mg

758. Veggie Tofu Instant Pot Stir Fry

Preparation Time: 5 minutes | **Cooking Time:** 15 minutes | **Servings:** 4

Ingredients:

3 tablespoons olive oil	1 block firm tofu, sliced
2 cloves garlic, minced	1 1-inch ginger, sliced thinly
2 fresh red chilis, chopped	½ head broccoli, cut into florets
4 baby corn, sliced	2 tablespoons soy sauce
black pepper to taste	½ cup of water
1 tablespoon cornstarch + 2 tablespoons water	3 tablespoons sesame seeds
2 tablespoons cashew nuts	

Directions:

Press the Sauté button and heat the olive oil. Once the oil is hot, sear the tofu on all edges until lightly golden. This takes about 5 minutes.

Once the tofu is golden, sauté the garlic and ginger until fragrant.

Add the broccoli and corn. Season with soy sauce and black pepper. Pour in enough water.

Close the lid and set the vent to the Sealing position.

Press the Pressure Cook or Manual button and adjust the cooking time to 6 minutes.

Do quick pressure release.

Once the lid is open, press the Sauté button and stir in the cornstarch slurry. Simmer for 3 minutes until the sauce thickens.

Sprinkle with sesame seeds and cashew nuts before serving;

Nutrition:
Calories 296, Total Fat 24g, Saturated Fat 4g, Total Carbs 8g, Net Carbs 5g, Protein 16g, Sugar: 2g, Fiber: 3g, Sodium: 138mg, Potassium: 278mg, Phosphorus: 231mg

759. Green Dream Noodles

Preparation Time: 5 minutes | **Cooking Time:** 25 minutes | **Servings:** 4

Ingredients:

1 tablespoon olive oil	3 cloves garlic, minced
1 1-inch ginger, sliced thinly	½ cup sliced mushrooms
1 sachet miso paste	1 ½ cups vegetable broth
1 cup broccoli florets	1 handful sugar snap peas
2 cup of rice noodles	A handful of fresh coriander leaves

Directions:
Press the Sauté button on the Instant Pot and heat the oil. Sauté the garlic and ginger for a minute or until fragrant.
Stir in the mushrooms and add the miso paste and vegetable broth.
Simmer for 3 minutes.
Stir in the broccoli florets, peas, and noodles.
Close the lid and set the vent to the Sealing position.
Press the Soup/Broth button and cook for 20 minutes.
Do natural pressure release.
Garnish with coriander leaves before serving.

Nutrition:
Calories 131, Total Fat 4g, Saturated Fat 0.5g, Total Carbs 22g, Net Carbs 21g, Protein 2g, Sugar: 0.1g, Fiber: 1g, Sodium: 21mg, Potassium: 39mg, Phosphorus: 30mg

760. Slow Cook Glazed Carrots and Parsnips

Preparation Time: 5 minutes | **Cooking Time:** 5 hours | **Servings:** 4

Ingredients:

2 large carrots, peeled and cut into thick strips	1 large parsnip, peeled and cut into thick strips
¼ cup maple syrup	salt and pepper to taste

Directions:
Place all ingredients in the Instant Pot and give a good stir.
Close the lid but do not seal the vent.
Press the Slow Cook button and adjust the cooking time to 5 hours.
Halfway through the cooking time, stir the vegetables.

Nutrition:
Calories 102, Total Fat 0.2g, Saturated Fat 0g, Total Carbs 25g, Net Carbs 22g, Protein 0.8g, Sugar: 15g, Fiber: 3g, Sodium: 10mg, Potassium: 298mg, Phosphorus: 48mg

761. Sweet Potato, Squash, Coconut, And Cardamom

Preparation Time: 10 minutes | **Cooking Time:** 12 minutes | **Servings:** 4

Ingredients:

2 tablespoons coconut oil	3 cloves garlic, minced
1 onion, chopped	1 1-inch thick ginger
3 cardamom pods	1 cup diced sweet potatoes
1 cup diced kabocha squash	1 14-ounce coconut milk
salt and pepper to taste	

Directions:
Press the Sauté button on the Instant Pot. Heat the oil and sauté the garlic and onion for 1 minute or until translucent.
Add the ginger and cardamom pods until fragrant.
Stir in the rest of the ingredients.

Close the lid and set the vent to the Sealing position.

Press the Pressure Cook or Manual button and adjust the cooking time to 10 minutes.

Do natural pressure release.

Nutrition:
Calories 102, Total Fat 7g, Saturated Fat 6g, Total Carbs 9g, Net Carbs 6g, Protein 2g, Sugar: 4g, Fiber: 3g, Sodium: 109mg, Potassium: 392mg, Phosphorus: 49mg

762. Jersey Royals with Wild Garlic

Preparation Time: 5 minutes | **Cooking Time:** 5 hours | **Servings:** 2

Ingredients:

5 tablespoons olive oil	½ pound Jersey royal potatoes scrubbed clean and cut into wedges
A handful of garlic leaves	A few sprigs of rosemary
salt and pepper to taste	

Directions:
Place all ingredients in the Instant Pot. Stir to combine everything.

Close the lid but do not seal the vent.

Press the Slow Cook button and adjust the cooking time to 5 hours.

Stir the potatoes halfway through the cooking time.

Nutrition:
Calories 386, Total Fat 34g, Saturated Fat 5g, Total Carbs 20g, Net Carbs 17g, Protein 2g, Sugar: 0.8g, Fiber: 3g, Sodium: 7mg, Potassium: 478mg, Phosphorus: 65mg

763. Miso-Glazed Eggplants

Preparation Time: 5 minutes | **Cooking Time:** 5 minutes | **Servings:** 2

Ingredients:

4 medium eggplants, sliced into 1-inch pieces	2 cloves garlic, minced
1 teaspoon miso paste	1 teaspoon brown sugar
1 teaspoon soy sauce	1 teaspoon sesame oil
Salt and pepper to taste	1 teaspoon toasted sesame seed

Directions:
Place all ingredients except for the toasted sesame seeds in the Instant Pot and give a good stir.

Close the lid and set the vent to the Sealing position.

Press the Pressure Cook or Manual button. Adjust the cooking time to 5 minutes.

Do natural pressure release.

Garnish with sesame seeds before serving.

Nutrition:
Calories 324, Total Fat 6g, Saturated Fat 1g, Total Carbs 68g, Net Carbs 35g, Protein 12g, Sugar: 41g, Fiber: 33g, Sodium: 117mg, Potassium: 2540mg, Phosphorus: 286mg

764. Butternut Squash and Thyme

Preparation Time: 5 minutes | **Cooking Time:** 6 minutes | **Servings:** 4

Ingredients:

2 tablespoons olive oil	2 cloves of garlic, minced
1 sprig of thyme	½ medium butternut squash, peeled and sliced
½ cup vegetable broth	salt and pepper to taste

Directions:
Press the Sauté button on the Instant Pot and heat the oil.

Sauté the garlic for 30 seconds until fragrant.

Stir in the rest of the ingredients.

Close the lid and set the vent to the Sealing position.

Press the Pressure Cook or Manual button and cook on high for 5 minutes.

Do natural pressure release.

Nutrition:
Calories 120, Total Fat 7g, Saturated Fat 1g, Total Carbs 15g, Net Carbs 12g, Protein 1g, Sugar: 3g, Fiber: 3g, Sodium: 74mg, Potassium: 446mg, Phosphorus: 44mg

765. Lemony Artichokes with Olives Pasta

Preparation Time: 10 minutes | **Cooking Time:** 12 minutes | **Servings:** 4

Ingredients:

6 ounces linguine pasta	4 cups of water
2 tablespoon olive oil	1 onion, minced
2 cloves garlic, minced	1 14-ounce can artichoke hearts, drained and halved
Salt and pepper to taste	1 tablespoon grated lemon zest
3 tablespoons lemon juice	½ cup green olives, pitted and chopped
1 teaspoon red pepper flakes	2 tablespoon parsley, chopped

Directions:

Place the pasta and water in the Instant Pot.
Close the lid and set the vent to the Sealing position. Press the Pressure Cook or Manual button and adjust the cooking time to 6 minutes. Do quick pressure release. Once the lid is open, drain the pasta then set it aside. Clean the inner pot.
Press the Sauté button on the Instant and heat olive oil. Sauté the onion and garlic for a minute or until lightly golden.
Stir in the artichokes and season with salt and pepper to taste. Stir for 3 minutes.
Add in the rest of the ingredients.
Stir for 3 minutes or until everything is combined.

Nutrition:

Calories 184, Total Fat 8g, Saturated Fat 1g, Total Carbs 28g, Net Carbs 17g, Protein 5g, Sugar: 3g, Fiber: 11g, Sodium: 68mg, Potassium: 371mg, Phosphorus: 118mg

766. One-Pot Curried Butternut Squash

Preparation Time: 5 minutes | **Cooking Time:** 5 minutes | **Servings:** 4

Ingredients:

1 14-ounce coconut milk	1 1-inch ginger, sliced
1 onion, minced	2 cloves garlic, minced
½ butternut squash, peeled and sliced	1 tablespoon turmeric powder
1 tablespoon garam masala powder	2 tablespoons lemon juice
salt and pepper to taste	

Directions:

Place all ingredients in the Instant Pot. Give a good stir.
Close the lid and set the vent to the Sealing position.
Press the Pressure Cook or Manual button.
Adjust the cooking time to 5 minutes.
Once the timer sets off, do natural pressure release.

Nutrition:

Calories 42, Total Fat 0.3g, Saturated Fat 0g, Total Carbs 9g, Net Carbs 7g, Protein 1g, Sugar: 4g, Fiber: 2g, Sodium: 106mg, Potassium: 354mg, Phosphorus: 38mg

767. Steamed Eggplant Salad

Preparation Time: minutes | **Cooking Time:** minutes | **Servings:** 2

Ingredients:

1 cup of water	4 medium-sized Chinese eggplants
½ cup chopped tomatoes	1 red onion, chopped
1 tablespoon grated ginger	Juice from ½ lemon, freshly squeezed
1 tablespoon chopped green onions	salt and pepper to taste

Directions:

Pour water into the Instant Pot and place a steamer basket or trivet inside.
Place the Chinese eggplants on the basket.
Close the lid and set the vent to the Sealing position.
Press the Steam button. Cook for 10 minutes.
Do natural pressure release.
Once the lid is open, take the eggplants out and allow them to cool.
Once cool, shred with two forks. Place in a bowl and add the rest of the ingredients.

Nutrition:
Calories 309, Total Fat 2g, Saturated Fat 0.5g, Total Carbs 73g, Net Carbs 39g, Protein 12g, Sugar: 42g, Fiber: 34g, Sodium: 27mg, Potassium: 2708mg, Phosphorus: 291mg

768. Plain Spaghetti Squash

Preparation Time: 5 minutes | **Cooking Time:** 10 minutes | **Servings:** 2

Ingredients:

1 cup of water	1 spaghetti squash, cut lengthwise and seeds removed
Salt and pepper to taste	

Directions:
Pour water into the Instant Pot and place a steamer basket or trivet inside.
Season the spaghetti squash with salt and pepper.
Place on the steamer basket.
Close the lid and set the vent to the Sealing position.
Press the Steam button cook for 10 minutes.
Do natural pressure release.
Once the lid is open, remove the squash and fluff using a fork.

Nutrition:
Calories 9, Total Fat 0.05g, Saturated Fat 0g, Total Carbs 2g, Net Carbs 1.7g, Protein 0.5g, Sugar: 1g, Fiber: 0.3g, Sodium: 4mg, Potassium: 77mg, Phosphorus: 10mg

769. Korean Braised Potatoes

Preparation Time: 5 minutes | **Cooking Time:** 30 minutes | **Servings:** 4

Ingredients:

1-pound baby potatoes scrubbed clean	3 tablespoons soy sauce
2 tablespoons sugar	3 cloves garlic, minced
1 cup of water	Sesame seeds for garnish

Directions:
Place all ingredients except for the sesame seeds in the Instant Pot.

Close the lid and set the vent to the Sealing position.
Press the Meat/Stew button and adjust the time to 20 minutes.
Once the timer sets off, do a quick pressure release to open the lid.
Once the lid is open, press the Sauté button and allow the sauce to simmer until it has reduced to a glaze. Stir constantly.
Garnish with sesame seeds before serving.

Nutrition:
Calories 141, Total Fat 2g, Saturated Fat 0.4g, Total Carbs 28g, Net Carbs 25g, Protein 3g, Sugar: 7g, Fiber: 3g, Sodium: 188mg, Potassium: 518mg, Phosphorus: 83mg

770. Broccoli and Rice

Preparation Time: 5 minutes | **Cooking Time:** 8 minutes | **Servings:** 6

Ingredients:

1 teaspoon coconut oil	2 cloves garlic, minced
3 cups broccoli florets	8 ounces shiitake mushrooms
10 ounces pre-cooked or leftover rice	1 cup roasted cashews
3 tablespoons soy sauce	pepper to taste
3 tablespoons toasted sesame oil	

Directions:
Press the Sauté button on the Instant Pot and heat the coconut oil.
Stir in the garlic and sauté for 30 seconds until fragrant.
Add in the broccoli and shiitake mushrooms.
Cook for 3 minutes until the broccoli has wilted.
Add in the leftover rice and cashew and season with soy sauce and pepper to taste.
Stir for 3 minutes.
Drizzle with sesame oil before serving.

Nutrition:
Calories 428, Total Fat 32g, Saturated Fat 6g, Total Carbs 33g, Net Carbs 30g, Protein 8g, Sugar: 7g, Fiber: 3g, Sodium: 264mg, Potassium: 301mg, Phosphorus: 212mg

771. Vegetable Paella

Preparation Time: 10 minutes | **Cooking Time:** 35 minutes | **Servings:** 6

Ingredients:

3 tablespoons olive oil	1 onion, chopped finely
6 cloves garlic, minced	2 teaspoons smoked paprika
1 15-ounces diced tomatoes	2 cups short-grain rice
1 can chickpeas	3 cups vegetable broth
½ cup dry white wine	½ teaspoon saffron threads
salt and pepper to taste	1 14-ounce artichoke, drained
½ cup Kalamata olives pitted and halved	½ cup frozen peas
2 red bell peppers, seeded and cut into strips	2 tablespoons lemon juice
¼ cup fresh parsley, chopped	

Directions:

Press the Sauté button on the Instant Pot and heat the oil. Sauté the onion and garlic until fragrant. Stir in the paprika, tomatoes, rice, and chickpeas. Stir for 2 minutes. Add in the broth, white wine, and saffron. Stir to combine or until the liquid is simmering. Season with salt and pepper to taste.

Arrange the artichokes, olives, peas, and bell pepper on top. Drizzle with lemon juice.

Close the lid and set the vent to the Sealing position.

Press the Rice button and cook on low until the timer sets off.

Do natural pressure release.

Garnish with parsley before serving.

Nutrition:

Calories 546, Total Fat 13g, Saturated Fat 3g, Total Carbs 93g, Net Carbs 81g, Protein 18g, Sugar: 8g, Fiber: 12g, Sodium: 339mg, Potassium: 908mg, Phosphorus: 306mg

772. Cauliflower in Cashew Chipotle Sauce

Preparation Time: 5 minutes | **Cooking Time:** 6 minutes | **Servings:** 4

Ingredients:

1 cup cashew nut, soaked overnight and drained	3 tablespoons nutritional yeast
2 tablespoons lime juice	3 tablespoons adobo or chipotle hot sauce
2 tablespoons olive oil	salt and pepper to taste
1 large head cauliflower, cut into florets	1 cup of water

Directions:

In a blender, place the cashew nuts, water, nutritional yeast, lime juice, adobo or chipotle sauce, and olive oil. Season with salt and pepper to taste. Pulse until smooth. Set aside.

Place the cauliflower and water in the Instant Pot and pour over the cashew chipotle sauce.

Close the lid and set the vent to the Sealing position.

Press the Pressure Cook or Manual button and adjust the cooking time to 6 minutes.

Once the timer sets off, do a quick pressure release.

Nutrition:

Calories 294, Total Fat 22g, Saturated Fat 4g, Total Carbs 17g, Net Carbs 13g, Protein 10g, Sugar: 4g, Fiber: 4g, Sodium: 615mg, Potassium: 733mg, Phosphorus: 220mg

773. Slow-Cooked Veggie Enchilada Casserole

Preparation Time: 5 minutes | **Cooking Time:** 5 hours | **Servings:** 5

Ingredients:

½ medium head of cauliflower, cut into florets	1 large sweet potato, peeled and cubed
2 red bell peppers, cut into squares	3 tablespoons extra virgin olive oil
1 teaspoon ground cumin	8 ounces red salsa

salt and pepper to taste
½ cup fresh cilantro
2 handful baby spinach leaves
9 corn tortillas, halved

Directions:
Place the cauliflower, sweet potato, bell peppers, olive oil, cumin, and salsa in the Instant Pot. Season with salt and pepper to taste. Add in the baby spinach on top.

Close the lid but do not seal the vent.

Press the Slow Cook function and adjust the cooking time to 5 hours.

Once cooked, serve with cilantro and tortillas.

Nutrition:
Calories 94, Total Fat 4g, Saturated Fat 0.5g, Total Carbs 14g, Net Carbs 11g, Protein 2g, Sugar: 6g, Fiber: 3g, Sodium: 416mg, Potassium: 456mg, Phosphorus: 58mg

774. Bok Choy With Mushrooms

Preparation Time: 5 minutes | **Cooking Time:** 10 minutes | **Servings:** 4

Ingredients:
3 tablespoons olive oil
1 small yellow onion, chopped

2 cloves garlic, minced
5 ounces fresh shiitake mushrooms

1 red bell pepper, seeded and sliced into strips
1-pound bok choy, torn

1 cup vegetable broth
2 tablespoons soy sauce

salt and pepper to taste
1 tablespoon sesame seed oil

1 tablespoon cornstarch + 2 tablespoons water

Directions:
Press the Sauté button on the Instant Pot. Heat the oil and sauté the onion and garlic for 30 seconds or until fragrant.

Stir in the mushrooms and red bell pepper. Sauté for 3 minutes.

Add in the bok choy and vegetable broth. Season with soy sauce, salt, and pepper to taste.

Close the lid and set the vent to the Sealing position.

Press the Pressure Cook or Manual button and adjust the cooking time to 3 minutes.

Do quick pressure release.

Once the lid is open, press the Sauté button and stir in the sesame oil and cornstarch slurry. Stir for 3 minutes until the sauce thickens.

Nutrition:
Calories 138, Total Fat 11g, Saturated Fat 2g, Total Carbs 10g, Net Carbs 8g, Protein 3g, Sugar: 4g, Fiber: 2g, Sodium: 131mg, Potassium: 447mg, Phosphorus: 63mg

775. Stuffed Acorn Squash

Preparation Time: 10 minutes | **Cooking Time:** 20 minutes | **Servings:** 4

Ingredients:
1 cup of water
2 medium acorn squash

2 tablespoons olive oil
½ cup quinoa, rinsed

¼ cup dried cranberries, chopped
¼ cup raw pepitas

¼ cup chopped green onions
1 tablespoon lemon juice

salt to taste

Directions:
Pour water into the Instant Pot and place a steamer basket or trivet on top.

Cut the squash lengthwise and scoop out the seeds. Set aside.

Prepare the filling by mixing in a bowl the quinoa, cranberries, pepitas, green onions, and lemon juice. Season with salt to taste.

Scoop the filling inside the hollowed part of the acorn squash. Do this on all squash halves.

Place the squash on the trivet.

Close the lid and set the vent to the Sealing position.

Press the Steam button and cook for 20 minutes.

Do natural pressure release.

Nutrition:
Calories 277, Total Fat 12g, Saturated Fat 2g, Total Carbs 40g, Net Carbs 35g, Protein 7g, Sugar: 2g, Fiber: 5g, Sodium: 10mg, Potassium: 939mg, Phosphorus: 263mg

776. Lacto-Vegetarian Caramelized Veggies

Preparation Time: 5 minutes | **Cooking Time:** 5 hours | **Servings:** 4

Ingredients:

1-pound small potatoes

3 tablespoons olive oil

A sprig of sage

5 tablespoons butter

½ pounds of frozen mixed vegetables

A sprig of rosemary

A sprig of thyme

salt and pepper to taste

Directions:

Place all ingredients in the Instant Pot.

Stir to combine.

Close the lid but do not Seal the vent.

Press the Slow Cook function and adjust the cooking time to 5 hours.

Stir halfway through the cooking time for even browning.

Nutrition:

Calories 341, Total Fat 25g, Saturated Fat 11g, Total Carbs 27g, Net Carbs 22g, Protein 4g, Sugar: 3g, Fiber: 5g, Sodium: 141mg, Potassium: 578mg, Phosphorus: 98mg

777. One-Pot Spicy Tomato Spaghetti

Preparation Time: 5 minutes | **Cooking Time:** 15 minutes | **Servings:** 4

Ingredients:

1 tablespoon olive oil

1 fresh red chili, chopped

4 plum tomatoes, chopped

4 tablespoons nutritional yeast

1 bunch fresh basil leaf, chopped

2 cloves garlic, minced

salt and pepper to taste

6 ounces dry spaghetti

1 cup of water

Directions:

Press the Sauté button on the Instant Pot and heat the oil. Sauté the garlic and red chili until fragrant.

Stir in the tomatoes and season with salt and pepper to taste. Sauté for 3 minutes until the tomatoes are wilted.

Add in the spaghetti, nutritional yeast, and water. Stir to combine.

Close the lid and set the vent to the Sealing position.

Press the Pressure Cook or Manual button and adjust the cooking time to 10 minutes.

Do natural pressure release.

Once the lid is open, stir in the basil leaves last.

Nutrition:

Calories 264, Total Fat 4g, Saturated Fat 0.5g, Total Carbs 47g, Net Carbs 44g, Protein 10g, Sugar: 12g, Fiber: 3g, Sodium: 545mg, Potassium: 521mg, Phosphorus: 107mg

778. Aubergine And Tomato Rogan Josh

Preparation Time: 5 minutes | **Cooking Time:** 15 minutes | **Servings:** 2

Ingredients:

1 tablespoon olive oil

2 cloves garlic, minced

2 big ripe tomatoes, chopped

½ cup of water

Juice from ½ lemon

1 bunch fresh coriander

1 shallot, chopped

2 teaspoons Rogan Josh spice paste or garam masala

1 large aubergine, chopped

salt and pepper to taste

½ cup pistachios shelled

Directions:

Press the Sauté button on the Instant Pot and heat the olive oil.

Sauté the shallot and garlic for 30 seconds or until fragrant.

Toast the garam masala or Rogan Josh spice paste for a minute until fragrant.

Add in the tomatoes and stir for 3 minutes.

Stir in the aubergine and water. Season with salt and pepper to taste. Drizzle with lemon juice.

Close the lid and set the vent to the Sealing position.

Press the Pressure Cook or Manual button and adjust the cooking time to 8 minutes.

Do natural pressure release.

Once the lid is open, stir in the pistachios and coriander.

Nutrition:
Calories 281, Total Fat 22g, Saturated Fat 3g, Total Carbs 19g, Net Carbs 14g, Protein 9g, Sugar: 3g, Fiber: 5g, Sodium: 53mg, Potassium:915mg, Phosphorus: 238mg

779. Instant Pot Roasted Root Vegetables

Preparation Time: 5 minutes | **Cooking Time:** 5 hours | **Servings:** 6

Ingredients:

1-pound medium-sized potatoes, scrubbed and quartered	2 large carrots, peeled and roughly chopped
1 large parsnip, peeled and roughly chopped	1 bulb garlic, smashed
½ bunch fresh rosemary	3 tablespoons olive oil
salt and pepper to taste	

Directions:
Place all ingredients in a mixing pot and toss to coat all ingredients with the oil and seasoning.
Place into the Instant Pot.
Close the lid but do not seal the vent.
Press the Slow Cook function and adjust the cooking time to 5 hours.
Halfway through the cooking time, carefully stir the vegetables for even browning.
Cook until done.

Nutrition:
Calories 144, Total Fat 7g, Saturated Fat 1g, Total Carbs 19g, Net Carbs 16g, Protein 2g, Sugar: 3g, Fiber: 3g, Sodium: 23mg, Potassium: 478mg, Phosphorus: 67mg

780. Tomato Curry

Preparation Time: 5 minutes | **Cooking Time:** 15 minutes | **Servings:** 4

Ingredients:

2 tablespoons olive oil	4 cloves garlic, minced
1 1-inch ginger, sliced thinly	1 ½ pounds mixed tomatoes
A pinch of saffron	½ cup almond meal
2 fresh red chilis, chopped	5 curry leaves
1 tablespoon garam masala	1 14-ounce can coconut milk
2 teaspoon mango chutney (optional)	salt and pepper to taste

Directions:
Press the Sauté button on the Instant Pot and heat the oil.
Sauté the garlic and ginger until fragrant.
Stir in the tomatoes and saffron for 2 minutes.
Add in the rest of the ingredients.
Close the lid and set the vent to the Sealing position.
Press the Manual button and adjust the cooking time to 10 minutes.
Do natural pressure release.

Nutrition:
Calories 113, Total Fat 7g, Saturated Fat 1g, Total Carbs 11g, Net Carbs 8g, Protein 3g, Sugar: 3g, Fiber: 3g, Sodium: 176mg, Potassium: 625mg, Phosphorus:75 mg

781. Potato and Artichoke Al Forno

Preparation Time: 5 minutes | **Cooking Time:** 5 hours | **Servings:** 5

Ingredients:

½ pound baby potatoes scrubbed clean	2 large fennel bulbs, peeled and sliced thinly
1 14-ounce artichoke hearts in oil	1 cup double cream
Salt and pepper to taste	

Directions:
Place all ingredients in the Instant Pot and give a good stir.
Close the lid and do not seal the vent.
Press the Slow Cook button and adjust the cooking time to 5 hours.

Nutrition:
Calories 258, Total Fat 16g, Saturated Fat 7g, Total Carbs 26g, Net Carbs 16g, Protein 6g, Sugar: 7g, Fiber: 10g, Sodium: 115mg, Potassium: 876mg, Phosphorus: 168mg

782. Mushroom Bourguignon

Preparation Time: 5 minutes | **Cooking Time:** 5 minutes | **Servings:** 6

Ingredients:

2 tablespoons olive oil	2 cloves garlic, minced
12 shallots, chopped	16 ounces dried porcini mushrooms, soaked in water overnight then drained
4 portobello mushrooms, sliced	16 ounces shiitake mushrooms, sliced
16 ounces chestnut mushrooms, sliced	1 medium carrot, sliced
1 sprig fresh thyme	2 bay leaves
1 cup red wine	2 tablespoons tomato paste
Salt and pepper to taste	

Directions:

Press the Sauté button on the Instant Pot and heat the oil.

Sauté the garlic and shallots until fragrant. Stir in the mushrooms and sauté for 3 minutes.

Add in the rest of the ingredients.

Close the lid and set the vent to the Sealing position.

Press the Pressure Cook or Manual button and adjust the cooking time to 5 minutes.

Do natural pressure release.

Nutrition:

Calories 346, Total Fat 6g, Saturated Fat 0.8g, Total Carbs 76g, Net Carbs 64g, Protein 12g, Sugar: 9g, Fiber: 12g, Sodium: 26mg, Potassium: 1662mg, Phosphorus: 337mg

783. Aubergine Penne Arrabbiata

Preparation Time: 5 minutes | **Cooking Time:** 15 minutes | **Servings:** 6

Ingredients:

2 tablespoons olive oil	4 cloves garlic, minced
12 fresh mixed color chilis, chopped	2 aubergines, sliced
6 ounces dried whole wheat penne	1 14-ounce can plum tomatoes
3 tablespoons nutritional yeast	½ cup of water
salt and pepper to taste	

Directions:

Press the Sauté button on the Instant Pot and heat the olive oil.

Sauté the garlic and chilis for 1 minute until lightly toasted.

Stir in the aubergines for 2 minutes.

Add in the rest of the ingredients and scrape the bottom to remove the brown bits at the bottom.

Close the lid and set the vent to the Sealing position.

Press the Pressure Cook or Manual button and adjust the cooking time to 10 minutes,

Do natural pressure release.

Nutrition:

Calories 291, Total Fat 8g, Saturated Fat 2g, Total Carbs 40g, Net Carbs 35g, Protein 17g, Sugar: 16g, Fiber: 5g, Sodium: 1044mg, Potassium: 579mg, Phosphorus: 290mg

784. Green Beans Ala Trapanese

Preparation Time: 5 minutes | **Cooking Time:** 14 minutes | **Servings:** 4

Ingredients:

1 cup blanched almond	2 tablespoons olive oil
1 clove of garlic, minced	2 cups ripe cherry tomatoes, chopped
2 cups green beans	salt and pepper to taste
½ cup pecorino cheese	1 bunch fresh basil
1 cup rocket arugula	

Directions:

Press the Sauté button on the Instant Pot and toast the almond for 3 minutes until lightly golden. Set aside to cool. Once cool, place in a plastic bag and crush with a rolling pin.

With the Sauté button still on, heat the oil and sauté the garlic until fragrant.

Stir in the tomatoes for 3 minutes or until wilted.

Add in the green beans and season with salt and pepper to taste.

Close the lid and set the vent to the Sealing position.

Press the Pressure Cook or Manual button and adjust the cooking time to 6 minutes.

Do quick pressure release.

Once the lid is open, press the Sauté button and stir in the pecorino cheese, basil, arugula, and ground almond. Cook for another 3 minutes.

Nutrition:
Calories 128, Total Fat 11g, Saturated Fat 3g, Total Carbs 5g, Net Carbs 3g, Protein 4g, Sugar: 1g, Fiber: 2g, Sodium: 118mg, Potassium: 137mg, Phosphorus: 81mg

785. Indian Spinach

Preparation Time: 5 minutes | **Cooking Time:** 7 minutes | **Servings:** 2

Ingredients:

1 tablespoon olive oil	1 teaspoon black mustard seed
1 teaspoon cumin seeds	1 onion, chopped
1 1-inch ginger, sliced	1 teaspoon curry powder
½ cup coconut cream	1-pound baby spinach
Juice from ½ lemon	salt and pepper to taste

Directions:
Press the Sauté button on the Instant Pot and heat the oil. Toast the mustard seeds and cumin seeds. Stir in the onion and ginger until fragrant. Add in the rest of the ingredients.
Close the lid and set the vent to the Sealing position.
Press the Pressure Cook or Manual button and adjust the cooking time to 5 minutes.
Do natural pressure release.

Nutrition:
Calories 348, Total Fat 29g, Saturated Fat 19g, Total Carbs 20g, Net Carbs 12g, Protein 10g, Sugar: 4g, Fiber: 8g, Sodium: 187mg, Potassium: 1596mg, Phosphorus: 219mg

786. Veggie Feijoada

Preparation Time: 5 minutes | **Cooking Time:** 30 minutes | **Servings:** 5

Ingredients:

2 tablespoons olive oil	2 red onions, chopped
3 cloves garlic, minced	1 teaspoon ground coriander
1 teaspoon smoked paprika	4 ripe tomatoes, chopped
1 cup of brown rice	1 cup diced sweet potatoes
1 red bell pepper, seeded and sliced	½ zucchini, diced
Juice from ½ lemon	A bunch of chopped coriander for garnish
salt and pepper to taste	2 cups of water

Directions:
Press the Sauté button on the Instant Pot and heat the oil. Sauté the onions and garlic until fragrant.
Add in the coriander and paprika and stir for another minute until fragrant.
Stir in the tomatoes and brown rice. Stir for another minute.
Add in the rest of the ingredients.
Close the lid and set the vent to the Sealing position.
Press the Pressure Cook or Manual button and adjust the cooking time to 25 minutes.
Do natural pressure release.

Nutrition:
Calories 95, Total Fat 6g, Saturated Fat 0.8g, Total Carbs 11g, Net Carbs 8g, Protein 2g, Sugar: 5g, Fiber: 3g, Sodium: 9mg, Potassium: 390mg, Phosphorus: 52mg

787. Creamy Asparagus

Preparation Time: 5 minutes | **Cooking Time:** 8 minutes | **Servings:** 4

Ingredients:

2 tablespoons olive oil	2 shallots, minced
2 tablespoon chives	12 ounces asparagus, trimmed and quartered
salt and pepper to taste	1 cup of water

Directions:
Press the Sauté button on the Instant Pot and heat the oil.
Sauté the shallots for a minute until translucent.
Add the chives and asparagus. Season with salt and pepper to taste.
Add the rest of the ingredients.

Close the lid and set the vent to the Sealing position.
Press the Pressure Cook or Manual button and adjust the cooking time to 5 minutes.
Do quick pressure release.
Once the lid is open, pour contents into a blender and pulse until smooth.

Nutrition:
Calories 77, Total Fat 7g, Saturated Fat 1g, Total Carbs 3g, Net Carbs 1g, Protein 2g, Sugar: 2g, Fiber: 2g, Sodium: 2mg, Potassium: 176mg, Phosphorus: 45mg

788. Instant Pot Maple Glazed Carrots

Preparation Time: 5 minutes | **Cooking Time:** 8 minutes | **Servings:** 4

Ingredients:

1 cup of water	2 large carrots, peeled and julienned
1 tablespoon oil	1 clove garlic, minced
1 shallot, minced	¼ cup maple syrup
Salt and pepper to taste	

Directions:
Pour water into the Instant Pot and place the trivet or steamer basket inside.
Place carrots in the steamer basket.
Close the lid and set the vent to the Sealing position.
Press the Steam button and cook for 5 minutes.
Do quick pressure release. Remove the carrots from the steamer basket then set them aside.
Clean the inner pot.
Press the Sauté button on the Instant Pot and heat the oil.
Sauté the garlic and shallots.
Stir in the steamed carrots and maple syrup.
Stir for 2 minutes. Season with pepper and salt.
Serve and enjoy.

Nutrition:
Calories 97, Total Fat 4g, Saturated Fat 0.5g, Total Carbs 17g, Net Carbs 16g, Protein 0.4g, Sugar: 14g, Fiber: 1g, Sodium: 27mg, Potassium: 160mg, Phosphorus: 14mg

789. Cider-Glazed Brussels Sprouts

Preparation Time: 5 minutes | **Cooking Time:** 10 minutes | **Servings:** 8

Ingredients:

1 cup apple cider	½ cup dried cranberries
2 pounds Brussels sprouts	salt to taste
2 tablespoons extra virgin oil	

Directions:
Place the apple cider in the Instant Pot. Press the Sauté button and bring it to a boil.
Add the cranberries and Brussels sprouts. Season with salt.
Press the Cancel button and close the lid. Set the vent to the Sealing position.
Press the Pressure Cook or Manual button. Adjust the cooking time to 5 minutes.
Do quick pressure release.
Once the lid is open, drizzle with extra virgin olive oil.

Nutrition:
Calories 94, Total Fat 4g, Saturated Fat 0.6g, Total Carbs 14g, Net Carbs 9g, Protein 4g, Sugar: 6g, Fiber: 5g, Sodium: 29mg, Potassium: 458mg, Phosphorus: 80mg

790. Instant Pot Ratatouille

Preparation Time: 10 minutes | **Cooking Time:** 10 minutes | **Servings:** 4

Ingredients:

1 ½ tablespoon extra-virgin olive oil	1 tablespoon minced garlic
1 cup chopped red onion	1 cup chopped red bell pepper
2 14-ounce cans diced tomatoes	1 large zucchini, sliced into 1inch pieces
1 large yellow squash, sliced into 1-inch pieces	1 small eggplant, peeled and slice into 1-inch pieces
1 tablespoon red wine vinegar	½ teaspoon smoked paprika
salt to taste	2 tablespoons fresh basil leaves

Directions:

Press the Sauté button on the Instant Pot and heat the oil. Sauté the garlic, onion, and bell pepper until fragrant.

Stir in the tomatoes and cook for another 3 minutes.

Add in the zucchini, yellow squash, and eggplant.

Season with red wine vinegar, paprika, and salt. Top with basil.

Close the lid and set the vent to the Sealing position.

Press the Pressure Cook or Manual button and adjust the cooking time to 5 minutes.

Do natural pressure release.

Nutrition:

Calories 354, Total Fat 7g, Saturated Fat 0.8g, Total Carbs 58g, Net Carbs 45g, Protein 15g, Sugar: 13g, Fiber: 13g, Sodium: 558mg, Potassium: 891mg, Phosphorus: 321mg

791. Summer Vegetable Dinner

Preparation Time: 5 minutes | **Cooking Time:** 15 minutes | **Servings:** 8

Ingredients:

4 large ears of corn, shucked and cleaned	1 cup of water
3 cups potatoes, cut into chunks	4 cups summer squash, sliced thickly
4 cups kale	

Directions:

Arrange the corn in the Instant Pot and pour water.

Arrange the potato pieces on top of the corn. Toss in the squash and add in the kale last.

Close the lid and set the vent to a sealing position.

Press the Pressure Cook or Manual button and cook on high. Adjust the cooking time to 15 minutes.

Do natural pressure release.

Nutrition:

Calories 123, Total Fat 1g, Saturated Fat 0g, Total Carbs 27g, Net Carbs 22g, Protein 4g, Sugar: 4g, Fiber: 5g, Sodium: 23mg, Potassium: 573mg, Phosphorus: 126mg

792. Instant Pot Vegetable Soup

Preparation Time: 10 minutes | **Cooking Time:** 19 minutes | **Servings:** 8

Ingredients:

1 teaspoon canola oil	1 onion, diced
2 teaspoons minced garlic	2 teaspoons Italian seasoning mix
1-pound potatoes, chopped	3 large carrots, peeled and chopped
2 celery ribs, sliced	1 ½ cups fire-roasted diced tomatoes
1 cup green beans	salt and pepper to taste
6 cups vegetable broth	1 cup spinach

Directions:

Press the Sauté button on the Instant Pot and heat the oil.

Sauté the onion and garlic for 30 seconds until fragrant.

Add in the Italian seasoning mix and stir for another 30 seconds.

Add the potatoes, carrots, celery, tomatoes, and beans. Season with salt and pepper to taste.

Pour in the broth.

Close the lid and set the vent to the Sealing position.

Press the Pressure Cooker or Manual button and cook on high. Adjust the cooking time to 15 minutes.

Do quick pressure release. Once the lid is open, press the Sauté button and stir in the spinach. Continue cooking for 3 minutes.

Nutrition:

Calories 101, Total Fat 1g, Saturated Fat 0g, Total Carbs 17g, Net Carbs 14g, Protein 6g, Sugar: 3g, Fiber: 3g, Sodium: 743mg, Potassium: 566mg, Phosphorus: 213mg

793. Vegetables in Tomatoes

Preparation Time: 5 minutes | **Cooking Time:** 24 minutes | **Servings:** 4

Ingredients:

1 tablespoon olive oil	2 cloves of garlic
1 large onion, chopped	1 cup diced carrots
½ cup peas	32 ounces vegetable broth

1 cup broccoli florets

2 tablespoons fresh basil

salt and pepper to taste

1 14-ounce can diced tomatoes

3 cups of water

Directions:
Press the Sauté button on the Instant Pot and heat the oil. Sauté the garlic and onion until fragrant for 30 seconds or until fragrant.
Stir in the carrots and peas and stir for 2 minutes.
Add in the rest of the ingredients. Give a good stir.
Close the lid and set the vent to the Sealing position.
Press the Broth/Soup button and cook on high. Adjust the cooking time to 20 minutes.
Do natural pressure release.

Nutrition:
Calories 77, Total Fat 4g, Saturated Fat 0.5g, Total Carbs 10g, Net Carbs 6g, Protein 2g, Sugar: 6g, Fiber: 4g, Sodium: 142mg, Potassium: 363mg, Phosphorus: 48mg

794. Vegetarian Mushroom Soup

Preparation Time: 5 minutes | **Cooking Time:** 6 minutes | **Servings:** 4

Ingredients:

8 ounces sliced cremini mushrooms

1 onion, chopped

½ cup of water

1 ½ cup of coconut milk

salt to taste

½ cup cilantro, chopped

1 cup frozen peas

1 14-ounce diced tomatoes

½ teaspoon ground cumin

1 tablespoon grated ginger

1 tablespoon sugar

Directions:
In the Instant Pot, combine the mushrooms, peas, onions, tomatoes, water, cumin, coconut milk, and ginger. Season with salt, and sugar.
Close the lid and set the vent to the Sealing position. Press the Pressure Cook or Manual button and adjust the cooking time to 6 minutes.
Do natural pressure release.

Once the lid is open, stir in the cilantro before serving.

Nutrition:
Calories 240, Total Fat 7g, Saturated Fat 5g, Total Carbs 35g, Net Carbs 28g, Protein 12g, Sugar: 13g, Fiber: 7g, Sodium: 440mg, Potassium: 930mg, Phosphorus: 310mg

795. Lemon Veggie Risotto

Preparation Time: 10 minutes | **Cooking Time:** 25 minutes | **Servings:** 4

Ingredients:

1 bunch asparagus, sliced thin

1 cup fresh peas

1 onion, diced

2 garlic, cloves

1 teaspoon fresh thyme

4 cups vegetable broth

½ bunch chives, chopped

1 teaspoon lemon zest

1 cup broccoli, florets

1 tablespoon + 2 tablespoons olive oil

1 cup leek, diced

salt and pepper to taste

1 ½ cups arborio rice

1 cup spinach

¼ teaspoon red pepper flakes

2 tablespoons lemon juice

Directions:
Preheat the oven to 4000F and line a baking sheet with parchment paper. To the baking sheet, add the asparagus, broccoli, and peas. Drizzle with oil and place in the oven for 20 minutes until the vegetables are tender. Set aside.
In the Instant Pot, press the Sauté button and heat the remaining oil. Sauté the onion, leeks, and garlic for 30 seconds or until fragrant.
Add rice and continue stirring for 2 minutes until lightly toasted.
Stir in the broth and season with salt and pepper. Press the Cancel button and close the lid. Make sure that the vent is set to the Sealing position.
Press the Pressure Cook or Manual button and cook on high for 7 minutes.
Once the timer sets off, do a quick pressure release.
Once the lid is open, press the Sauté button and add the rest of the ingredients including the roasted vegetables.

Serve warm.

Nutrition:
Calories 204, Total Fat 13g, Saturated Fat 2g, Total Carbs 30g, Net Carbs 19g, Protein 7g, Sugar: 3g, Fiber: 11g, Sodium: 18mg, Potassium: 827mg, Phosphorus: 774mg

796. Steamed Asian Brussels Sprouts

Preparation Time: 10 minutes | **Cooking Time:** 10 minutes | **Servings:** 4

Ingredients:

1 cup of water	2 tablespoons sesame oil
4 teaspoons soy sauce	2 teaspoon rice vinegar
1 ½ cups Brussels sprouts, thinly sliced	salt to taste
2 tablespoons chopped peanuts, toasted	

Directions:
Pour water into the Instant Pot and place a steamer basket or trivet inside.
In a heat-proof dish, mix all ingredients except for the peanuts. Toss to coat the Brussels sprouts with the ingredients.
Place the dish with the Brussels sprouts on the trivet.
Close the lid and set the vent to the Sealing position.
Press the Steam button and cook for 10 minutes.
Do natural pressure release to open the lid.
Garnish with toasted peanuts before serving.

Nutrition:
Calories 137, Total Fat 11g, Saturated Fat 2g, Total Carbs 8g, Net Carbs 6g, Protein 4g, Sugar: 3g, Fiber: 2g, Sodium: 137mg, Potassium: 205mg, Phosphorus: 63mg

797. Mushroom, Vegetable, And Rice Curry

Preparation Time: 5 minutes | **Cooking Time:** 33 minutes | **Servings:** 6

Ingredients:

1 tablespoon olive oil	2 cloves garlic, minced
1 onion, chopped	1 fresh chili, chopped
1 teaspoon turmeric powder	1 teaspoon fenugreek seeds
1 teaspoon black mustard seeds	1 teaspoon curry powder
½ pounds mixed mushrooms sliced	½ pounds of mixed vegetables
½ cup brown basmati rice	1 14-ounce coconut milk
salt and pepper to taste	½ cup of water
A bunch of fresh coriander, chopped	

Directions:
Press the Sauté button on the Instant Pot and heat the oil. Sauté the garlic and onion for a minute. Stir in the chili, turmeric powder, fenugreek seeds, mustard seeds, and curry powder. Stir for another minute or until toasted. Stir in the mushrooms and stir for 3 minutes or until wilted.
Stir in the rest of the ingredients except for the coriander.
Close the lid and do not seal the vent.
Press the Rice button and cook using the pre-set cooking time.
Once cooked, stir in the coriander last.

Nutrition:
Calories 174, Total Fat 10g, Saturated Fat 2g, Total Carbs 23g, Net Carbs 15g, Protein 7g, Sugar: 7g, Fiber: 8g, Sodium: 147mg, Potassium: 968mg, Phosphorus: 450mg

798. Smoky Veggie Chili

Preparation Time: 5 minutes | **Cooking Time:** 37 minutes | **Servings:** 5

Ingredients:

1 tablespoon olive oil	2 onions, chopped
1 teaspoon cumin seeds	2 teaspoons smoked paprika
2 teaspoons cocoa powder	1 tablespoon peanut butter
1 fresh chili, chopped	3 mixed color peppers, seeded and chopped
3 large tomatoes, chopped	2 sweet potatoes, peeled and cubed
8 small jacket potatoes	1 bunch fresh coriander, chopped

salt and pepper to taste

1 cup of water

Directions:

Press the Sauté button on the Instant Pot and heat the oil.

Sauté the onions and cumin until fragrant.

Stir in the paprika, cocoa powder, peanut butter, chili, peppers, tomatoes, and potatoes.

Season with salt and pepper and pour in water.

Close the lid and set the vent to the Sealing position.

Press the Meat/Stew button and cook using the preset cooking time.

Do natural pressure release.

Nutrition:

Calories 586, Total Fat 4g, Saturated Fat 0.7g, Total Carbs 126g, Net Carbs 108g, Protein 15g, Sugar: 14g, Fiber: 18g, Sodium: 123mg, Potassium: 3131mg, Phosphorus: 426mg

799. Sicilian Aubergine Stew

Preparation Time: 5 minutes | **Cooking Time:** 25 minutes | **Servings:** 5

Ingredients:

2 tablespoons olive oil	1 small onion, chopped
3 cloves garlic, minced	1 large aubergine, chopped
2 large tomatoes, chopped	1 tablespoons caper
8 green olives, pitted	1 tablespoon red wine vinegar
½ cup couscous	salt and pepper to taste
3 cups of water	1 tablespoon flaked almonds

Directions:

Press the Sauté button and heat the olive oil.

Sauté the onion and garlic until fragrant.

Stir in the aubergine and tomatoes for three minutes until slightly wilted.

Add the capers, olives, red wine vinegar, and couscous. Season with salt and pepper to taste.

Pour water.

Close the lid and set the vent to the Sealing position.

Press the Meat/Stew button and adjust the cooking time to 20 minutes.

Do natural pressure release.

Once the lid is open, sprinkle with flaked almonds.

Nutrition:

Calories 161, Total Fat 10g, Saturated Fat 1g, Total Carbs 9g, Net Carbs 7g, Protein 10g, Sugar: 3g, Fiber: 2g, Sodium: 131mg, Potassium: 323mg, Phosphorus: 99mg

800. Aubergine Dip

Preparation Time: 10 minutes | **Cooking Time:** 10 minutes | **Servings:** 2

Ingredients:

1 large aubergine	1 clove garlic, minced
1 fresh green chili, minced	1 tablespoon extra-virgin olive oil
Juice from ½ lemon	½ teaspoon smoked paprika
salt and pepper to taste	

Directions:

Pour water into the Instant Pot and place a trivet or steamer basket inside.

Place the aubergine inside.

Close the lid and set the vent to the Sealing position.

Press the Steam button and cook for 10 minutes.

Do natural pressure release.

Remove the aubergine from the Instant Pot and allow it to cool.

Once cooled, peel the aubergine and place it in a food processor.

Add the rest of the ingredients. Pulse until smooth.

Serve with crackers.

Nutrition:

Calories 102, Total Fat 4g, Saturated Fat 0.5g, Total Carbs 18g, Net Carbs: 9 g, Protein 3g, Sugar: 10g, Fiber: 9g, Sodium: 66mg, Potassium: 662mg, Phosphorus: 72mg

Conclusion

There are so many powerful and persuasive reasons to make a positive change and switch over to a plant-based diet. A plant-based diet will improve your quality of life, give you more energy and vitality, help you lose unwanted body fat, and it may even lengthen your years on this beautiful planet. As a bonus, by making the change you will be making a real and significant difference to our planet Earth's future. So much energy and fossil fuels are wasted by sourcing meat and other animal products, transporting them from place to place across miles and miles of road, and processing all of these animal products.

By switching to a plant-based diet, you will be greatly decreasing your carbon footprint and ensuring that fewer animals have to suffer at the hands of humans. And isn't that a good feeling?

Considering all the ethical reasons for switching to a plant-based diet, the enormous health benefits and improved quality of life are the icings on an already extremely appealing cake.

Thank you for reading!

Made in the USA
Middletown, DE
20 February 2021

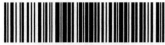